CONTENTS

To
Elaine
and to
Matthew
Emma Jane
Nicholas
Katy Thi
and
Lucy

Practical Genetic Counselling

Sixth edition

Peter S. Harper MA DM FRCP
Professor of Medical Genetics
University of Wales College of Medicine
Consultant in Medical Genetics
and Consultant Physician
University Hospital of Wales, Cardiff

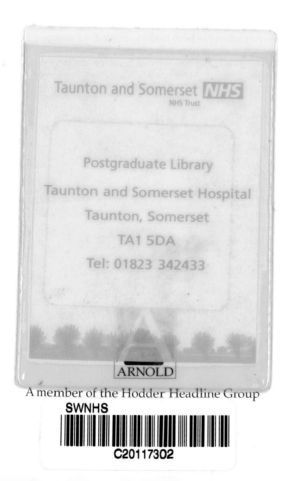

ARNOLD

A member of the Hodder Headline Group

First published in Great Britain in 1981 by Butterworth-Heinemann Ltd
Reprinted 1982
Second edition 1984
Third edition 1988
Reprinted 1991
Fourth edition 1993
Fifth edition 1998
Reprinted in 2001 by Arnold
This sixth edition published in 2004 by
Arnold, a member of the Hodder Headline Group,
338 Euston Road, London NW1 3BH

http://www.arnoldpublishers.com

Distributed in the United States of America by
Oxford University Press Inc.,
198 Madison Avenue, New York, NY10016
Oxford is a registered trademark of Oxford University Press

British Library Cataloguing in Publication Data
A catalogue record for this book is available from the British Library

Library of Congress Cataloging-in-Publication Data
A catalog record for this book is available from the Library of Congress

ISBN 0340 81196 X

1 2 3 4 5 6 7 8 9 10

Commissioning Editor: Joanna Koster
Development Editor: Sarah Burrows
Production Controller: Lindsay Smith
Cover Design: Sarah Rees

Typeset in 9/12, Palatino by Charon Tec Pvt. Ltd, Chennai, India
Printed and bound in Malta.

What do you think about this book? Or any other Arnold title?
Please send your comments to feedback.arnold@hodder.co.uk

The advances in our understanding of genetic disorders since the previous edition of this book have been even greater than between earlier editions, so a complete reassessment, and often rewriting, of the entire text has been needed to keep it up to date. At the same time, however, I have been struck by how much has not changed; this applies especially to the general principles and underlying philosophy of genetic counselling, where many aspects have increasingly been adopted by others outside medical genetics who are involved with inherited disorders. Even for specific disorders and risk estimates, though, many of the older data have not been superseded by newer information based on molecular evidence from the human genome project and elsewhere.

I should like to highlight here three areas where changes of special significance have occurred during the past 5 years. The first relates to the rapid development of cancer genetics as a field of medical practice, now of the greatest value in terms of both genetic counselling and disease prevention. A knowledge of this field is becoming essential for all in medicine, not just those specializing in the field.

A second major advance, still at an early stage, has been the identification of the molecular basis of developmental disorders, not just individual syndromes, but also broader underlying pathways that are now begining to allow clinicians involved with dysmorphic syndromes to understand their full aetiology, as well as increasingly providing laboratory confirmation of a suspected diagnosis.

A final advance to highlight is the realization that the genetics of most common disorders, apart from the important mendelian subsets, is going to be extremely complex, with involvement and interaction of numerous genetic and other factors. Thus, in contrast to single gene conditions, it is unlikely that molecular or other tests for genetic susceptibility are going to play an important role in clinical practice or genetic counselling in the near future; new advances in this field are more likely to be small steps towards a fuller understanding, rather than of immediate practical significance.

I have tried to keep the length of this new edition about the same as the previous one, since its small size and portability are, I suspect, the main reasons for a continued demand. I shall be most grateful, though, to be informed of any errors or major omissions.

Finally, I should like to acknowledge here my debt to many people, especially all my Cardiff colleagues, nurse counsellors, clinicians and scientists, who have not only made particular suggestions, but have supported my work over the years; much of what appears in this book reflects their own good practice. Specifically, I thank Hayley Archer, Angus Clarke, Merryl Curtis, Selwyn Roberts and Peter Thompson for comments on individual chapters, Buddug Williams for help with web sources, and Audrey Budding and Michele Matthews for the organizing and typing of the text.

Peter Harper
Cardiff, February 2004

PART I

General aspects of genetic counselling

CHAPTER I

Genetic counselling: an introduction

WHAT DO WE MEAN BY 'GENETIC COUNSELLING'?

Although most people working in the field of medicine are familiar with the term 'genetic counselling' and have some idea what it means, it is surprisingly rare to see it actually defined. Closer enquiry among patients and colleagues shows a wide variation in people's concepts of what the process of genetic counselling actually entails. Some envisage an essentially supportive – even psychotherapeutic – role, akin to that of counselling processes in the social field; others see genetic counselling as primarily concerned with special diagnostic tests in inherited disease; yet others regard it as a complex mathematical process involving the estimation of risk.

All these views of genetic counselling contain a considerable element of truth, but none fully identifies what the overall process of genetic counselling actually involves. Even within the group of professionals for whom genetic counselling is a major activity, there are varied opinions as to its proper role and scope, but the following definitions include what the author believes to be the essential features. The first is the definition that has been used in successive editions of this book:

> Genetic counselling is the process by which patients or relatives at risk of a disorder that may be hereditary are advised of the consequences of the disorder, the probability of developing or transmitting it and the ways in which this may be prevented, avoided or ameliorated.

Table 1.1 Genetic counselling: the main elements

Diagnostic and clinical aspects
Documentation of family and pedigree information
Recognition of inheritance patterns and risk estimation
Communication and empathy with those seen
Information on available options and further measures
Support in decision-making and for decisions made

A second definition of genetic counselling is given by Kelly in his valuable book *Clinical Genetics and Genetic Counselling* (see 'Further reading'):

An educational process that seeks to assist affected and/or at risk individuals to understand the nature of the genetic disorder, its transmission and the options open to them in management and family planning.

From these definitions, it can be seen that all three aspects mentioned in the opening paragraph are indeed involved – a diagnostic aspect, without which all advice has an insecure foundation; the actual estimation of risks, which may be simple in some situations and complex in others; and a supportive role ensuring that those given advice actually benefit from it and from the various management and preventive options that may be available. The complexity of the process makes the definitions sound cumbersome and a clearer idea is perhaps given by listing the main elements involved (Table 1.1). This chapter outlines these main elements, which are then dealt with in more detail in subsequent sections of the book. It is the satisfactory synthesis of these various aspects which makes up genetic counselling as a specific process. A thoughtful and valuable discussion of the process of genetic counselling is given by Clarke (see 'Further reading').

THE DEVELOPMENT OF GENETIC COUNSELLING

The study of human genetics was already well developed by the early decades of the twentieth century; a graphic and comprehensive historical account of its evolution is given by McKusick (see 'Further reading'). From a more medical viewpoint, Charles Davenport of the Eugenics Records Office in New York State began to give genetic advice as early as 1910. However, genetic counselling did not emerge as a recognized procedure until much later, as outlined by Reed (see 'Further reading'). During the 1920s and 1930s, the development of 'eugenic' policies in both totalitarian Germany and in North America, accompanied by discriminatory laws prohibiting marriage of those with particular diseases, brought the subject of eugenics into disrepute; the abuse of genetics in the guise of eugenics is discussed further in the final chapter. It was not until the time of the Second World War that the first genetic counselling clinics were opened in America, in Michigan in 1940 and in Minnesota in 1941. In the UK, the Hospital for Sick Children in Great Ormond Street, London, developed the first such clinic in 1946. By 1955 there were over a dozen centres in North America and there has been a steady development since that time. As with many pioneering developments, the early centres were often the work of far-sighted eccentrics. Sheldon Reed, in his book *Counselling in Medical Genetics*, first published in 1955, gives a delightful description of Edward Dight, responsible for founding the Dight Clinic in Minneapolis, who lived in a house built in a tree and who failed to file income tax returns. Francis Galton, who originated what was to become the Galton Laboratory in London, was another individualist, although a more scientific one; like Davenport he was associated uncomfortably closely with the development of eugenics.

Reed's book gives a vivid picture of the main areas covered in the early stages of genetic counselling, and it was Reed himself who first introduced the term. Many of the problems are unchanged today and his examples of individual cases show that the fears and concerns of families have altered little. In other respects, there have been profound changes in the 50 years since the book was written. Carrier detection was almost non-existent and prenatal diagnosis entirely non-existent, so the options open to patients at risk were limited; either they took the risk or they did not. An even more important change has been that of the general climate of opinion among the public and the medical profession, in particular a greater openness in relation to family disorders.

Reed's case histories illustrate the background of ignorance and prejudice with which his patients had to cope, and it is no wonder that he found them grateful, even when he could only give them pessimistic advice.

It is of interest that the most common cause of referral to the Dight Clinic was regarding skin colour and whether a child for adoption would 'pass for white'. Several other problems among the 20 most common causes for referral listed by Reed are infrequently encountered today, including eye colour, twinning and rhesus haemolytic disease. The last of these provides a real example of advance in treatment and prevention; the others reflect changes in social attitudes. Many other of Reed's most common problems remain equally important today, including mental handicap, schizophrenia, facial clefting, neural tube defects and Huntington's disease.

CONSTRUCTING A FAMILY TREE

Collecting genetic information is the first and most important step in genetic counselling, and is best achieved by drawing up a family tree or pedigree. The use of clear and consistent symbols allows genetic information to be set out much more clearly than does a long list of relatives. Drawing a satisfactory pedigree is not difficult, although it is remarkable how rarely those clinicians without an interest in genetics will attempt the process. A clearly drawn pedigree has a certain aesthetic appeal, but its chief value is to provide an unambiguous and permanent record of the genetic information in a particular family. Although computer programs exist, they are no substitute, in the author's view, for a clearly drawn pedigree constructed by hand at the time of the interview.

Figure 1.1 shows the main symbols used in constructing pedigrees. The symbols shown for the sexes ($\square$, $\bigcirc$) are preferred to the alternatives ($\male$, $\female$), which tend to be confused at a distance. Heterozygous carriers can be denoted by half-shaded symbols or, in the case of an X-linked disorder, by a central dot. Although the sign for an early abortion (spontaneous or induced) can also be used for a stillbirth, it is preferable to denote the sex of the

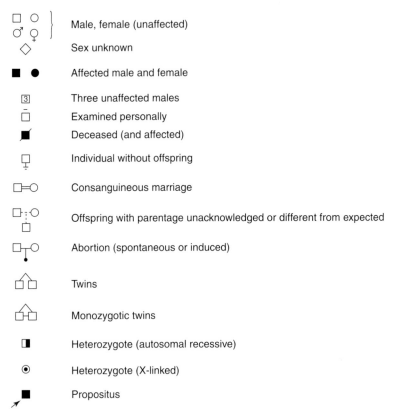

Figure 1.1 Symbols used in drawing a pedigree.

latter with an appropriate symbol and indicate that it was a stillbirth beneath. The previous use of a broken line for an offspring from outside marriage is no longer appropriate. 'Illegitimacy' is no longer a meaningful concept in most Western societies, but employing a broken line in a pedigree is still useful to represent the situation where parentage is unknown or unacknowledged.

The proband – also called the propositus (male) or proposita (female) – should be clearly indicated with an arrow. The proband is the individual through whom the family is ascertained. Large families will commonly have several probands. The proband is generally an affected individual, but the person primarily seeking advice may well not be affected. The term 'consultand' is conveniently used for this individual.

Multiple marriages and complex consanguinity can cause problems in constructing a pedigree, and artistry will have to be sacrificed for accuracy in such cases. It is usually wise to start near the middle of the pedigree sheet and to leave more room than one thinks will be needed, so that particularly prolific family branches do not become crowded out. Figure 1.2 shows examples of the 'working pedigree', one simple and one more complex.

The following practical points deserve emphasis:

• Enquire specifically about infant deaths, stillbirths and abortions. These may be highly relevant, especially if structural abnormalities prove to have been present; the fact that the information had not been volunteered may be significant. Thus two

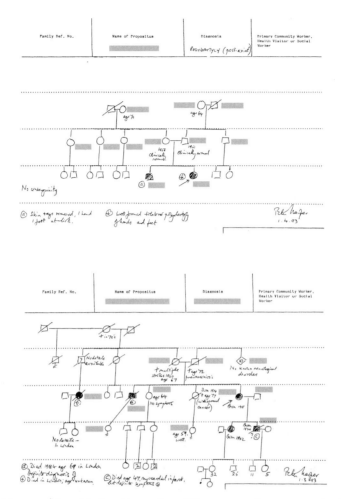

Figure 1.2 Two examples of the 'working pedigree'. These two pedigrees – one simple, the other more extensive – show how family data can be easily and clearly recorded at the time of the interview. A simple lined sheet is used; more detailed information on individuals can be recorded at the foot of the pedigree or on the back. Identifying details have been deleted.

children 'lost at birth' by the mother of a woman seen for counselling proved to have both had spina bifida, a fact that considerably altered the risks.

- Consanguinity should be directly asked about and may be the clue that suggests autosomal recessive inheritance (see Chapter 9).
- Mistaken or unacknowledged paternity must be borne in mind, especially in a puzzling situation. A family doctor or nurse, particularly in a small community, may well be able to clarify this possibility, but increasingly families are more open about it, recognizing its importance in the context of genetic risk. Definitive tests of paternity based on DNA (see Chapter 5) can help to resolve these problems more easily, but DNA-based diagnostic tests may equally produce new difficulties by the detection of unsuspected non-paternity.
- Always take at least basic details about both sides of the family, even in a dominantly inherited disorder clearly originating from one side. Unexpected findings may emerge.

The family that insists that there is 'nothing on our side' should be regarded with suspicion until this is verified. Taking details about both sides may also help to avoid feelings of guilt or blame resting exclusively on one member of a couple, always an important factor, but particularly in some cultural and social situations.

- Record dates of birth where possible rather than ages. Note the date when the pedigree was drawn up.
- Record maiden names of women; this is especially significant for X-linked disorders, where the surname of affected members is likely to change with each generation.
- Note the addresses of key relevant members – this may prove invaluable in obtaining hospital records or in later contact with relatives.

Most of the above points are obvious, yet it is surprising how often vital information is not obtained unless a systematic approach is used.

In constructing a pedigree, it is not generally necessary to trace a person's ancestry back more than three or four generations; medical details often become inaccurate at this early period. Sometimes, though, it may be important to link kindreds or to establish a common ancestor, in which case genealogical records will be useful. These are surprisingly abundant in many European countries, especially Scandinavia. In the UK, a useful guide has been produced to the different sources (see Bevan and Duncan, 'Further reading'). Even in mobile populations such as America, the growth in interest in family history has considerably increased people's knowledge of their ancestors.

DIAGNOSTIC INFORMATION

It has already been emphasized that a clear diagnosis is the essential basis for accurate genetic counselling. Unfortunately, this basis is all too often a shaky one, and one of the principal tasks of anyone involved in genetic counselling is to ensure that it is made as firm as possible before risk estimates are given to those seeking advice. Common reasons for lack of a clear diagnosis include the following:

- *The affected individual may have lived a considerable time ago, when relevant diagnostic investigations were not available.* There is little that can be done about this, but it is surprising how much detailed information may be obtained by questioning close relatives who were involved in caring for the patient. Even if an exact diagnosis cannot be established, it may be possible to exclude a disorder. Thus a man with muscular dystrophy who lived to the age of 40 years clearly would not have had the Duchenne type.
- *The affected individual may have died without essential investigations having been done, or without autopsy being performed.* This is all too often the case and is inexcusable. Reasons usually offered are reluctance to trouble the parents in distressing circumstances, or the fact that investigations would not have altered the patient's management; but frequently the real reason is that those involved have not taken the trouble to undertake the studies, or to make arrangements with those who can undertake them. The recent sharp reduction in the frequency of autopsy has made the situation worse. The tragic consequences of such inertia only become apparent when the question of risk to further family members arises.

- *A firm diagnosis cannot be reached even with the affected individual living*. This is inevitable in some cases, since our knowledge of many genetic disorders remains very incomplete, but a considerable degree of help can be obtained by enlisting the efforts of colleagues, even at a distance. Photographs, radiographs and samples of urine, blood, DNA and cultured skin fibroblasts can all be sent to distant parts of the world for experts to study, and developments in 'telemedicine' now extend greatly the scope of what can be done in this way, especially for imaging. Presentation of puzzling cases at clinical meetings may often result in a diagnosis being provided. Even if it does not, one can feel happier that one is not overlooking a recognizable disorder if one has sought the advice of those most likely to know and families also appreciate these efforts. Wherever possible, one should store (with consent) appropriate samples for future biochemical or DNA analysis.
- *The diagnosis may be wrong*. This is a much more dangerous situation than when the diagnosis is uncertain, as it may lead to false confidence. It is extremely difficult to know how far to rely on other people's diagnoses and how far to insist on confirming them oneself. Clearly, neither a medical geneticist nor any other clinician can be an expert diagnostician in every speciality, and one will frequently have to rely on colleagues' advice. Nevertheless, it is essential for all clinicians involved in genetic counselling to have a wide range of diagnostic ability, to know their limitations – and those of their colleagues – and to develop a healthy scepticism in diagnostic matters and a sensitivity for where error may lie. For non-medical genetic counsellors, it is essential to work in the closest cooperation with clinical geneticists if major problems are to be avoided.

Bearing in mind the foregoing problems, how can one ensure that diagnostic information is as extensive and accurate as possible? There is no simple answer, but the following points may be helpful:

- Always arrange to see the affected individual or individuals where possible, even if they have already been fully investigated. How detailed an examination should be made will depend on circumstances.
- Always examine asymptomatic members at risk (after careful explanation of why this is important and the potential consequences), to exclude mild or early disease. This is especially important with variable dominantly inherited disorders or where there is a possibility of new mutation. Beware of the person who insists that there is no need for them to be examined because they know they are normal!
- Warn families in advance that the full answers to their questions may not be possible on the initial visit, and ask them to bring as much relevant information as possible about affected individuals, especially those not in the same household as themselves. A preliminary visit, or at least telephone contact, by a co-worker will be extremely valuable in this respect, as well as giving a general preparation for the clinic visit, as discussed further in Chapter 10.
- Be prepared to interview older or more distant relatives who may have valuable information on deceased individuals. A home visit may be very useful here. Such relatives will almost always be happy to help, but the part of the family requesting advice should be told beforehand if other branches are going to be approached and asked whether any members are likely to be upset by this. It is preferable for initial contact to be made by family members themselves.

- When arranging a follow-up appointment for genetic counselling, allow adequate time for obtaining records and other information. Specific written permission should always be sought before requesting medical records of living relatives.
- A variety of special investigations may prove necessary, including radiological, biochemical and genetic studies, and sometimes biopsy diagnosis. Most studies can be performed on an outpatient basis, but occasionally it is extremely helpful to have facilities for in-patient investigation. It frequently happens that the affected individual on whom investigations are needed is already under the care of a clinical colleague; obviously, careful liaison prior to seeing such a person is essential if confusion or duplication of investigations is to be avoided and good working relationships with colleagues maintained.

GENETIC RISK ESTIMATION

Having taken a careful pedigree, documented the various details of affected individuals and examined relevant family members, one is now in a position to attempt to answer the questions that gave rise to the request for genetic counselling and to estimate and transmit to the family concerned the risks of particular members, born or unborn, developing the particular disorder. The fact that the process of recording information will probably have taken a considerable time is in some ways an advantage, particularly if the family is not under one's regular care but is being seen specifically for genetic counselling. From the way in which information is given (or not given) and from the reaction to questions, much can be learned about the general attitude of the individuals being counselled to the family disorder. Did they themselves initiate the request for genetic counselling, or did someone else? Is there an unspoken and perhaps exaggerated fear of the disorder? Do feelings of guilt or hostility exist between parents? Is the rest of the family supportive, or are there tensions between the generations? Is an affected child valued and loved, or regarded as a burden? Much information on these and other important issues can be obtained by a person who is sensitive and observant, without the need for direct questioning.

It is also possible during this preliminary stage to assess the way in which information is to be most suitably transmitted. Some couples will be unable to grasp more than the simplest concepts of 'high risk' or 'low risk', while others will require a precise risk figure and even a detailed explanation of the mode of inheritance.

Information on genetic risks is rarely an absolute 'yes' or 'no', and in medical genetics, more perhaps than in any other branch of medicine, one thinks and works almost entirely in terms of probabilities or odds. Colleagues frequently find this unsatisfactory, preferring to accept only a 'definite' conclusion. Yet when examined closely, there is often as much, if not more, uncertainty in the apparently 'definite' specialities than there is in medical genetics. Thus the chance that a definitely inflamed appendix will be found at appendicectomy is far from 100 per cent, while the entire process of clinical diagnosis is based on the combination of numerous pieces of information, each with a degree of uncertainty, although this is often unappreciated by those involved. The same applies to the 'normal ranges' of most laboratory investigations. It is perhaps only because uncertainty is well recognized in genetics that methods of measuring it and defining its limits have generally been used, as exemplified in genetic counselling. More recently, other areas of medicine have started to use these approaches.

Table 1.2 Risk estimates: conversion table between odds and percentages

Odds	Percentage	Percentage	Odds
I in 2	50	50	I in 2
3	33	40	2.5
4	25	30	3.3
5	20	25	4
6	17	20	5
7	14	15	6.7
8	12	12	8.3
9	II	10	10
10	10	9	II
12	8	8	12.5
14	7	7	14
16	6	6	17
18	5.5	5	20
20	5.0	4	25
25	4.0	3	33
30	3.3	2	50
35	2.9	I	100
40	2.5	0.5	200
50	2.0	0.25	400
60	1.7	0.1	1000
70	1.4		
80	1.3		
90	1.1		
100	1.0		

Risk figures in genetic counselling may be given either as odds or as percentages. Some people prefer to use odds and to quote risks as 1 in 10, 1 in 50, 1 in 100, etc. Others prefer to use such figures as 10 per cent, 2 per cent, 1 per cent. The author admits to inconsistency in this, both in practice and in this book, and for this reason, and because others are equally inconsistent, a table of conversions is given (Table 1.2), which should allow ready exchange between the two approaches. It is often necessary to adapt whichever is used to a particular situation, for some people simply do not understand odds, while others are more confused with percentages. It also needs to be borne in mind that the margins of error for many risk figures are very high and that using precise figures can give a spurious impression of exact knowledge. In such a situation, the author often prefers not to give a precise figure at all.

Whatever method is used, there are pitfalls in interpretation that must be avoided, as described below, and this may require much patience:

- Odds refer to the future, not the past. Thus, a 1 in 4 risk, as seen with autosomal recessive inheritance, does not mean that because the previous child was affected the next three will be guaranteed normal. Nor does having two affected children in succession make it less (or more) likely that the next will be affected. That 'chance has no memory'

Table 1.3 Risk of abnormalities in the 'normal' population (approximate)

Risk of a child being born with some congenital abnormality	1 in 30
Risk of child being born with a serious physical or mental handicap	1 in 50
Risk of a pregnancy ending in a spontaneous abortion	1 in 8
Risk of perinatal death*	1 in 120
Risk of a child dying in the first year of life after the first week*	1 in 300
Risk that a couple will be infertile	1 in 10

*Figure for 'developed' countries; there is great geographical variation.

may require repeated explanation, since couples may accept the correct situation intellectually, yet retain an emotionally powerful view based on erroneous ideas.

- It is embarrassingly easy for odds to be reversed. Thus a patient seen by the author with one spina bifida child, having been correctly advised by her obstetrician that there was a 1 in 20 recurrence risk, came seeking termination of her next pregnancy because she considered that 'a chance of 1 in 20 of a normal child was far too low'.
- Odds of 1 in 2 (1/2) are not the same as 1 to 2 (1/3); this may be misinterpreted by those used to betting. Fortunately, the difference is only considerable for the highest risks.
- Many people do not have a clear idea of what constitutes a high or low risk. Thus some couples who are given a low risk (e.g. 1 in 200) express the view that this is far too high to be acceptable, whereas others seen by the author have been greatly relieved by a risk of 50 per cent. Clearly the nature and severity of the disorder will determine what risk is acceptable, but it is helpful to be able to give some kind of reference point for comparison, such as the fact that one child in 50 in the population is born with a serious disability, or that the population frequency of the disorder in question is, say, 1 in 2000. Some useful data of this type are summarized in Table 1.3.

THE BASIS OF RISK ESTIMATION

The ways in which risks can be estimated and the results of these estimates form the basis of this book and are considered in detail in later chapters. It is important from the outset, though, to recognize that not all risk estimates are of the same type. They may be based on different sorts of information and may be of greater or lesser reliability. The main categories discussed below can be recognized.

Empiric risks

Here the estimate is based on observed data rather than theoretical predictions (Figure 1.3; see also Chapter 3); this is the form of risk estimate available for most of the more common non-mendelian or chromosomal disorders. The information is usually reliable provided it has been collected in an unbiased manner (often not easy), and provided that the population from which the individual receiving genetic counselling comes is comparable to the one on which the data were established. Sadly, there is a dearth of recent empiric risk studies and the use of older ones is often made more complex as the result of changes in classification following recognition of genetic heterogeneity or identification of specific genes, as well as by genuine biological changes in disease frequency (e.g. neural tube defects).

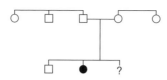

Figure 1.3 Empiric risk estimate: one child is affected with spina bifida. The risk of a subsequent child being affected by a neural tube defect is around 3 per cent in an area of high risk (e.g. south Wales) and with no other affected family members. The risk estimate would be different in an area of low incidence and would be altered by the presence of other affected relatives. It has also changed with time, being less than in earlier surveys 30 years ago.

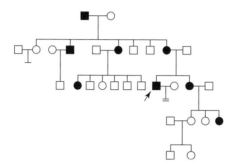

Figure 1.4 Mendelian risk estimate: a family with myotonic dystrophy (an autosomal dominant disorder). The risk for the offspring of affected individuals is 50 per cent regardless of the incidence of the disorder and the number of affected individuals in the family (see Chapter 11 for the relevance of genetic instability to this disorder).

Mendelian risks

Mendelian risk estimates can only be given when a clear basis of single gene inheritance can be recognized for a disorder (Figure 1.4; see Chapter 2). They are perhaps the most satisfactory form of risk estimate because they commonly allow a clear differentiation into categories of negligible risk (e.g. offspring of healthy sibs in a rare autosomal recessive disorder) and high risk (e.g. offspring of an individual affected with an autosomal dominant disorder). There often remains the problem of achieving greater certainty in the individual at high risk (e.g. a person at 50 per cent risk of developing Huntington's disease), and information from the next two risk categories may be helpful in this situation.

Modified genetic risks

Non-geneticists may find modified genetic risk estimates (Figure 1.5) difficult to use initially; they are particularly applicable in X-linked recessive inheritance, where fully worked-out examples are given (see Chapter 2). The essential feature is that a 'prior' genetic risk, based usually on mendelian inheritance, may be modified by 'conditional' information, usually genetic, but sometimes from other sources. Thus the modified risk of a man developing Huntington's disease whose grandparent was affected is not the same as the prior risk of 1 in 4, but is reduced by his own age and by the fact that the intervening parent was unaffected. It may also be reduced by the number of unaffected sibs, if

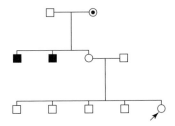

Figure 1.5 Modified risk estimate: Duchenne muscular dystrophy. The grandmother of the individual seeking advice (consultand) is an obligatory carrier; prior risks of the mother and the consultand being carriers are thus 50 per cent and 25 per cent, respectively. These risks are, however, greatly reduced by the fact that the mother has had four healthy sons and no affected sons (see Chapter 2 for further details).

these have reached an advanced age. Such modifying information may drastically alter the risk estimate and should always be used when available, especially if presymptomatic or prenatal genetic tests are being considered.

Risk estimates from independent evidence

Where special investigations can be utilized, these may greatly alter the risk estimates. Thus a normal serum immunoreactive trypsin test in an infant having a sib with cystic fibrosis will considerably reduce the chance of the disorder being present.

Carrier detection in such disorders as haemophilia and Duchenne muscular dystrophy provides comparable information, as do linked DNA markers in many mendelian disorders. However, a strong caution must be given here: the results of these investigations are rarely so clear-cut that they can be used in isolation; they require combination with the prior genetic risk, along with other modifying information. Failure to appreciate this may lead to serious error, especially when investigations are being applied as screening procedures in situations of low prior risk. Thus, in the example given of cystic fibrosis, the final risk, and very possibly the actions taken, would depend very much on whether there was a close family history of cystic fibrosis or whether the abnormality resulted from a screening test.

Composite risks

Most empiric risks really fall into this category, but in some instances it is obvious that one is dealing with a mixed situation which cannot be satisfactorily resolved. Thus a disorder such as osteogenesis imperfecta congenita is composed of a large number of cases representing new dominant mutations, with a very small recurrence risk to sibs, and a small number of autosomal recessive cases, with a recurrence risk of 1 in 4. Because the two situations cannot always be reliably distinguished, one ends up with an intermediate risk depending on the relative frequency of the two groups. Obviously this intermediate risk does not really exist at all – the family must represent one or other of the extreme positions. Such a composite risk estimate is an unsatisfactory one and should be regarded as a temporary measure. With improved resolution of genetic heterogeneity, to which molecular analysis is now contributing, it may be possible to distinguish the individual components, while even within a single family, additional information may resolve the situation. Thus the birth of a further affected child in the example given of osteogenesis imperfecta would make it almost certain that autosomal recessive inheritance (or possibly gonadal mosaicism) is operating in this family, with at least a 1 in 4 risk for further children. The recognition of mendelian subsets within a disorder generally considered to be 'multifactorial' (e.g. congenital heart disease, breast cancer) is also proving important, as discussed in Chapter 3.

COMMUNICATION AND GENETIC COUNSELLING

No matter how well one may have confirmed a genetic diagnosis, utilized appropriate genetic tests and established an accurate risk estimate, all this will count for little if one cannot communicate satisfactorily with the family that one is seeing. The constant and unending variety provided by the interactions inherent in genetic counselling is one of the chief reasons why those involved find it such a rewarding activity, but even the most 'natural' communicators need training to optimize their skills, while a basic knowledge of the main theoretical aspects underpinning counselling skills is also of the greatest help. As indicated later in the chapter, these skills can also help to turn what may start out as an essentially information-giving interview into one which is also therapeutic in nature.

GENETIC COUNSELLING AND NON-DIRECTIVENESS

It will have been noted that the emphasis so far has been placed on ensuring that a correct diagnosis and risk estimate have been reached and that those being counselled have correctly understood the situation. Nothing has been said about recommending a particular line of action or of advising couples against having children in high-risk situations, and it may surprise some readers to learn that the author, in common with most professionals involved in genetic counselling, rarely if ever adopts a 'directive' approach. A survey of American genetic counselling centres has shown that a similarly non-directive approach was almost universal, although this has not always been the case in eastern Europe until recently, and may be difficult to apply in relation to some cultural and ethnic groups used to a more authoritarian situation.

This may appear all the more surprising since many doctors with little experience of genetics do frequently give directive advice. Remarks such as 'We were told not to have further children' or 'The doctors said I must have it terminated' are still commonly heard at genetic counselling clinics, and in many cases great distress has been caused to the couples involved, particularly because the advice has not been accompanied by an explanation of why it has been given or how great the risk really is.

The author's view is that it is not the duty of a doctor to dictate the lives of others, but to ensure that individuals have the facts to enable them to make their own decisions. This includes not simply a knowledge of the genetic risks, but a clear appreciation of the consequences, long-term as well as short-term, that may result from a particular course of action. In any case, it seems likely (although not proven) that directive counselling may be counterproductive. Intelligent couples may resent being told what to do in a situation where they have already spent much troubled thought over the alternatives. Among the less privileged, there is often a strong resentment of being dictated to by authority and the author's experience with Huntington's disease suggests that some individuals in this situation may deliberately embark on a pregnancy as a gesture of defiance.

By contrast, some couples seen for genetic counselling will plead for direction. 'What would you do if you were in my place?' is a common question. It is tempting to give a clear direction in these circumstances, but frequently these are the very couples for whom this may be most inadvisable. Such a plea often indicates an unwillingness to face up to the consequences of a serious situation, or a serious disagreement between marriage partners, and for the physician to take on the responsibility that can only really be taken by the couple themselves may have serious long-term consequences.

It would be wrong to pretend that those engaged in genetic counselling never give directive advice. One's own views are likely to be expressed in the way one approaches the subject, whether the more serious or the milder aspects of a disease have been stressed and whether one holds out the possibility of future treatment. Even the way a risk estimate is phrased can vary – for example, in the case of an autosomal recessive condition with a 1 in 4 recurrence risk, it is possible to make it appear quite encouraging if one states that there are three chances out of four that the child will be healthy! The type of society in which one lives and practises will also inevitably influence the way in which genetic counselling is given, and this is discussed further in the final chapter of this book. Clarke (see 'Further reading') points out clearly the limitations involved.

Since 'non-directiveness' has become a somewhat central tenet of genetic counselling, it is important that it should not be used as an excuse for being vague or appearing detached, or for presenting so many apparent options that it becomes difficult for those seen to reach a clear decision. People will often need support for a tentative decision, as indicated later in this chapter; the importance of non-directiveness lies in allowing the decisions to be taken by the individuals involved, not by the person giving genetic counselling.

It is particularly important that couples realize that, in general, there is no 'right' or 'wrong' decision to be made, but that the decision should be the right one for their own particular situation. It is also important that those giving genetic counselling (and those evaluating genetic services) do not judge 'success' or 'failure' in terms of a particular outcome, and that they give support to families whatever their decisions may be.

ADVICE AT A DISTANCE

The less one is able to verify a situation oneself, the greater is the possibility of error. However, the person who refuses to give any advice unless able to do everything personally is going to be of limited benefit to patients and colleagues. The author is in no doubt that one of the most valuable roles of a medical geneticist – and the same applies to any clinician with a particular interest in genetic counselling – is to act as a focal point and source of information for colleagues in a variety of specialities who need someone to turn to for advice. A high proportion of telephone and postal enquiries from colleagues do not require actual referral of the patient; frequently, one is simply confirming what is already thought to be the case. In other instances, one may be able to advise that prenatal or other special investigations are available; in a small proportion of enquiries, however, the advice has to be that one cannot give a reliable opinion without seeing the patient oneself.

One soon learns to recognize the small number of colleagues who attempt to use indirect or 'casual' advice as a substitute for a proper referral, as well as the enquiries 'on behalf of a friend' that can disguise a serious personal genetic problem requiring a full referral and thorough assessment.

Actual genetic counselling by post or other indirect means is an entirely different matter, and the author's policy regarding enquiries from patients and relatives is to arrange a clinic appointment, via their family doctor wherever possible. The same policy applies to enquiries from health visitors, social workers and other paramedical personnel. Not only is there a serious risk that erroneous information may be given or risk figures misinterpreted, but without directly seeing those requesting advice, it is often impossible to decide what the real problem leading to their enquiry is and whether there are additional or underlying factors that have not been mentioned.

E-mail enquiries coming directly from patients or family members, are increasingly frequent, particularly if one has expertise in a specific disorder or is closely involved with lay groups. In this case, one can usually help best by directing the enquirer to useful information sources or a local centre. Although it may be tempting to try to provide detailed help, especially if there seems to be no local facility, this is almost always unwise in the author's opinion. By contrast, carefully organized and appropriately selected remote video-conferencing consultations may be of real value in difficult geographical situations.

THE BACK-UP TO GENETIC COUNSELLING

It has already been emphasized that genetic counselling does not simply consist of giving risk figures, and that it must often be preceded by a considerable diagnostic effort, in comparison with which the estimation of risks may be a relatively simple matter. Similarly, genetic counselling does not stop with the giving of risks, but must include a variety of other actions if it is to be fully effective.

In the first instance, it must be established as clearly as possible that the individuals counselled have really understood what they have been told. This includes not only the risk estimate, but the nature of the disorder and what other measures are available for prevention and treatment. It is often possible to get an approximate idea of how well information has been understood at the time of the interview, but it is well worthwhile, and often a salutary experience, to have this checked by an independent observer. A skilled genetics nurse or similar co-worker can often do this while discussing other matters with the family after the consultation, and, surprisingly, will often find that part or all of the information has been forgotten or misinterpreted before the couple has even left the clinic. A system of regular follow-up is useful both to check on this and to support the genetic counselling that has been given at the initial interview. For the same reason, it is important to provide a letter summarizing the main points of the consultation, including the risk estimates; a copy of the letter to the referring doctor may be appropriate in some cases, but in general the author prefers to write a separate letter specifically to the individual or family seen.

Where information has been seriously misinterpreted or forgotten, this may be for various reasons. Some individuals have genuinely poor memories, while others may have been seen at an inappropriate time, such as soon after the death of a child; yet others may have come to the clinic encumbered with small and active children and been preoccupied in restraining their activities rather than in listening to what has been said. Most commonly, one has probably not taken sufficient time and effort to ensure that the information has really been absorbed and it is important to be aware of one's failures in this respect. The author has on several occasions seen couples who have acquired grossly erroneous ideas of risk and has wondered who could possibly have misinformed them so completely, only to find that it was he himself who had seen them some years previously!

An essential accompaniment to genetic counselling is that those being counselled should have full and accurate knowledge of the various other measures that may be available. In many cases, these require application as an integral part of counselling – thus an assessment of the risk of a woman having a child affected by Duchenne muscular dystrophy or haemophilia is likely to be incomplete without carrier detection tests (see Chapter 7). In other cases, the risk may not be altered, but the consequences may be. Thus, where prenatal diagnosis is available (see Chapter 8), many couples will be prepared to embark on a high-risk pregnancy when they would not have considered doing so in the absence of such diagnostic facilities. Similarly, the development of treatment fundamentally alters attitudes to genetic counselling. Most couples with a phenylketonuric child diagnosed in the newborn period and developing normally with treatment are happy to risk another affected child; where treatment is less satisfactory and the outcome less certain, the attitude may be very different.

Further 'back-up' measures that may be required are contraception and sterilization, as well as the exploration of other possible options such as adoption, artificial insemination by donor or ovum donation. These aspects are discussed later (see Chapter 9), but it cannot be too strongly emphasized that their consideration is an integral part of genetic counselling.

SUPPORT IN THE CONTEXT OF GENETIC COUNSELLING

Many couples coming for genetic counselling require active support in one way or another. Sometimes the actual information given in genetic counselling may be of such grave consequence as to require support if serious problems are not to arise. Huntington's disease (see Chapter 12) is perhaps the most striking example, but a severe depressive reaction is not uncommon in women who have recently lost a child after a chronic illness and who have to be told that the risk for other children is high. A sympathetic family doctor to whom the couple can turn is probably the best safeguard in this situation, but a skilled social worker can often accurately judge those families particularly in need of support.

Support may also be required for problems quite unrelated to the genetic aspects. Thus in genetic counselling for a chronic disease, it is frequently found that an affected individual is receiving no medical attention at all, that practical aids such as wheelchairs are not being provided, or that social service benefits of various kinds are not being claimed. It is sometimes argued that such matters are not part of genetic counselling; this may theoretically be so, but as a physician the author feels strongly that genetic counselling is an integral part of the overall management of patients and their families, that basic supportive measures may be as important as, or even more important than, the actual information regarding genetic risks, and that it is one's duty to see that the necessary measures are taken, if not by oneself then by an appropriate colleague.

Finally, while genetic counselling is largely distinct from psychotherapeutic counselling and does not have therapy as a specific aim, there is no doubt that it does have the potential for containing a strong therapeutic element. Most medical and other staff involved in genetic counselling have relatively little specific training in psychotherapy and related fields, but from working closely with such a colleague the author has learned not only how it can contribute to interviewing skills and the handling of family dynamics, but also how much of the 'ordinary' activity of genetic counselling can be therapeutic for those seen, if the interview is undertaken with sensitivity and experience.

There is little doubt that the time taken in genetic counselling is an important factor, as is the need for empathy with those being seen, but it is reassuring to know that it is possible for a person not fully trained in psychological aspects to make a contribution of this nature. It is also immensely helpful to have a colleague who is expert in this area for referral of those with serious psychological problems.

FURTHER READING

Introductory books

Connor JM, Ferguson Smith MA (1997). *Essential Medical Genetics*. Oxford, Blackwell.
Gelehrter RD, Collins FS (1998). *Principles of Medical Genetics*. Baltimore, Williams and Wilkins.
Kingston H (2002). *ABC of Medical Genetics*. London, BMJ Publishing.
Korf B (2000). *Human Genetics: a Problem-based Approach*. Oxford, Blackwell.
Mueller RF, Young ID (2001). *Emery's Elements of Medical Genetics*. Edinburgh, Churchill Livingstone.
Nussbaum R, McInnes J, Willard H (2001). *Thompson and Thompson's Genetics in Medicine*. Philadelphia, Saunders.
Skirton H, Patch C (2002). *Genetics for Healthcare Professionals*. Oxford, BIOS.

General textbooks

King R, Stansfield WD (2002). *A Dictionary of Genetics*. Oxford, University Press.
Mange AP, Mange EJ (1996). *Genetics: Human Aspects*. New York, Sinaver.
Snustaad DP, Simmonds MJ (1997). *Principles of Genetics*. New York, Wiley.
Vogel F, Motulsky AG (1996). *Human Genetics. Problems and Approaches*. Berlin, Springer – still the most detailed and rigorous textbook on the scientific basis of human genetics.

Genetic counselling

Baker D, Schuette J, Uhlmann W (eds) (1998). *A Guide to Genetic Counselling*. New York, Wiley.
Clarke A (ed.) (1994). *Genetic Counselling: Practice and Principles*. Routledge, London.
Clarke A (1997). The process of genetic counselling: beyond non-directiveness. In: Harper PS, Clarke A, eds. *Genetics, Society and Clinical Practice*. Oxford, BIOS, pp. 179–200.
Evers-Kiebooms G, Fryns J-P, Cassiman J-J, van den Berge H (1992). *Psychological Aspects of Genetic Counselling*. New York, Wiley-Liss.
Greenwood Genetic Center (2002). *Genetic Counseling Aids*, 4th edn. Greenwood, SC, Greenwood Genetic Center.
Kelly TE (1986). *Clinical Genetics and Genetic Counseling*. Chicago, Year Book.

Reference works

Cooper DN (ed.) (2003). *Nature Encyclopedia of the Human Genome*. London, Nature Publishing Group.

Gardner RJM, Sutherland GR (2003). *Chromosome Abnormalities and Genetic Counselling*. Oxford, Oxford University Press.

King RA, Rotter JI, Motulsky AG (2002). *The Genetic Basis of Common Diseases*. Oxford, University Press – a most valuable source for information on all disorders of complex inheritance.

Jameson LJ (ed.) (1998) *Principles of Molecular Medicine*. New Jersey, Humana.

McKusick VA (1998). *Mendelian Inheritance in Man*, 12th edn. Baltimore, Johns Hopkins University Press – see also online version below.

Rimoin DL, Connor JM, Pyeritz RE, Korf B (eds) (2002). *Emery and Rimoin's Principles and Practice of Medical Genetics*. Edinburgh, Churchill Livingstone – the individual chapters of this book provide a wealth of detailed information on specific groups of genetic disorders.

Scriver CR, Beaudet AL, Sly WS, Valle D (2001). *The Metabolic and Molecular Bases of Inherited Disease*. New York, McGraw Hill – see online version and CD-Rom, below.

Historical approaches

Harper PS (ed.) (2004). *Landmarks in Medical Genetics: Classic Papers with Commentaries*. New York, Oxford University Press.

McKusick VA (2002). History of medical genetics. In: Rimoin DL, Connor JM, Pyeritz RE, Korf B, eds. *Emery and Rimoin's Principles and Practice of Medical Genetics*, Edinburgh, Churchill Livingstone, pp. 1–30.

Books for lay people

Bennet RL (1999). *The Practical Guide to the Genetic Family History*. New York, Wiley.

Bevan A, Duncan A. (1992). *Tracing your Ancestors in the Public Record Office*. London, HMSO.

Milunsky A (1992). *Heredity and your Family's Health*. Baltimore, Johns Hopkins University Press.

Modell B, Modell M (1992). *Towards a Healthy Baby. Congenital Disorders and the New Genetics in Primary Health Care*. Oxford, Oxford University Press.

Zallen DT (1997). *Does it Run in the Family? A Consumer's Guide to DNA Testing for Genetic Disorders*. New Brunswick, NJ, Rutgers University Press.

Computer-based sources

Cooper DN, Krawczak M. Human Gene Mutation Database – *http://www.hgmd.org*

GeneReviews – *http://www.genetests.org* – a new internet-based source of information on genetic disorders, still only partially complete, but should become extremely useful. Linked to GeneTests (see Chapter 5).

The Metabolic and Molecular Bases of Inherited Disease – *http://genetics.accessmedicine.com* – an updated version of Scriver *et al.* (2001) (above); CD-Rom also available.

National Organization for Rare Disorders (NORD) – *http://www.rarediseases.org* – a valuable source of both professional information and support groups (US) details for rare conditions.

OMIM (Online Mendelian Inheritance in Man) – *http://www.ncbi.nlm.nih.gov/omim* – a continually updated version of McKusick's reference book; CD-Rom also available. An essential companion to all working in the field.

POSSUM. CD-Rom. Melbourne, Australia, Murdoch Children's Research Institute – a valuable database of malformation syndromes; informaiton on *http://www.possum.net.au/*

Schinzel A. *Human Cytogenetics Database*. CD-Rom. Oxford, Oxford University Press.

Winter RM, Baraitser M. *London Dysmorphology Database*. CD-Rom. Oxford, Oxford University Press.

Winter RM, Baraitser M. *London Neurogenetics Database*. CD-Rom. Oxford, Oxford University Press.

Genetic counselling in mendelian disorders

When assessing the clinical and genetic information available for a family with a particular disorder, the primary question requiring an answer is: does the disorder follow mendelian inheritance? If the answer is 'yes', it is likely that precise and well-established risks can be given regarding its occurrence in other family members; if the answer is 'no', then the information that can be given is usually much less certain, although fortunately the risks are also likely to be lower than for mendelian inheritance. If, as is often the case, the answer is not clear, the correct initial course may be to attempt to obtain further evidence rather than to give risks which may require radical revision. This is particularly the case for those common disorders known to have a significant mendelian subset (see Chapter 3).

Mendelian inheritance may be established in several ways, and the more independent evidence one has supporting the same conclusion, the more confident one can be that the risks one has given are correct. In some cases, the pattern of transmission of the disorder in the family may be conclusive, even if the diagnosis is unknown, or proves to be erroneous. Thus the pedigrees shown in Figures 2.1 and 2.2 could hardly be anything other than autosomal dominant and X-linked recessive, respectively. Nevertheless, one can be mistaken even in what appears to be a classic pattern, as in Figure 2.3, where the inclusion of data from both parental lines in a disorder not known to follow regular mendelian inheritance makes a polygenic origin more likely.

More commonly, mendelian inheritance is established by a combination of clinical diagnosis with a compatible (but not in itself conclusive) pedigree pattern. Thus the pedigree shown in Figure 2.4 is suggestive of autosomal dominant inheritance, but could be a chance concentration of cases of a non-mendelian – or even non-genetic – disorder. The knowledge that the diagnosis in the family was Huntington's disease would remove all doubt and allow genetic counselling to be given accordingly.

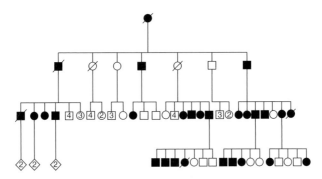

Figure 2.1 Typical autosomal dominant inheritance (a south Wales kindred with Huntington's disease). The disorder is transmitted by affected individuals to around half of their offspring. Both sexes transmit and develop the condition equally. The only unaffected individual to transmit the disorder died young and would presumably have developed it herself at a later date. (From Harper PS (1976). *J R Coll Phys Lond* **10**, 321–332.)

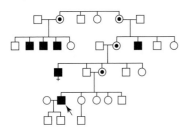

Figure 2.2 Typical X-linked recessive inheritance in a south Wales kindred with Becker (late onset X-linked) muscular dystrophy. In each generation the disorder has been transmitted by healthy females, but only males are affected. The propositus has not transmitted the disorder to his sons.

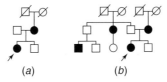

(a)   (b)

Figure 2.3 Polygenic inheritance simulating a mendelian pattern. Manic-depressive illness. (a) The superficial pedigree, with two generations affected, suggests dominant inheritance (autosomal or X-linked). (b) The recognition of affected individuals in both parental lines makes polygenic inheritance more likely than mendelian. (Pedigree details have been modified for illustration purposes.)

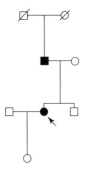

Figure 2.4 Pedigree pattern compatible with but not conclusive of autosomal dominant inheritance. Without a specific diagnosis it would be difficult to give more than approximate risks in this situation. In fact the pedigree is of a family with proven Huntington's disease, so confident advice as for autosomal dominant inheritance is possible.

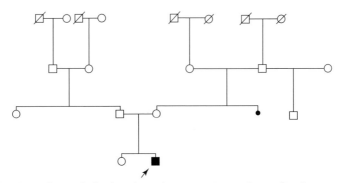

Figure 2.5 A 'sporadic case' of a disorder – the most common form of pedigree seen in genetic counselling. The affected individual could be the result of a non-genetic process, the family could represent autosomal dominant, autosomal recessive or X-linked inheritance, or a chromosomal or polygenic disorder. The absence of other affected family members does *not* mean that the disorder is not genetic.

Not infrequently the pedigree information is entirely unhelpful and one is completely dependent on the clinical diagnosis. Nowhere is this seen more clearly than in the 'sporadic case', as shown in Figure 2.5, where there are the following possibilities:

- the disorder is largely or entirely non-genetic, with insignificant recurrence risk
- the disorder is polygenic or chromosomal in basis, with a definite (usually low to moderate) recurrence risk depending on the disorder
- inheritance may be autosomal recessive, with a 1 in 4 recurrence risk to further children of either sex
- the disorder may represent a new dominant mutation, with negligible recurrence risk to sibs, but a high (50%) risk for offspring of the affected individual
- inheritance might be X-linked recessive, with a risk of recurrence in future sons of the healthy sister.

Clearly the conclusion reached (if any) will depend on the accuracy of diagnosis and whether it is known that the disorder constantly follows a mode of mendelian inheritance. Thus, if the diagnosis were classic achondroplasia, one could confidently predict that the case represented a new dominant mutation, whereas with some complex and atypical malformation syndromes, no definite conclusion might be possible.

Although such an example may be regarded as extreme, reduction in family size means that the 'isolated case' is rapidly becoming the typical one for genetic counselling, a trend that will certainly continue. It is no more logical in genetic counselling to await the occurrence of a classic pedigree pattern in a family than it would be to delay the diagnosis of a disorder by waiting until the full clinical picture had developed.

A warning should be given at this point not to regard mendelian inheritance as a rigid and unvarying mechanism following a fixed set of rules. As will be seen in the following pages, variability and exceptions are frequently found, often resulting in difficulties for genetic counselling. One of the most fascinating developments of recent years has been the discovery of the biological mechanisms underlying these variations and the increased understanding that this has brought to the field of genetics as a whole. As a result, we now have a much more flexible concept of genes and of mendelian inheritance than was the case even a few years ago.

AUTOSOMAL DOMINANT INHERITANCE

Although, in theory, autosomal dominant inheritance is the simplest mode for genetic counselling, in practice it provides some of the most difficult problems, with traps for the unwary that require special mention.

An autosomal dominant disorder or trait can be defined as one that is largely or completely expressed in the heterozygote. The homozygous state is either unknown or excessively rare in dominantly inherited disorders, but when it does occur it is usually much more severe than the normal heterozygous form (e.g. familial hypercholesterol-aemia) or lethal (e.g. achondroplasia). In Huntington's disease, however, the homozygote appears to be little different from the heterozygote.

In its fully developed form, the pattern of autosomal dominant inheritance is characteristic (see Figure 2.1) and allows precise risks to be given, as illustrated in Figure 2.6. The risk to offspring of affected members will be one-half, regardless of sex and regardless of whether the disease is fully developed or preclinical. The risk for offspring and more distant descendants of unaffected family members is not increased over the general population risk, provided that the individual really is unaffected.

Problems arise from the variability of gene expression that is seen in many dominantly inherited disorders and which, until recently, has not been understood to any significant extent. The uncovering of the molecular basis of this variability is proving to be one of the most interesting fields of human genetics, as well as helping to resolve the practical problems encountered in genetic counselling.

LATE OR VARIABLE ONSET

Late or variable onset of a disorder such as Huntington's disease or adult polycystic kidney disease can be a major problem. Here genetic counselling for an *affected* person provides no problems in risk estimation, but the question of how old family members have to be before they can be certain of not developing the disorder may be extremely difficult to answer. The best approach is to use a 'life table' such as that for Huntington's disease given on page 175. Unfortunately, for most disorders there is either insufficient information

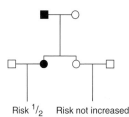

Risk ¹/₂   Risk not increased

Figure 2.6 Genetic risks in classic autosomal dominant inheritance.

or too much variation in families; while for others, such as myotonic dystrophy, the discrepancy between age at onset and first detection of the disease may be extreme. More prospective data need to be collected to answer this question for other late-onset autosomal dominant disorders.

INCOMPLETE PENETRANCE

A small but important group of dominantly inherited disorders may show no evidence of disease, even at an advanced age, in individuals known to possess the gene by reason of an affected parent and offspring. This is termed 'incomplete penetrance' of the gene. Figure 2.7 shows an example of lack of penetrance in one such disorder, hereditary pancreatitis. In part, this is determined by how hard one looks for minor or subclinical signs, and what biochemical or other diagnostic tests are available. Thus, careful biochemical study of family members in acute porphyrias will show some who are biochemically affected but who have never had clinical features. Age is also a relevant factor; thus the mutation for Huntington's disease, once established in a family, is close to 100 per cent penetrant at age 70 years, but only about 50 per cent or so at age 40 years (see Chapter 12). Conversely, penetrance may decrease with age, as with petit mal epilepsy, where the proportion of family members that can be shown to be affected clinically or by electroencephalography (EEG) decreases after adolescence. Some disorders, of which retinoblastoma is the most notable, show lack of penetrance unrelated to age or other detectable factors.

As our understanding of gene expression increases, the different mechanisms underlying lack of penetrance are becoming clearer. In the case of familial retinoblastoma, it is now clear that a mutation inherited in the heterozygous state must be accompanied by a somatic mutation involving the remaining normal allele in developing retinal tissue if a tumour is to occur.

It is possible to relate in a general way the degree of penetrance to risks for the offspring of an apparently healthy relative; the risk for children of a healthy sib never exceeds 10 per cent, even at the peak of 60 per cent penetrance (see 'Further reading'). The basis for this is that, when penetrance is high, it is unlikely that a healthy relative will have the mutant gene; when penetrance is low, the chance of actually being affected will be small, even though the mutation is present.

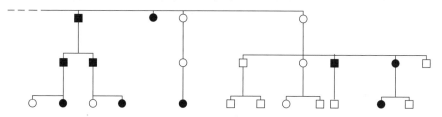

Figure 2.7 Lack of penetrance in autosomal dominant inheritance. Part of a large kindred with hereditary pancreatitis. Three apparently normal individuals have transmitted the disorder to their descendants. (Courtesy of Dr J. Sibert.) A specific mutation in cationic trypsinogen is now known in this kindred.

VARIATION IN EXPRESSION

Variation in expression refers to the degree to which the disorder is expressed in an individual (unlike penetrance, which is an index of the proportion of individuals with the gene who show it). Although some disorders (e.g. achondroplasia) are expressed with little variation, this is the exception rather than the rule for dominantly inherited disorders, so that it is wise never to assume a family member is unaffected without careful examination. In some disorders, variability is so marked that special care is needed and radiological and other tests may be required; tuberous sclerosis and myotonic dystrophy are notable examples. Apparent inconsistencies such as 'skipped generations' may be explained in this way.

Variation in expression also produces another problem in genetic counselling. Because those individuals who reproduce tend to be the least severely affected, the severity of a variable disorder is likely to be greater in the child than in the parent and this must be made clear to potential parents. Tuberous sclerosis provides a striking example of this. In addition, one may have to consider parent-of-origin effects, with severity in the children dependent on the sex of the transmitting parent, as in Huntington's disease and myotonic dystrophy. Genomic imprinting may provide a molecular explanation for some parental influences, while 'anticipation' due to unstable mutations is now recognized as a true phenomenon, as discussed below, and is involved in the two disorders mentioned.

THE BASIS OF VARIABILITY IN MENDELIAN DISORDERS

The variability that is characteristic of so many genetic disorders, notably but not exclusively those following autosomal dominant inheritance, has so far been discussed as a practical problem encountered in genetic counselling, without attempts to explain its basis. Until recently, we have had no direct evidence as to what the factors involved might be, but this is now changing rapidly and we already have a series of specific mechanisms that have been shown to operate in different situations, and which must be considered when unexplained variability is encountered. Table 2.1 summarizes those most clearly identified so far.

Genomic imprinting

The term **genomic imprinting** has been given to the process underlying differences in expression of a gene or genetic disorder according to which parent has transmitted it. On the basis of classical mendelian inheritance, it should make no difference which parent transmits a disease gene, but several striking instances exist where a disorder apparently following autosomal dominant inheritance is only fully expressed when transmitted by one particular sex. Examples include Beckwith–Wiedemann syndrome, Albright's hereditary osteodystrophy (maternal transmission) and familial glomus tumours (only clinically expressed if paternally transmitted).

These observations would not necessarily imply a special and similar underlying mechanism were it not for the fact that the genes involved lie in regions where experimental studies (mostly in mice) show a marked difference between paternal and maternal gene expression. This 'imprinting' influence of the parental genome is reversible and may be

Table 2.1 Factors underlying variability in mendelian disorders (see text for details)

Factor	Effect
Genomic imprinting	Phenotype varies according to parent of origin
Anticipation due to unstable DNA	More severe phenotype in successive generations
Mosaicism	Mild or non-penetrant phenotype
Modifying alleles	Influence of unaffected parent
Somatic mutation also required (e.g. familial cancers)	Variable penetrance

related to the degree of methylation of the DNA, something that can provide a practical test of whether this effect is operating in the human examples. To what extent imprinting is also involved in more minor variation remains to be seen, since parental effects have often not been looked for carefully in family studies.

Imprinting is important not only in mendelian disorders but in chromosome abnormalities, since it is only if the parental origin of a chromosome or chromosomal region is significant that the phenomenon of **uniparental disomy**, in which both copies of a particular chromosome or chromosomal segment are received from the same parent, will be clinically relevant. This important and increasingly recognized occurrence is described further in Chapter 4 and is a further example of how our concepts of mendelian inheritance are becoming more flexible.

Recent concern has arisen over whether there may be an increase in disorders related to genetic imprinting in children born as a result of assisted reproduction techniques, such as intracytoplasmic sperm injection (ICSI). In animals created by cloning of adult cells, there are clear problems related to this.

Anticipation and unstable DNA

The concept of a genetic disease worsening with successive generations is far from new and, indeed, was used by the early eugenicists as an argument for preventing reproduction of those with mental illness and mental handicap. While the basis for this was soon discredited, the phenomenon of anticipation persisted in relation to variable dominantly inherited disorders, notably myotonic dystrophy, where a striking progression through the generations in both age at onset and severity was difficult to explain without a special mechanism. It was over half a century until the true biological explanation emerged, which is that the myotonic dystrophy mutation is an unstable one, characterized by a DNA triplet repeat sequence that expands in successive meioses, and whose size correlates closely with the severity of the disorder. A comparable unstable sequence had already been found to underlie fragile-X mental retardation and the same has now been shown for Huntington's disease and several types of dominant spinocerebellar ataxia, forming a group of 'trinucleotide repeat disorders', mainly neurological in nature.

The details relevant to these diseases are described in Chapters 11–13; so far no other diseases have been found to have such striking instability underlying their variation, but the discovery of this previously unknown and unsuspected mechanism shows how careful one must be before dismissing phenomena for which one has no obvious explanation.

Other modifying influences

If variations in penetrance and expression reach more than a certain level, it becomes meaningless to consider the disorder as following mendelian inheritance. Nevertheless, there are numerous influences that can modify a basic autosomal dominant pattern, including sex (as in familial breast cancer), drugs (as in the acute porphyrias) and diet (as in familial hypercholesterolaemia). Variations in the normal allele may also exert an effect.

THE NEW MUTATION

The dangers of assuming that an isolated case of a dominantly inherited disorder represents a new mutation have already been mentioned. It is important to establish this accurately because if it is a new mutation, the risk of recurrence in a sib is generally low or very low (Figure 2.8). The proportion of cases of a disorder resulting from new mutations will be directly related to the degree to which the disease interferes with reproduction, i.e. its genetic fitness. Thus, almost all cases of Apert syndrome, where reproduction is rare, are new mutations, whereas in Huntington's disease, with onset most commonly in later life, the proportion is very small.

Evidence from simpler experimental species has for many years indicated the range of alterations in DNA that might underlie human disease mutations, but, visible chromosomal rearrangements apart, it is only recently that we have begun to gain insight into this for many of the important genetic disorders considered in this book. The practical importance of this new information, considered more fully in Chapter 5, is twofold. First, it is often possible to correlate the nature and site of the mutation with the severity or characteristic clinical features of the disease; this allelic or mutational heterogeneity is proving to underlie much of the phenotypic variation encountered in mendelian disorders, recessive as well as dominant, while the identification of a specific mutation in a family often makes it possible to predict, at least within broad limits, the range and severity of disease features that might occur in those at risk. Secondly, the detection of a specific mutation in a patient who appears to be a new mutant allows this to be tested directly; if neither parent shows the defect, then the presumption of a new mutation having occurred is confirmed. Clearly, this is especially relevant for those variable disorders where it is difficult to rule out the gene being present in one or other apparently healthy parent as a result of the phenomena described above.

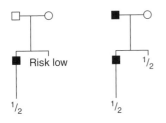

New mutation   Transmitted case

Figure 2.8 Autosomal dominant inheritance. Genetic risks for a new mutation and for a transmitted case.

However, before the low or minimal risks already indicated as appropriate to the new dominant mutation can be given confidently, one further factor, mosaicism, must be considered.

MOSAICISM AND MUTATION

Mosaicism denotes the occurrence in a single individual of cells or tissue of more than one genetic constitution. The term is confined to differences that have originated after fertilization (the term **chimaera** is used for those rare situations where an individual originates from more than one fertilized egg). Mosaicism results from mutations occurring in early development so that a significant part of the body cells or germ line carries the mutation. Visible chromosomal mosaicism has been long recognized (see Chapter 4), but only since the development of molecular analysis has the importance of its occurrence for other types of mutation been demonstrated.

Somatic mutation of later life, while of the greatest importance in relation to cancer and other degenerative disorders, is not relevant here to genetic risks. The importance of mosaicism from early embryonic mutation is that it may involve the germ line (gonadal or germinal mosaicism) in an individual who is otherwise healthy. If an affected child is born to such a person, there is a serious risk of this being attributed to a new mutation when a significant proportion of eggs or sperm are in fact carrying the mutation, with a considerable risk of recurrence.

Such a possibility has long been recognized to be likely in exceptional situations, but it has now become clear that it is a widespread phenomenon, and one that is far from rare in both dominant and X-linked disorders. For some conditions (e.g. Duchenne muscular dystrophy, tuberous sclerosis), it may give an appreciable risk of recurrence in a situation that would otherwise have been attributed to an isolated new mutation. For other conditions (e.g. osteogenesis imperfecta, achondroplasia), it is well documented but infrequent. For practical purposes, it is probably wise to regard a recurrence risk of around 1 per cent to be likely for any apparent new dominant mutation, unless a more specific estimate is available.

Gonadal mosaicism must also be considered as an alternative to autosomal recessive inheritance where two affected offspring have been born to healthy parents, especially where the disorder is normally dominant in inheritance. A number of such cases of osteogenesis imperfecta and other disorders of collagen, thought previously to be recessive in origin, have now been shown to be the result of previously unsuspected mosaicism.

HOMOZYGOSITY IN AUTOSOMAL DOMINANT DISEASE

Almost all patients seen with autosomal dominant conditions will be heterozygotes, having inherited their disorder from only one side of the family or representing new mutations. Homozygosity requires both parents to have transmitted the gene; this is most unlikely to happen unless one of the following is the case:

- the gene is common and relatively mild or late onset in its effects
- two affected individuals have married one another.

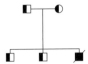

Figure 2.9 Homozygosity for an autosomal dominant disorder, achondroplasia. The parents and the two surviving children all have classic achondroplasia; they are represented by half shading to indicate that they are heterozygotes. The third child received the achondroplasia gene from both parents and had the lethal homozygous form of the disease, dying from respiratory insufficiency soon after birth. The pedigree is analogous to that commonly seen with autosomal recessive inheritance except that the heterozygotes are affected, not carriers.

Familial hypercholesterolaemia provides an example of the first situation; the heterozygote frequency may be as high as 1 in 500, so one might expect chance marriages between such individuals to occur with a frequency of 1 in 250 000. Since only a quarter of the offspring of such a couple would be homozygous, one would expect the frequency of homozygotes to be only 1 in 10^6, and they are indeed exceedingly rare. Consanguinity would, of course, increase the chance of homozygosity, exactly as in autosomal recessive inheritance.

The situation more likely to be met in a genetic counselling clinic is where two individuals with the same disorder marry preferentially. This is seen not infrequently in achondroplasia (Figure 2.9); the risks for the offspring in such a situation will be: one-quarter homozygous affected; one-half heterozygous achondroplastic; one-quarter unaffected.

In achondroplasia, the affected homozygote usually dies rapidly after birth on account of the constricted chest; in most other dominant disorders the homozygous condition is likewise very severe or lethal. In the case of Huntington's disease, no such differences have been observed, even though a number of marriages between heterozygotes are recorded; molecular analysis of the offspring has now confirmed that the homozygote may be indistinguishable from the heterozygote. An even more unusual possibility has recently been suggested for open-angle glaucoma, where homozygotes for the abnormal mutation are clinically normal.

A somewhat similar (though rare) situation may occur when marriage partners have different, but allelic, disorders. The child may then receive both abnormal alleles and will appear as a 'genetic compound'. This has been recorded with achondroplasia and the milder dysplasia hypochondroplasia. The resulting child was more severely affected than either parent, but less severely affected than the homozygote for achondroplasia.

AUTOSOMAL RECESSIVE INHERITANCE

The principal difficulty with autosomal recessive inheritance is to be sure that this is indeed the mode of inheritance in a particular family. The great majority of cases of an autosomal recessive disorder are born to healthy but heterozygous parents, with no other affected relatives. Vertical transmission, so characteristic of dominant inheritance, is rarely seen (Figure 2.10) and with the small families of the present time, it is unusual to see more than one (at most two) affected sibs. Thus autosomal recessive disorders, even more than autosomal dominant disorders, usually have to be detected from the isolated case, with little or no genetic information to help.

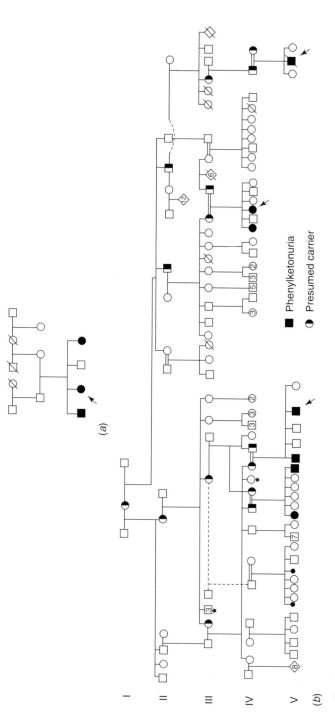

Figure 2.10 Patterns of autosomal recessive inheritance. Although many cases of autosomal recessive disease are isolated ones, a characteristic pedigree pattern is seen with large or inbred families. (a) A family with cystic fibrosis. The disorder is confined to a single sibship, with parents and more distant relatives entirely healthy. Both sexes are affected. (b) Phenylketonuria in an inbred Welsh gypsy kindred. The affected individuals have been born to healthy but heterozygous parents in this highly inbred kindred. The gene can be traced back to a single ancestral heterozygote. The origin of the gene has subsequently been confirmed by use of the phenylalanine hydroxylase gene probe.

Where the diagnosis makes this mode of inheritance certain, or in the minority of families where the genetic pattern is clear, risk prediction is relatively simple (Figure 2.11). In the great majority of instances, the only significant increase in risk is for sibs of the affected individual, for whom the risk is 1 in 4. Unless the disorder is especially common or there is consanguinity, the risks for half-sibs and children, and in particular for children of healthy sibs, is only minimally increased over that for the general population. The precise risk will depend on the frequency of heterozygotes in the population, since it will be necessary for both partners to contribute the abnormal gene for a child to be affected. It is thus important to know how to estimate the chance of being a carrier for an autosomal recessive disorder, both for family members and for the general population, and this is outlined below.

RISK OF BEING A CARRIER

The parents and children of a patient with an autosomal recessive disorder are obligatory carriers, while second-degree relatives (uncles, aunts, nephews, nieces, half-sibs, grandparents) will have a 50 per cent chance of being a carrier (Figure 2.12). Each further step will reduce the risk by 50 per cent, so that it is relatively simple to estimate the chance of any relative being a carrier if their closeness to the patient is known (see also p. 132). Sibs provide a special case: although the chance that the child of two carrier

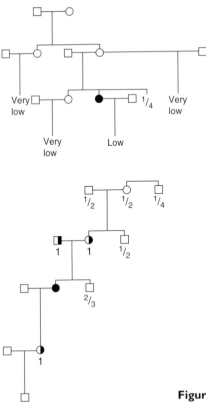

Figure 2.11 Genetic risks in autosomal recessive inheritance.

Figure 2.12 Risks of being a carrier in autosomal recessive inheritance (obligatory carriers are half shaded).

parents will be a carrier is 2 out of 4, the chance of a healthy sib being a carrier is 2 out of 3, because the affected category of individuals has been removed from consideration.

When calculating the risks for a family member being a carrier, the possibility of new mutation can be ignored because it is excessively rare in relation to the other risks. Likewise, although the general population risk must in theory be added, this is insignificant except for the most common disorders.

POPULATION RISK

It is rare for the population frequency of carriers for an autosomal recessive disease to be known by direct observation, but fortunately it can be estimated from the disease frequency by the relationship known as the Hardy–Weinberg equilibrium. In the few cases where direct observations are available, they agree closely with the predicted frequencies, so it seems reasonable to rely on them at least as an approximation.

The basis of the Hardy–Weinberg equilibrium and the possible reasons for variation from it are covered fully in genetics textbooks and are not given here. What the clinician needs to know is that the gene frequency and heterozygote frequency can be predicted, provided that the frequency of the affected homozygote is known. For the usual situation where one has two alleles, the more common 'normal' allele with frequency p, and the rarer 'disease' allele with frequency q (the combined frequency of the two must equal 1), the proportions of the different categories are as follows:

q^2 abnormal homozygotes (=disease frequency)
p^2 normal homozygotes
$2pq$ heterozygotes (carriers)

The starting point is the disease frequency, which is often known. The square root of this gives the 'abnormal' gene frequency q. From this one can obtain p, which must be $(1 - q)$. This allows one to work out the carrier frequency, $2pq$.

In practice p (the 'normal' gene frequency) is close to 1 except for exceedingly common diseases, so $2pq$ differs little from $2q$; i.e. for rare recessive disorders, the carrier frequency is twice the square root of the disease frequency.

If the above over-simplification helps non-genetically minded clinicians, it will be more than worth any retribution the author receives from his fellow geneticists!

Returning to the practicalities of genetic counselling, the risk for offspring of patients with a recessively inherited disease, and for their sibs and other relatives, can now readily be estimated. Table 2.2 gives the risks for a range of gene frequencies. It can be seen that only for the most common of recessive disorders do the risks become considerable, so that whether a relative is or is not a carrier is not of critical importance unless they are themselves marrying a close relation (see also Chapter 9).

CONSANGUINITY

The estimation of genetic risks in relation to consanguinity is discussed fully in Chapter 9, but needs a mention here in relation to autosomal recessive inheritance, because it is

Table 2.2 Risk of transmitting an autosomal recessive disorder in relation to disease incidence (the spouse is assumed to be healthy and unrelated)

Disease frequency (q^2) (per 10 000)	Gene frequency (q) (%)	Carrier frequency (2pq) (%)	Risk for offspring of affected homozygote (%)	Risk for offspring of healthy sib (%)
100	10.1	18.0	9.0	3.0
50	7.1	13.2	6.6	2.2
20	4.5	8.6	4.3	1.4
10	3.2	6.2	3.1	1.0
8	2.8	5.4	2.7	0.9
6	2.4	4.7	2.3	0.78
5	2.2	4.3	2.1	0.72
4	2.0	3.9	2.0	0.65
2	1.4	2.8	1.4	0.46
1	1.0	2.0	1.0	0.33
0.5	0.71	1.4	0.70	0.23
0.1	0.32	0.64	0.32	0.11
0.05	0.22	0.44	0.22	0.07
0.01	0.10	0.20	0.10	0.03

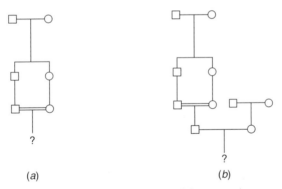

(a)   (b)

Figure 2.13 (a) Consanguinity involving both parental lines is relevant to the genetic risk. (b) Consanguinity not relevant to offspring of the marriage in question.

this category of disorders that is principally influenced by it. Several points need to be emphasized:

- Consanguinity is only relevant to genetic risks if it involves both parental lines, not just one, as shown in Figure 2.13.
- Two brothers marrying two sisters (or similar combinations), as shown in Figure 2.14, do not constitute consanguinity.
- The rarer the disorder, the higher will be the proportion of affected individuals resulting from consanguineous marriages.

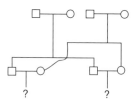

Figure 2.14 Marriage of two brothers to two sisters does not constitute consanguinity.

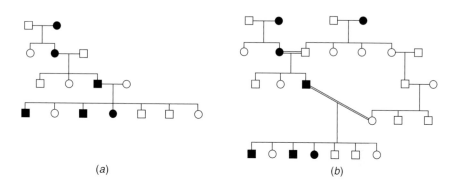

(a)   (b)

Figure 2.15 (a) An incomplete pedigree showing quasidominant inheritance of alkaptonuria. (b) The complete pedigree showing that consanguinity accounts for the pedigree pattern simulating autosomal dominant inheritance.

- The presence of consanguinity in relation to a syndrome of uncertain inheritance favours, but does not prove, autosomal recessive inheritance.
- Consanguinity must be seen in the context of the particular community; thus, in a population where 30 per cent of marriages are between cousins, an apparent relationship of a particular disorder with consanguinity is much less certain than in a population where there is only 1 per cent of cousin marriages.
- Extensive consanguinity can give the appearance of autosomal dominant inheritance, with vertical transmission resulting from an affected person marrying a carrier, as shown in Figure 2.15.

OTHER PROBLEMS WITH AUTOSOMAL RECESSIVE DISEASE

Once one is confident that the mode of inheritance is indeed autosomal recessive, the difficulties in genetic counselling are much less than those encountered in autosomal dominant disorders. In particular, lack of penetrance is rarely encountered and variation in expression is much less. Genetic heterogeneity, in terms of both more than one locus and multiple alleles at a single locus, is probably the major cause of variation within an apparently single entity; sometimes this can be recognized biochemically, as in many of the inborn errors of metabolism, while in other conditions it must be inferred from family data. An example of the practical importance of recognizing such heterogeneity is seen in the different types of recessively inherited polycystic kidney disease, in which sibs show close concordance in age of onset and death (see Chapter 21); similarly in the spinal muscular atrophies (see Chapter 11), where the classic Werdnig–Hoffman disease shows close similarity between sibs, whereas the later-onset forms show a much broader scatter. Information of this type, which may influence the likely prognosis, is just as important for parents contemplating another pregnancy as is the actual risk of recurrence.

A further factor of particular relevance for autosomal recessive disorders is the availability of prenatal diagnosis in many cases, especially those where the underlying biochemical defect is known. This is discussed in Chapter 8. The use of donor insemination, or more rarely donor ovum *in vitro* fertilization, is also relevant in recessive disorders, because the risk of an unrelated donor being a carrier for the same gene is small.

A final factor, again related to the fact that an autosomal recessive disorder necessitates both parents being carriers, is the outlook for parents remarrying. With the frequency of divorce at its current level in most of Europe and America, this must be a serious consideration when sterilization is being considered in either parent. It is, however, a difficult subject to discuss with parents, particularly when the burden of caring for an affected child is likely to be a major factor in the break-up of a marriage.

In cultures where the status of women is low and where the recognition that the genetic risks are for a particular marriage partnership could have major implications, considerable sensitivity is needed in addressing the issues.

Conversely, the necessary contribution of both parents to an autosomal recessive disorder in a child can be a positive feature in genetic counselling. It is frequently found that one parent (commonly the mother) is assuming the burden of guilt for the occurrence of the disorder, and this may be reinforced by the views (spoken or tacit) of other relatives. The realization that 'one side of the family' is not solely to blame, and that everyone carries at least one harmful genetic factor, is frequently a great relief to couples to whom a child with an autosomal recessive disorder has been born.

MARRIAGES BETWEEN AFFECTED INDIVIDUALS

Marriage between two affected individuals has already been discussed for autosomal dominant disorders, and is seen rather more frequently with those showing autosomal recessive inheritance. The usual reason is preferential marriage between similarly affected people, particularly those with blindness or deafness, who may be educated together and have a common social bond. Albinism and severe congenital deafness provide the two best-documented examples.

If the two individuals with the same disorder (e.g. the severe form of oculocutaneous albinism) marry, all offspring must be affected, since each parent can only transmit an abnormal gene, as shown in Figure 2.16.

It is crucial, however, to be sure that genetic heterogeneity does not exist, because if the parents' disorders are controlled by different loci, all offspring will be unaffected, although carriers at both loci (Figure 2.17); a greater potential for erroneous counselling cannot be imagined.

In the case of albinism, careful clinical study will usually distinguish the different forms (see Chapter 16). In severe congenital deafness, however, this is impossible, so that advice must be based on knowledge of the number and relative frequency of the different types, and on whether the couple concerned have already had affected or normal children. This situation is one of many in genetic counselling where the recognition of genetic heterogeneity is of extreme importance. Identification of the specific molecular

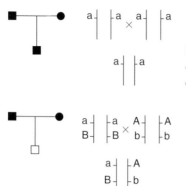

Figure 2.16 Marriage of two individuals with the same disorder; all offspring must be affected since the parents can only transmit the abnormal gene 'a'.

Figure 2.17 Marriage of two individuals with the same disorder; here the abnormal genes occur at different loci so the offspring are unaffected.

defects in the different types of both albinism and congenital deafness (see Chapters 16 and 18, respectively) is helping to resolve these problems.

X-LINKED DISORDERS

Since virtually no serious human diseases are known to be borne on the Y chromosome, sex linkage is equivalent to X linkage, so far as genetic counselling is concerned. X linkage produces some unusual problems which are of considerable practical importance, and as a result X-linked disorders occupy a much more prominent place in a genetic counselling clinic than would be expected from the relative contribution of the X chromosome to the human genome.

Over 100 definitely X-linked human disorders or traits have been recognized, and a list of the more important ones is given in Table 2.3.

McKusick's *Mendelian Inheritance in Man*, with its on-line version OMIM, (see 'Further reading') is the fullest source for rare conditions. The great majority are classed as X-linked recessive, with a much smaller number as dominant and a few as dominant but lethal in the hemizygous male. The terms 'dominant' and 'recessive' must be used with caution in X-linked disease, because a much greater degree of variability in the heterozygous female is seen than is the case with autosomal disorders. This is largely the result of X-chromosome inactivation (the Lyon hypothesis), which appears to affect almost the entire X chromosome in the human female, except for a few specific sequences. One of the two X chromosomes is randomly inactivated in early embryonic life and becomes visible as the 'sex chromatin' or 'Barr body' under the nuclear membrane. Because the descendants of each cell retain the same inactivated X chromosome, it follows that a female heterozygous for an X-linked disorder or trait will be a mosaic, with two populations of cells, one of which has the 'normal' and the other the 'abnormal' X chromosome functioning.

There is a considerable amount of direct evidence for X-chromosome inactivation in human diseases, which may be expressed in several ways. Some disorders show 'mosaic' or 'patchy' changes in heterozygotes; thus patchy retinal changes are seen in carriers for X-linked retinitis pigmentosa and choroideraemia, and patchy muscle biopsy changes may be found in carriers for Duchenne muscular dystrophy. More commonly, variability in X inactivation can result in a milder and more variable expression of clinical and biochemical changes. Thus in X-linked hypophosphataemic rickets, generally considered to be an X-linked dominant condition, affected females have milder or even subclinical disease; conversely, in haemophilia A, usually classed as an X-linked recessive condition, some carriers show a mild bleeding tendency in addition to reduced levels of factor VIII. The implications for tests of carrier detection in X-linked diseases are discussed in Chapter 7.

Table 2.3 Important mendelian disorders following X-linked inheritance

Addison's disease with cerebral sclerosis	Hypophosphataemic rickets
Adrenal hypoplasia (one type)	Ichthyosis (steroid sulphatase deficiency)
Agammaglobulinaemia, Bruton type	Incontinentia pigmenti*
(sometimes also Swiss type)	Kallmann syndrome
Albinism, ocular	Keratosis follicularis spinulosa
Albinism–deafness syndrome	Lesch–Nyhan syndrome (hypoxanthine-
Aldrich syndrome	guanine-phosphoribosyl transferase deficiency)
Alport syndrome (some kindreds)	Lowe (oculocerebrorenal) syndrome
Amelogenesis imperfecta (two types)	Macular dystrophy of the retina (one type)
Anaemia, hereditary hypochromic	Menkes syndrome
Angiokeratoma (Fabry's disease)	Mental retardation, with or without fragile
Cataract, congenital (one type)	site (numerous specific types)
Cerebellar ataxia (one type)	Microphthalmia with multiple anomalies
Cerebral sclerosis, diffuse	(Lenz syndrome)
Charcot–Marie–Tooth peroneal	Mucopolysaccharidosis II (Hunter syndrome)
muscular atrophy (one type)	Muscular dystrophy (Becker, Duchenne
Choroideraemia	and Emery–Dreifuss types)
Choroidoretinal degeneration	Myotubular myopathy (one type)
(one rare type)	Night blindness, congenital stationary
Coffin–Lowry syndrome	Norrie's disease (pseudoglioma)
Colour blindness (several types)	Nystagmus, oculomotor or 'jerky'
Deafness, perceptive (several types)	Ornithine transcarbamylase deficiency
Diabetes insipidus, nephrogenic	(type I hyperammonaemia)
Diabetes insipidus, neurohypophyseal	Orofaciodigital syndrome (type I)*
(some families)	Phosphoglycerate kinase deficiency
Dyskeratosis congenita	Phosphoribosylpyrophosphate (PRPP)
Ectodermal dysplasia, anhidrotic	synthetase deficiency
Ehlers–Danlos syndrome, type V	Reifenstein syndrome
Faciogenital dysplasia (Aarskog syndrome)	Retinitis pigmentosa (one type)
Focal dermal hypoplasia*	Retinoschisis
Glucose-6-phosphate dehydrogenase	Rett syndrome*
deficiency	Spastic paraplegia (one type)
Glycogen storage disease, type VIII	Spinal muscular atrophy (one type)
Gonadal dysgenesis (XY female type)	Spondyloepiphyseal dysplasia tarda
Granulomatous disease (chronic)	Testicular feminization syndrome
Haemophilia A	Thrombocytopenia, hereditary (one type)
Haemophilia B	Thyroxine-binding globulin, absence
Hydrocephalus (aqueduct stenosis, one type)	Xg blood group system

* X-linked dominant, male lethal.

Although X-chromosome inactivation applies to almost all the human X chromosome, there are a few loci where it does not apply, including those for the Xg blood group and steroid sulphatase. The terminal region of the short arm also has homology with part of the Y chromosome and is involved in pairing between the sex chromosomes at meiosis. The process of X inactivation is itself controlled by a different region of the X chromosome, the X-inactivation centre on the proximal long arm.

THE RECOGNITION OF X LINKAGE

Recognition of an X-linked pedigree pattern is crucial to correct genetic counselling and is surprisingly often overlooked. The following criteria apply regardless of whether the disorder is recessive, dominant or intermediate in expression (some examples are given in Figures 2.18–2.23):

- Male-to-male transmission never occurs, because a man does not pass his X chromosome to his son.
- All daughters of an affected male will receive the abnormal gene, i.e. they will all be affected if the inheritance is X-linked dominant, and will all be carriers if it is X-linked recessive.
- Unaffected males never transmit the disease to descendants of either sex. A notable but so far solitary exception to this is fragile-X mental retardation (see Chapter 13), where normal transmitting males can carry a premutation.
- The risk to sons of women who are definite carriers (or affected in the case of an X-linked dominant) is 1 in 2.
- Half the daughters of carrier women will themselves be carriers. In the case of an X-linked dominant, half the daughters of affected women will be affected and twice as many females as males will generally be affected.
- Affected homozygous females are exceptional in X-linked recessive disorders, and will only occur when an affected male marries a carrier female.

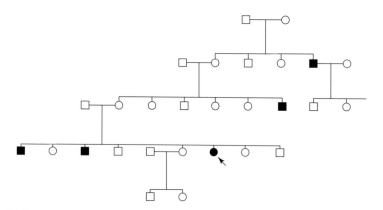

Figure 2.18 Where an affected girl is found to have a rare and clearly X-linked disorder, a sex chromosome abnormality such as Turner (45,X) syndrome should be considered. This proved to be the case in this family with X-linked cerebellar ataxia reported by Shokeir (1970), X-linked cerebellar ataxia. *Clin Genet* 1, 225–231.

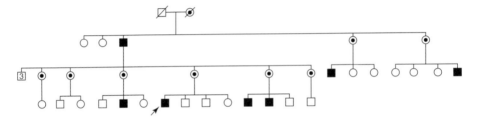

Figure 2.19 Typical X-linked recessive inheritance (haemophilia A). Note that *all* sons of an affected male are healthy, while *all* daughters are carriers. The disorder is transmitted by healthy females and is confined to males, but these features are less critical than the lack of male-to-male transmission in establishing or disproving X linkage.

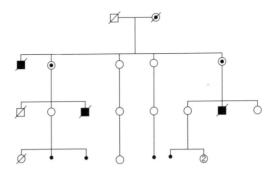

Figure 2.20 Presumed X-linked inheritance. Duchenne muscular dystrophy in a south Wales kindred. Although the disorder is confined to males and is transmitted by healthy females, as expected with X-linked recessive inheritance, the lack of reproduction by affected males means that the crucial test of lack of male-to-male transmission cannot be seen. Genetic linkage data and isolation of the gene have now confirmed X linkage.

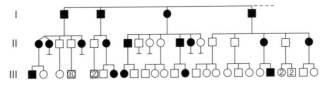

Figure 2.21 X-linked dominant inheritance in a family with familial hypophosphataemia (vitamin D-resistant rickets). The pattern is superficially similar to autosomal dominant inheritance but when the offspring of affected males are considered it becomes clear that all daughters are affected, but that the disorder is never transmitted from father to son. (After Mckusick VA (1969). *Human Genetics*, London, Prentice-Hall.)

These simple guidelines will cover most genetic counselling problems and will allow a definite decision to be made in most instances as to whether the disorder is X-linked or not. It can be seen that the situation is essentially similar for X-linked recessive and X-linked dominant disorders, the heterozygous women in the latter group being affected rather than carriers. Apparent anomalies may be the result of chromosome disorders,

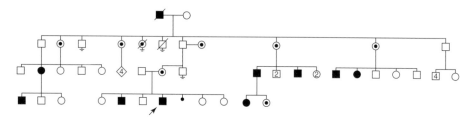

Figure 2.22 Intermediate X-linked inheritance. A south Wales kindred with hereditary oculomotor nystagmus. The pattern is recognized by examining the offspring of affected males. All sons are unaffected, but all daughters are either affected or proved to be carriers.

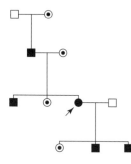

Figure 2.23 Occurrence of an affected homozygous female in a common X-linked recessive trait, red–green colour blindness.

e.g. occurrence of the disease in a 45,X female (see Figure 2.18), or of non-paternity. Very few genes are located on the pairing (pseudo-autosomal) parts of the X and Y chromosomes, giving an autosomal inheritance pattern in families. Some particular problems are shown in the following examples.

The classic X-linked recessive pattern

Figure 2.19 shows this in a family with haemophilia A.

Disorders where affected males do not reproduce
(Figure 2.20)

This may result from the severity of the disease (e.g. Duchenne muscular dystrophy) or from infertility (e.g. Kallmann syndrome). Here the test of male-to-male transmission cannot be applied, so, unless one has other genetic data (e.g. linkage markers, or occurrence in a 45,X female), X linkage is presumed rather than proven. The recognition of gene deletions and an increasing number of specific mutations on the X chromosome, including the examples mentioned, are now providing direct proof in such cases.

X-linked dominant inheritance (Figure 2.21)

The pattern may at first glance be mistaken for autosomal dominant inheritance, but if offspring of affected males are considered, all sons are unaffected and all daughters are affected. The excess of affected females can also be seen.

'Intermediate' X-linked inheritance

The blurred distinction between dominant and recessive in X-linked disease has already been mentioned. In a few conditions, heterozygotes may show the disease in one branch of a family, but not in another. Figure 2.22 shows an example of this. Although at first sight the pattern appears confusing, the situation is soon clarified if the offspring of affected males are considered – all sons are unaffected while the females either are affected or are carriers.

X-linked dominant inheritance with lethality in the male

Here the disorder is only seen in the heterozygous females, the affected (hemizygous) males being undetected or appearing as an excess of spontaneous abortions. It is difficult to prove this situation, but it has now been confirmed for several disorders, including Rett syndrome, focal dermal hypoplasia and incontinentia pigmenti. Genetic counselling requires some care: leaving aside spontaneous abortions, one-third of the offspring of an affected woman will be affected; all the live-born males will be unaffected, as will half of the females. Two-thirds of all offspring will be female. Fetal sexing with termination of female pregnancies may be considered. Where an affected child has been born to healthy parents, this is likely to represent a new mutation and the recurrence risk is likely to be low (most such patients will be female).

Common X-linked genes

Where an X-linked gene is common in a particular population, confusing pedigree patterns may be produced. This may be seen with colour blindness in European populations and with glucose 6-phosphate dehydrogenase deficiency in the Middle East. The marriage of affected males to heterozygous females is not infrequent and will result in homozygous females (see Figure 2.23), all of whose sons will be affected. A similar pattern can occasionally be seen with rarer disorders when there is consanguinity.

THE RISK OF BEING A CARRIER FOR AN X-LINKED DISORDER

Methods of carrier detection in X-linked disorders are discussed in Chapter 7, but it is clearly important to estimate the genetic risk of a female relative being a carrier so that information from carrier testing (if any) can be appropriately combined. The estimation of these risks is not always easy and is one of the situations where a mathematical approach is needed in genetic counselling. Young's *Introduction to Risk Calculation* (see 'Further reading') is strongly recommended for this and other areas of risk estimation.

Leaving aside the problems of new mutations, the situation can be approached as follows, using Figure 2.24 (the pedigree of a family with Duchenne muscular dystrophy) as an example.

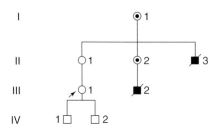

Figure 2.24 A family with Duchenne muscular dystrophy.

Table 2.4 A working table to combine risk information for the pedigree shown in Figure 2.24

	Consultand a carrier	Consultand not a carrier
Prior risk	1/4	3/4
Conditional risk (two normal sons)	1/2 × 1/2 (=1/4)	I
Joint risk	1/16	3/4 (=12/16)
Relative risk	I	12
Final risk	1/13	12/13

1. Obligatory carriers should be identified – these are I-1 and II-2.
2. The prior genetic risk of the individual requiring advice, sometimes referred to as the 'consultand' (arrowed), should be estimated. Here it is 1 in 4, since her mother's prior risk is 1 in 2.
3. Other relevant information must be incorporated. Here the relevant fact is that the consultand has had two normal sons; common sense tells us that this makes it less likely that she is a carrier – the question is, how much less likely? In fact, it can be estimated and combined with other information simply (using what is sometimes termed Bayes' theorem) by multiplying it with the corresponding prior risk. This is best done by constructing a table, which gives the chances of the two possibilities, as shown in Table 2.4.

The prior risks are clearly 1 in 4 and 3 in 4, respectively. The 'conditional' information resulting from the normal sons will give a change of 1 in 2 for this happening once if she is a carrier, and 1 in 4 (1/2 × 1/2 = 1/4) for both sons being normal if she is a carrier (three sons would give a risk of 1 in 8 and so on). The corresponding chance of two sons being normal if she is not a carrier is clearly 1 (100 per cent).

The joint risk is then obtained by multiplying the two columns and, if they are placed over the same denominator (giving 1/16 and 12/16), the relative risk can be seen to be 1 to 12 that the consultand is a carrier, or a final risk of 1 in 13.

Care must be taken to relate the 'conditional' information to the correct person. Thus, in Figure 2.25, showing another Duchenne family, the normal sons affect the chances of the mother of the consultand (II-1), being a carrier, and the risk must be worked out for her before proceeding to the daughter (III-1), whose prior risk (1 in 10) is half her mother's risk (1 in 5) (Table 2.5). If the daughter herself had normal sons, one could proceed as in the previous example but using the new prior risk of 1 in 10 as the starting point.

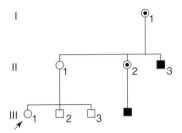

Figure 2.25 Carrier risks with an X-linked recessive disorder (Duchenne muscular dystrophy) (see Table 2.5 for calculations).

Table 2.5 Risk calculations, X-linked recessive disorder (see Figure 2.25)

	Carrier	Not a carrier
Risks for II-1		
Prior risk	1/2	1/2
Conditional risk	1/2 × 1/2 (=1/4)	1
Joint risk	1/8	1/2 (=4/8)
Relative risks	1	4
Final risk	1/5	4/5
Prior risk for III-1	1/10	

It can be seen that the use of genetic information in this way can substantially affect the risks given in genetic counselling, and in general with a methodical approach the estimations are not difficult. Incorporation of data from more distant relationships can become complex (computer programs are available to help), but rarely affects the risks to a great extent. It is important to recognize that not only genetic information may be used in this way, but also data on carrier detection, such as may be available in haemophilia and Duchenne muscular dystrophy. Some examples of this are given in Chapter 7.

A final caution should be given: because all these estimates are based on uncertainty, they may need to be modified in the light of future events. Thus the birth of an affected child to II-1 in Figure 2.25 would make her an obligatory carrier and all previous estimates would have to be discarded in the light of this. Likewise, the increasing feasibility of direct gene analysis may be a reason for reassessment.

THE ISOLATED CASE OF AN X-LINKED DISORDER

In autosomal dominant inheritance, new mutations can usually be clearly distinguished from transmitted cases; in autosomal recessive disorders, mutation plays an insignificant part in relation to transmitted genes and can be ignored in genetic counselling. In X-linked recessive disorders, however, it may be extremely difficult, if not impossible, to tell whether an isolated case represents a new mutation or whether the mother is a carrier. Since an accurate distinction is essential for correct genetic counselling, this situation needs careful consideration.

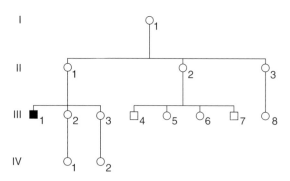

Figure 2.26 An isolated case of a lethal X-linked disorder (Duchenne muscular dystrophy). Is this a new mutation or not? (See text and following figures for the estimation of carrier risks in this difficult situation.)

When reliable methods of carrier detection exist, these should be employed. Unfortunately, the variability of gene expression in heterozygotes for X-linked disease makes carrier detection difficult in a proportion of women, even when tests exist. This is clearly seen in haemophilia A and Duchenne muscular dystrophy, where 20–30 per cent of known carriers show results of phenotypic carrier tests falling within normal limits (see Chapter 7).

The example shown in Figure 2.26 shows the practical aspects of the problem. Three possibilities exist to explain the occurrence of this isolated case of Duchenne muscular dystrophy:

- *The case III-1 is the result of a new mutation.* In this case none of the numerous female relatives is at significant risk of being a carrier.
- *The mother II-1 is a carrier, but is herself the result of a new mutation.* In this case, the daughters III-2 and III-3 are at 50 per cent risk of being carriers and their daughters IV-1 and IV-2 have a carrier risk of 25 per cent. However, none of the other female relatives is at risk.
- *The disorder has been transmitted through the mother from the grandmother I-1.* In this case, in addition to those already mentioned as being at risk, II-2 and II-3 are at 50 per cent prior risk, with a carrier risk of 25 per cent for their daughters III-5, III-6 and III-8.

Unfortunately, these three situations cannot always be distinguished with certainty by carrier testing, so one needs to approach the problems as follows:

1. The prior risk of II-1 and I-1 being carriers as opposed to III-1 resulting from a new mutation must be estimated. From this, the prior risk of other family members such as II-2 and II-3 can be estimated.
2. Conditional information (from normal sons and carrier testing results) can be tabulated as shows in the previous examples.
3. These pieces of information can be combined to give a final risk, as already shown.

The difficult problem is to decide what is the prior risk that this isolated case has resulted from mutation or has been transmitted. It has long been assumed that for an isolated case of an X-linked recessive disorder in which affected males do not reproduce and mutation rates in egg and sperm are equal, the proportions are as follows:

- new mutation (mother not carrier) – 1/3
- transmitted case (mother carrier but not grandmother) – 1/3
- transmitted case (mother and grandmother carriers) – 1/3

The derivation of this will not be given here, but using this information one can readily assign risks to the various women in the family, as shown in Figure 2.27. In Figure 2.27(b), the information from the normal sons of II-3 has also been incorporated, and it can be seen that the risks of III-5 and III-6 have been considerably lowered by the normal brothers. Carrier testing results would have produced further information which has been omitted for simplicity.

Unfortunately, there is considerable uncertainty as to whether the formula given above is generally applicable; it assumes equal mutation rates in the sexes, and in some disorders a higher proportion of mothers of isolated cases are carriers than the two-thirds expected, as is also the case for disorders where the affected males reproduce, such as the haemophilias and Becker muscular dystrophy. In the absence of other information, it is wise to assume that such a woman is a carrier rather than the reverse. For Duchenne dystrophy, the situation may vary according to whether the change is a deletion or a point mutation.

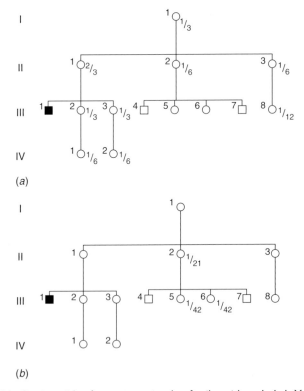

Figure 2.27 (a) Carrier risks for women in the family with a lethal X-linked disorder (Duchenne dystrophy) shown in Figure 2.26, assuming that a third of cases are due to a new mutation. (b) The same pedigree showing the modification of risks from the normal sons of II-2.

Fortunately, molecular tests are increasingly able to distinguish new mutations, though the relatively frequent occurrence of mosaicism, especially in Duchenne dystrophy, still provides problems for genetic counselling in the isolated case, as noted further in Chapter 11.

MITOCHONDRIAL INHERITANCE

While mitochondrial inheritance cannot be described in any sense as mendelian, it seems appropriate to describe it in this chapter, since it provides a characteristic pattern of transmission within families that must be compared with the equally distinctive patterns of mendelian transmission described above. The increasing identification of specific mitochondrial mutations makes it especially important to recognize this form of inheritance, which has major implications for genetic counselling.

The mitochondria are the principal cell components outside the nucleus to contain DNA, which is present in the form of a small, circular genome that can replicate and which is quite independent of the mechanisms controlling chromosomal DNA. The mitochondrial genome has been sequenced; it determines the proteins of a series of key oxidative enzymes involved in mitochondrial functions, although other such enzymes are produced by genes in the nucleus. Mitochondrial DNA is, for practical purposes, exclusively maternal in origin, with no process involving recombination and a negligible contribution from sperm.

It has long been recognized that any disorder following mitochondrial inheritance should be exclusively maternal in its transmission, as shown in Figure 2.28. While a number of individual families with differing disorders have in the past been claimed to fit the pattern, one disorder in particular, Leber's optic atrophy, has consistently done so and been predicted to be mitochondrial in origin, a conclusion now fully confirmed by the identification of mutations. Figure 2.29 shows a typical family with this disorder, which can be used, together with the preceding diagram, to summarize the general risks

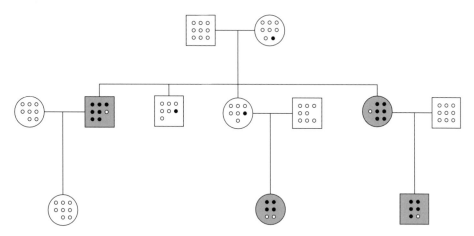

Figure 2.28 Mitochondrial inheritance (schematic pedigree). Normal mitochondria, ○; abnormal mitochondria, •. Since mitochondria are only transmitted through the ovum, not through sperm, affected individuals (shaded) are related through the maternal line. Whether an individual is clinically affected may reflect the proportion of abnormal mitochondria in the relevant tissue.

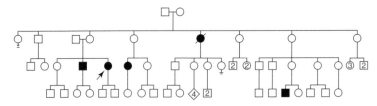

Figure 2.29 A family pedigree of a mitochondrial disorder, Leber's optic atrophy. All the affected individuals are related in the maternal line; no male family members, affected or unaffected, have transmitted the disorder. It can be seen that there are numerous females in the pedigree who are potentially at risk of developing or transmitting the disorder, as well as males who can be re-assured that they have no significant risk of transmitting it, whether or not they themselves are or become affected.

for family members relevant to genetic counselling, as follows (details specific for Leber's optic atrophy are given in Chapter 17):

- No transmission occurs to children or other descendants of males, whether they are affected or not. Nor are such descendants at risk of being gene carriers, a situation that contrasts with X linkage, where all daughters of an affected male are obligatory carriers.
- Both sexes may be affected, the precise sex ratio being dependent on the particular disorder and probably determined by other genetic and environmental factors. In Leber's optic atrophy males are more commonly affected in Europe but not in Japan.
- Females may be symptomless carriers (so may males, but this is irrelevant as they cannot transmit their mitochondria). All daughters of an affected or carrier female are themselves at risk of transmitting the disorder, as well as of becoming affected, while all sons are at risk of becoming affected.
- The precise proportion of offspring, male or female, who will become affected is vari-able (in Leber's optic atrophy this is around 50 per cent of sons and 30 per cent of daughters) and not determined by any fixed rule.

It can be seen from the above summary that the recognition of mitochondrial inher-itance is extremely satisfactory for the genetic counselling of males, since, whether they are affected or not, a confident reassurance can be given that their descendants will not be affected. For females the situation is unsatisfactory in the extreme, since there is some degree of risk to all offspring with none of the sharp demarcations and exclusions that are possible in mendelian inheritance.

A major advance during the past few years has been the identification of specific defects in mitochondrial DNA, both point mutations and large deletions, and the real-ization that such disorders are much more frequent than previously suspected. Table 2.6 lists some of the more important of these. Not all have a clearly defined phenotype, and the finding that subgroups of such common and heterogeneous disorders such as dia-betes and deafness may have an underlying mitochondrial defect is likely to pose logis-tical problems as to when a molecular defect should be searched for. It should be noted, in particular, that there are only genetic implications if the molecular defect is present in the germ line (more likely to be the case if found in DNA from a blood sample), not if the

Table 2.6 Disorders resulting from mitochondrial mutations

Leber's optic atrophy
MELAS (mitochondrial encephalopathy with lactic acidosis and stroke-like episodes)
MERFF (myoclonic epilepsy with ragged red fibres)
Kearns–Sayre syndrome
Pearson syndrome (lactic acidosis, pancreatic insufficiency, pancytopenia)
Deafness (antibiotic-induced and some forms of progressive nerve deafness)
Various poorly classified central nervous system degenerations
Diabetes mellitus (some familial types)

defect is confined to the target organ (e.g. muscle). Most large deletions of mitochondrial DNA are sporadic in nature.

It might be thought that once a molecular mitochondrial defect has been identified in a family, analysis of relatives at risk would help to resolve the genetic counselling problems described above. Unfortunately, this is not the case at all, since all those genetically at risk are likely to show at least some degree of the defect, often showing both mutant and normal mitochondrial DNA ('heteroplasmy'). We do not know at present whether there is any correlation between the proportion of abnormal mitochondria found (in blood) and the risk of developing or transmitting the disorder. Tests are also inconclusive in prenatal diagnosis for the same reason, although absence of the mutant line in a prenatal sample seems likely to indicate a low risk.

Thus the conclusion at present has to be that while the recognition of mitochondrial inheritance by pedigree pattern and molecular analysis is important in identifying genetic risks and in removing risk from descendants in the male line, it is extremely unhelpful in resolving the situation for those known to be at risk, and does not warrant testing of asymptomatic relatives. Looking to the future, the hope must be that effective therapeutic agents enhancing mitochondrial function will be developed that can be applied to those at risk before serious and irreversible clinical problems occur. A final point to be emphasized is that many mitochondrial enzymes are determined by nuclear genes; thus a mitochondrial disorder does not necessarily imply mitochondrial inheritance.

FURTHER READING

General (see also Chapter 1)

McKusick VA (1998). *Mendelian Inheritance in Man*, 12th edn. Baltimore, Johns Hopkins University Press – an invaluable resource on all aspects of mendelian disorders. A continuously updated on-line computer version (OMIM) is also available (*www.ncbi.nlm.nih.gov/omim*) as is a CD-Rom version.

Ostrer H (1998). *Non-Mendelian Inheritance in Humans*. Oxford, Oxford University Press – despite its title, this book gives a valuable account of the exceptions to mendelian inheritance.

Young ID (2000). *Introduction to Risk Calculation in Genetic Counselling*, 2nd edn. Oxford, Oxford University Press – a clearly explained and valuable guide to practical situations and to their underlying principles.

Mitochondrial disorders

Holt IJ (ed.) (2003). *Genetics of Mitochondrial Disease*. Oxford, Oxford University Press.
Suomalainen A (1997). Mitochondrial DNA and disease. *Ann Med* **29**, 235–246.
Wallace DC, Brown MD, Lott MT (2002). Mitochondrial genetics. In: Rimoin DL, Connor JM, Pyeritz RE, Korf B (eds), *Emery and Rimoin's Principles and Practice of Medical Genetics*. Edinburgh, Churchill Livingstone, pp. 277–332.

Mosaicism

Hall JG (1988). Somatic mosaicism: observations related to clinical genetics. *Am J Hum Genet* **43**, 355–363.

Imprinting

Clayton-Smith J (2003). Genomic imprinting as a cause of disease. *Brit Med J* **327**, 1121–1122.
Engel E, Antonorakis S (2002). *Genomic Imprinting and Uniparental Disomy in Medicine*. New York, Wiley-Liss.

Incomplete penetrance

Pauli RM, Motulsky AG (1981). Risk counselling in autosomal disorders with undetermined penetrance. *J Med Genet* **15**, 339–345.

Anticipation

Harper PS, Harley HG, Reardon W, Shaw DJ (1992). Anticipation in myotonic dystrophy: new light on an old problem. *Am J Hum Genet* **51**, 1016.
Richards K, Sutherland GR (1992). Heritable unstable DNA sequences. *Nat Genet* **1**, 7–9.

CHAPTER 3

Genetic counselling in common, non-mendelian disorders

The disorders to be considered here, in contrast to most mendelian conditions, will be encountered frequently by those working in all branches of medicine and in primary care. Arbitrarily, a population frequency of greater than 1 in 1000 (for the clinical disease, not for any predisposing genotype) will be taken as a working definition of what is common.

Most common disorders do not follow any of the clear patterns of mendelian inheritance outlined in the previous chapter. This applies not only to the commoner birth defects (e.g. neural tube defects, most congenital heart disease), but also to most common chronic disorders of later life (e.g. asthma, diabetes, hypertension, coronary heart disease, common cancers). Yet it has long been recognized that, to some degree, these conditions show a familial tendency, which may occasionally be striking. As a result of this, families in which such common disorders occur often seek genetic counselling, especially if multiple members have been affected. The recent general increase in awareness of genetic factors, often heightened by media attention, has increased this tendency, notably in the case of cancer.

The fact that many of these disorders are so common, at least by comparison with the mendelian disorders that form the basis of activity for most specialists in medical genetics, creates special challenges. It is quite clear that most genetic counselling for this group must, of necessity, be done by those in primary care or those involved directly in management of the particular field, since the sheer numbers would swamp the small number of available specialist clinical geneticists and their associated staff. On the other hand, available genetic risk information is often inadequate or variable and may be changing rapidly as advances in research alter classification and identify specific genetic factors.

This chapter examines some of these problems in the context of recent developments in attempting to identify the specific genes involved in common disorders. As will be seen, this is one of the most active areas of genetic research, but one where the practical applications of these advances in terms of risk estimation and genetic counselling remain extremely limited, as does the use of genetic tests.

THE GENETIC BASIS OF COMMON DISORDERS

The terms 'multifactorial' or 'polygenic' are frequently used to describe the genetic basis underlying the great majority of common disorders where there is no clear mendelian pattern. Of the two terms, multifactorial is the more appropriate since it recognizes that these disorders are the result of both environmental and genetic factors, and does not prejudge the relative role of either category. 'Polygenic' implies that a number of different genetic loci are involved rather than a single major gene.

The term 'heritability' is often encountered in relation to common disorders and refers to the proportion of variation, familial and other, that is determined by genetic factors, regardless of any pattern of inheritance. This can be assessed by a number of approaches, notably the comparison of monozygotic and dizygotic twin pairs where at least one twin has the disorder. Clearly the heritability will be one of the factors influencing recurrence risk in a family.

Our growing ability to map and isolate specific genes involved with common disorders, described later in this chapter and also in Chapter 5, has allowed two main categories to be defined, as follows:

- common disorders containing a significant mendelian subset, resulting from the action of a single major gene in a family
- common disorders where a number of genetic (and usually also environmental) factors are involved, each usually being of small or, at most, moderate influence.

MENDELIAN SUBSETS

This group is of particular importance in genetic counselling because the recognition of a mendelian (usually dominant) subset of cases gives extremely high risks for family members (or very low risk if the particular gene mutation can be excluded). The familial cancers provide a striking example, largely unrecognized until recently. Although very rare familial cancer syndromes have been recognized for many years (e.g. familial adenomatous polyposis as a cause of colon cancer), the identification of mendelian forms of breast and colon cancer that are not phenotypically distinct has had a major influence on both research and genetic counselling practice in these disorders, influences beginning to extend to most common cancers (see Chapter 25 for details). It is no longer sufficient to derive overall theoretical risks, as was done in early editions of this book, since the separation of the mendelian forms will affect the recurrence risks for those remaining. This dissection of the multifactorial basis of common diseases is not confined to cancer, but is proving relevant to a wide range of conditions where previously unsuspected or undefined mendelian families are proving to account for a significant proportion of recurrent cases.

POLYGENIC DISORDERS

In this second group, where clear mendelian forms are absent or very rare, some of the genetic factors primarily responsible for the genetic influence on the disorders are now also beginning to be identified. Much research here has focused on the HLA region of chromosome 6, long known to be a susceptibility locus for a variety of disorders with an immunological basis (Table 3.1) and it remains much the best documented susceptibility locus even after more than a decade of analysing wider genetic markers.

The past decade has seen intense research efforts into identifying the other genetic components, utilizing the existence of DNA markers across the whole genome and building on the striking success in mapping genes for mendelian disorders. Unfortunately, this important but difficult procedure has often been approached with considerable naivety. So far, only a handful of the original claims have been established beyond doubt (Table 3.2), and virtually none are sufficiently strong or reproducible to use in clinical practice or genetic counselling. It seem increasingly likely that, for many common disorders and for most normal characteristics, the genetic component results from a large number of individually small genetic effects, no one gene contributing more than a small part of the susceptibility.

A third type of genetic involvement in common disease requires a mention, although its importance outside the field of common cancers is not clear. This is where a specific gene, relatively rare in the population, has a moderate effect, insufficient to cause much family clustering but still significant in its contribution to the overall causation of the disorder.

Table 3.1 Non-mendelian disorders where the HLA region represents a significant susceptibility locus

Ankylosing spondylitis
Coeliac disease
Dermatitis herpetiformis
Diabetes (type 1)
Goodpasture syndrome
Haemochromatosis (see p. 287)
Idiopathic membranous nephropathy
Multiple sclerosis
Narcolepsy
Psoriasis
Reiter syndrome
Subacute thyroiditis

Table 3.2 Common non-mendelian diseases and DNA variations – consistently reproducible associations (excluding HLA region) (Based on Hirschhorn et al. (2002), Genet Med **4**, 45–61.)

Disease	Gene
Alzheimer's disease	ApoE
Creuzfeldt–Jakob disease	PRNP (prion protein gene)
Diabetes type 1	Ins (insulin gene)
Graves' disease	CTLA4
HIV infection	CCR5
Venous thrombosis	F5 (factor V Leiden)

Examples are seen in some types of cancer and in some congenital malformations, such as Hirschsprung's disease.

It must be emphasized strongly that the finding that a particular gene is involved in a common disorder does not convert the disorder (or even a subset of it) into a mendelian disorder. Of course, the gene itself will show mendelian segregation at the DNA level (it cannot do otherwise) but it is the disease phenotype that is relevant in terms of mendelian inheritance. This may seem an obvious point, but has been ignored by many who should know much better!

PERCEPTION AND THE GENETIC BASIS OF COMMON DISEASE

For clear-cut single gene disorders, there is rarely much doubt in the minds of professionals or the public that one is dealing with a 'genetic disorder', where environmental aspects are subsidiary to the inherited factor. For most common disorders, by contrast, the situation is far less clear, even though studies may have clearly identified an important genetic component. To a considerable extent, the perception of a disorder as 'genetic' or 'environmental' will depend on how successful workers have been in identifying specific factors; new discoveries may result in a radical change in perception – and in demand for genetic counselling.

To take two examples, peptic ulcer was regarded for many years as a largely genetic condition, with important familial influences, and with a large body of research on its genetic basis. Once an infective agent was identified, the genetic aspects rapidly became overshadowed and most people would now consider it as having a primarily environmental cause, with relatively little demand for genetic counselling.

Conversely, in breast cancer, genetic factors were considered of little relevance outside a few striking families until the BRCA genes were identified, which produced a rapid change in perception to this being a mainly 'genetic' disorder, despite the fact that these genes are responsible for only a small proportion of cases overall.

In both cases, the underlying facts and balance between genetic and environmental factors have not changed at all, but there has been a major and rapid shift in public and medical perception, reflected in the demand for, and uptake of, genetic services.

A final factor is that the degree to which a condition is seen as genetic may reflect the frequency of the environmental factors involved. Thus, for rare infectious disorders, contact with the agent itself will be the determining factor in most cases, while, if the infectious agent is ubiquitous, genetic susceptibility will have most influence.

GENERAL RULES FOR 'MULTIFACTORIAL' INHERITANCE

Since research for most common disorders is still at an early stage in resolving the number and nature of the genes involved, it is this second 'multifactorial' group where it is helpful to have some general rules that will influence risk prediction and genetic counselling.

These are summarized here, but it must be recognized that they will be largely super-seded when the specific genes involved become clear, or mendelian subgroups are identified.

The essential distinguishing factor from the mendelian disorders is that a single genetic locus cannot be held responsible for the condition; it is the result of the additive effect or interaction of a number of genetic loci and a number of external factors. The sum of these determines a person's liability to be affected with the particular disorder, and this liabil-ity can be expected to show a more or less 'normal' distribution in the population, with most people having an intermediate degree of liability and smaller numbers at each end of the distribution curve having unusually low or unusually high liability (Figure 3.1). The last group comprises those who are actually affected, whose liability is above a pos-tulated 'threshold' for the disorder.

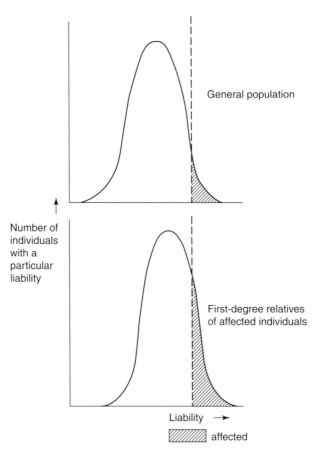

Figure 3.1 Number of individuals with a particular liability

General population

First-degree relatives of affected individuals

Liability →

▨ affected

Figure 3.1 Liability and genetic risks in multifactorial inheritance. The distribution of liability to the disorder in the general population follows an approximately normal distribution, with individ-uals exceeding a certain threshold value being affected. First-degree relatives have a similar nor-mal distribution of liability, but the curve is shifted to the right by the increased genetic component, so a greater proportion will exceed the threshold and be affected.

Table 3.3 Multifactorial inheritance: factors increasing risk to relatives

Close relationship to proband
High heritability of disorder
Proband of more rarely affected sex
Severe or early-onset disease in proband
Multiple family members affected

From this concept, it can be seen that even a person with an unusually high genetic liability may not be affected if environmental factors are favourable, and the converse will also apply. The degree to which liability is determined by genetic factors as opposed to environmental factors is often considered as the heritability of a disorder, although in practice familial but non-genetic factors may often be included in this. The liability of relatives of a patient with the disorder will also be normally distributed in a similar way to that of the general population, but the curve will be shifted towards higher liability because of the increased genetic component.

The 'threshold model' is not essential for the operation of multifactorial inheritance; for quantitatively distributed variables such as height or blood pressure, the same principles apply. It should also be noted that only a small number of genetic loci (as few as four or five) are required for the discrete patterns of mendelian inheritance to be transformed into a relatively smooth curve of distribution of liability.

Turning to the practical aspects, the following points are relevant (summarized in Table 3.3):

- Increased risk is greatest among closest relatives and decreases rapidly with distance of relationship. It is rare to find a significant increase in risk for relatives more distant than second degree; even here risks are usually small.
- The risk of recurrence will depend on the incidence of the disorder, unlike in mendelian inheritance. A useful approximation where specific figures are not available is that the maximum risk to first-degree relatives is approximately the square root of the incidence, i.e. where the incidence is 1 in 10 000, the recurrence risk would be 1 in 100.
- Dominance and recessiveness do not generally apply. Thus the risk for sibs is comparable to that for offspring. Risks for offspring are not yet available for many serious childhood disorders, but can usually be taken as approximately equivalent to the risks for sibs in the absence of further information, unless there is evidence of a significant proportion of isolated cases being the result of new dominant mutations.
- Where there is an unequal sex incidence, the risk is higher for relatives of a patient of the sex in which the condition is less common; for example, in pyloric stenosis (which is more common in males), the risk for brothers of a male index case is 3.8 per cent, but for brothers of a female index case it is 9.2 per cent (see Chapter 20). At first sight this may seem unexpected, but when it is considered that girls require a greater genetic liability to develop the disorder than do boys, it can readily be seen that relatives of an unaffected girl will also have a greater genetic liability than where the index case is a boy.
- The risk may be greater when the disorder is more severe. This is well shown in Hirschsprung's disease, where the risk for sibs of patients with long segment disease

is greater than for those with a short segment affected (see Chapter 20). Again, the greater severity reflects greater liability, part of which will be genetic and thus shared with relatives. For disorders of adult life, early onset in the proband will increase the risk for relatives (as in breast cancer). In part, this effect may result from inclusion of unrecognized mendelian cases in these severe or early-onset groups.

- The risk is increased when multiple family members are affected. This again results from the concentration of genetic liability in the particular family and is in contrast to the mendelian situation where the number of affected family members (leaving aside mutation) is irrelevant. The influence of more distant relatives is less easy to determine, although computer programs have been developed to combine the information. In general, one close (first-degree) relative outweighs several distant ones. Particular care must be taken in such families to be as certain as possible that one is not dealing with a mendelian subtype of the disorder.

EMPIRIC RISK DATA

This term, already mentioned in Chapter 1, is merely a statement of the fact that someone has actually looked at what happens in a particular situation. Data on the risks to relatives are available for a large number of non-mendelian disorders and, provided the study has been careful and as far as possible unbiased, such information provides the most satisfactory basis for counselling until the genetic basis can be resolved further. It has to be remembered, however, as stated in Chapter 1, that such risk figures are not universal in their application as are mendelian ratios. In particular:

- Data collected on one population may not be applicable to others where the incidence, and perhaps aetiology, of the disorder in terms of both genetic and environmental factors are different.
- Improved classification of disorders, in particular resolution of heterogeneity, identification of single gene subsets, or identification of specific causative factors, may require radical revision of risk estimates.
- Risks may depend not only on the diagnosis but also on individual factors such as sex, severity of disease and number of affected family members.

Empiric risk figures are given for as many disorders as possible in the specific sections of this book. Most are based on old, though thorough, studies, so there is a need for new data of this type using revised criteria.

THE MOLECULAR BASIS OF GENETIC SUSCEPTIBILITY

The way in which isolation of specific genes has increased our understanding of a disease has already been mentioned. The effects on our understanding of common disorders, though, are beginning to be much more profound, especially where single gene subsets are identified, and this forms one of the most exciting areas of current medical research generally. It has to be admitted that epidemiological and other approaches to detecting the environmental components have, for most disorders (with a few exceptions such as neural tube defects), been disappointing; thus the value of current genetic research is not so much that it shows the importance of genetic factors in common disorders but that it is starting to provide knowledge of their pathogenesis, which is equally relevant to the external factors. Colorectal cancer again provides an excellent example, with the series of tumour suppressor genes identified providing defined points on which environmental carcinogens can act. In diabetes, although the evidence remains far from secure, the identification of involvement of different susceptibility genes in types 1 and 2 reinforces the role of different external factors – probably infective in type 1 and nutritional in type 2.

These advances are likely to have major consequences in how we classify diseases and, in the future, how we approach therapy, which may well need different agents according to the underlying genetic changes. This prospect in part explains the high interest and involvement of major pharmaceutical firms in this field.

When it comes to using genetic susceptibility tests in risk prediction and genetic counselling, however, their use is at present of minimal help and potentially of considerable harm. The scientific basis of risk estimates applied to individuals, as opposed to large series, is generally very uncertain, with wide margins of error, complex interactions with other factors and differences between populations. Even the strongest associations (e.g. HLA B27 and ankylosing spondylitis) are far from definitive (see Chapter 14); although a normal result in a suspected patient may make the condition very unlikely, an 'abnormal' result in a healthy relative at risk is still much more likely to be associated with normality than with clinical disease. Most associations (e.g. ApoE4 and Alzheimer's disease) are much less strong and consequently of little use in genetic counselling, while, as mentioned earlier, the great majority of associations with particular genetic polymorphisms either fail to be confirmed or are of uncertain significance. As general population screening tools for susceptibility, they are likely to be positively harmful, creating needless worry without being able to resolve it.

Thus the main aims of genetic counselling for common disorders at present remain the identification (and exclusion) of the high-risk genetic subsets, along with the provision of risk estimates based on empiric studies and the general principles given above. With these points in mind, primary clinicians should be able to handle themselves most of the requests that they encounter and be able to refer on the relatively small number where unusual family patterns or clinical features point to a high-risk situation, where a specialist in clinical genetics may be able to be of real additional help.

FURTHER READING

Hirschhorn JN, Lohmueller K, Byrne E, Hirschhorn K (2002). A comprehensive review of genetic association studies. *Genet Med* **4**, 45–61.

King RA, Rotter J, Motulsky AO (eds) (2002). *The Genetics of Common Disorders*, 2nd edn. Oxford, Oxford University Press – a valuable and comprehensive book giving details on all major topics, as well as on general and theoretical aspects. Its often critical approach is especially valuable (e.g. the chapter on evolution of human genetic diseases by Diamond and King).

Ostrer H (1998). *Non-Mendelian Inheritance in Humans*. Oxford, Oxford University Press.

Weatherall DJ (2000). The role of nature and nurture and common diseases. Garrod's legacy. *The Harveian Oration*. London, Royal College of Physicians.

Wilkie AO (2003). Polygenetic inheritance and genetic susceptibility screening. In: Cooper DN, ed. *Nature Encyclopedia of the Human Genome*. London, Nature Publishing Group, pp. 596–601.

Young ID (2000). *Introduction to Risk Calculation in Genetic Counselling*, 2nd edn. Oxford, Oxford University Press – an extremely useful book for those needing risk estimates.

CHAPTER 4

Chromosome abnormalities

Chromosome disorders are relatively common as the cause of serious childhood malformations, but before describing the risks in specific groups of chromosomal disorders, there are two points worthy of mention that the clinician should bear in mind from the outset:

- The great majority of chromosomal disorders have an extremely low risk of recurrence in a family, especially where no abnormality is present in a parent.
- The great majority of disorders following mendelian inheritance, especially those of adult life, show no visible chromosomal abnormality.

Thus, not all patients with a genetic disorder need chromosome analysis; to request this uncritically is unnecessary, expensive and will prevent the laboratory from concentrating its resources on samples for which a detailed analysis may be essential. There may even be the danger of a family being given a falsely low genetic risk on the grounds of a normal chromosome result. However, since chromosomal disorders are poorly treatable but accurately detectable prenatally, it is essential that situations requiring cytogenetic analysis are recognized and that the small number of cases of chromosome abnormality giving high risks to relatives are clearly distinguished from the much larger number where these risks are low.

During the last few years, the separation between mendelian and chromosomal disorders has become less clear with the recognition of small chromosomal deletions in a number of different disorders, including some important malformation syndromes appearing to follow mendelian inheritance. Working from the other direction, molecular geneticists have shown that the mutational event involved in some cases of mendelian disorder is a deletion of genetic material rather than a specific base change. Additional recent developments include the recognition that parent-of-origin effects due to genetic imprinting and uniparental disomy, already mentioned in Chapter 2, are relevant to disorders of whole chromosomes or chromosomal regions.

Fortunately, a series of new technical developments, notably fluorescence in-situ hybridization (FISH), are now in diagnostic use, helping to resolve chromosome disorders that were previously confusing, as well as identifying others not recognizable by the use of earlier techniques.

CHROMOSOME TERMINOLOGY

All 23 pairs of human chromosomes can be distinguished microscopically from each other, and much fine detail within each chromosome can also be recognized (Figure 4.1). An agreed international system of nomenclature (Figure 4.2), reviewed at regular intervals, forms the basis of reports from laboratories. Although these reports will usually be

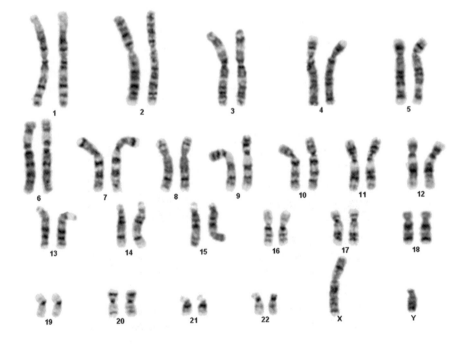

Figure 4.1 The normal human karyotype (male); trypsin–Giemsa preparation to show G-banding pattern. (Kindly provided by Selwyn Roberts and Merle Vaughan.)

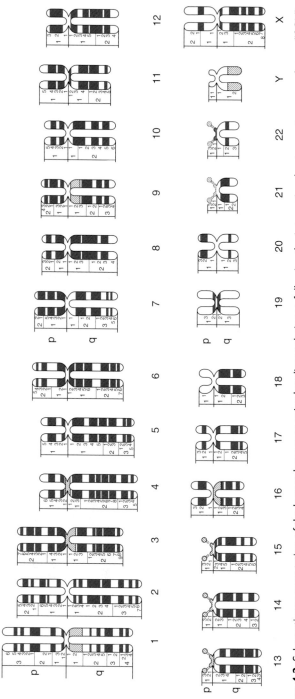

Figure 4.2 Schematic representation of the human karyotype using banding techniques, following the international cytogenetic nomenclature (ISCN).

accompanied by an explanatory letter, clinicians may be deterred by the terminology itself, so some brief notes are given here.

Take the following example:

46,XY,t(4;22)(q32;q12)

This denotes the fact that the individual has a balanced translocation between the long arms of chromosomes 4 and 22. Several points can be noted:

- The total chromosome number is given first. In this example there is the normal number of 46.
- The sex chromosome constitution comes next. Here the patient is chromosomally male (XY) as opposed to female (XX).
- A translocation is indicated by the letter 't' with details of the chromosomes involved in brackets. In this example, chromosomes 4 and 22 are involved.
- The arms of a chromosome are indicated by the letters 'p' for the short arm and 'q' for the long arm ('p' is for *petit*, reflecting the strong French influence in early cytogenetics). In our example, the long arms of the two chromosomes are involved in the translocation. The breakpoints are given in the second brackets, indicated by numbers corresponding to band designations at points of exchange, in this case bands q32 and q12 on chromosomes 4 and 22, respectively.

Gain or loss of an entire chromosome is indicated by a '+' or '−'. For example, a male infant with Down's syndrome resulting from trisomy 21 would have the karyotype designation 47,XY,+21.

For gain or loss of part of a chromosome, the terms 'add' (addition) or 'del' (deletion) are used. An example is 46,XY,del(5)(p15) (deletion of the short arm of chromosome 5), as seen in the cri-du-chat syndrome.

Further details in chromosome reports may deal with mosaicism (the presence of more than one cell line), inversions, ring chromosomes, the identification of particular bands on a chromosome and the use of FISH techniques. If in any doubt, the clinician should make personal contact with the cytogenetics laboratory. This will provide a more meaningful idea of the problem and will allow a better assessment of risks by discussion with cytogeneticist colleagues. Most laboratory cytogeneticists will be delighted by the opportunity to learn more specific details from the referring clinician, and may in turn be able to suggest further clinical investigations from their knowledge of the phenotype associated with particular chromosomal defects.

CYTOGENETIC TECHNIQUES

Cytogenetic techniques are not described here, but are covered by suggestions in the 'Further reading' section. It should be noted that techniques are evolving rapidly, and that a fusion of molecular and cytogenetic methods is allowing molecular applications to chromosomal disorders, notably FISH. It is also becoming possible to study interphase nuclei, a process that is beginning to have major implications for the early prenatal detection of Down's syndrome.

FREQUENCY OF CHROMOSOME ABNORMALITIES IN THE POPULATION

Four sources of information are available:

- studies of newborn populations
- studies of particular chromosomal disorders
- studies of abortions and stillbirths
- prenatal diagnosis series.

STUDIES OF UNSELECTED NEWBORN POPULATIONS

Table 4.1 summarizes the principal findings, based on studies which revised earlier estimates by using banding techniques. It can be seen that 9.2 per 1000 (or approaching 1 in 100) infants had recognizable chromosomal abnormalities, of which around three-quarters had autosomal abnormalities and a quarter had sex chromosome abnormalities. Although the numbers were insufficient to give accurate data on individual disorders, these newborn figures are a useful reference point with which to compare any increased risk. Table 4.2 gives data collected on the major specific chromosome disorders; these prevalence data do not exactly correspond with Table 4.1 because of mortality and ascertainment differences. In Tables 4.3 and 4.4, data on spontaneous abortions are summarized. It can be seen that live-born infants with chromosomal disorders represent only a fraction of those conceived with such abnormalities. Indeed, spontaneous abortion is the rule rather than the exception for most serious autosomal disorders, some of which (e.g. trisomy 16) are extremely common in abortuses, but never reach full term. The incidence of chromosomal abnormalities in abortions declines with increasing gestation, and studies of stillbirths have shown a frequency of around 5 per cent. Identification of a chromosomal abnormality in a stillbirth is of considerable practical importance, especially when multiple malformations are present, because it allows a possible rare mendelian disorder to be ruled out, and may also identify a familial translocation.

Table 4.1 Chromosome abnormalities in unselected newborns

Abnormality	Frequency (per 1000 births)
All abnormalities	9.1
Autosomal trisomies	1.4
Balanced autosomal rearrangements	5.2
Unbalanced autosomal abnormalities	0.6
Sex chromosome abnormalities:	
in phenotypic males	1.2
in phenotypic females	0.75

Based on Jacobs PA et al. (1992), J Med Genet **29**, 103–108.

Table 4.2 Population frequency of specific chromosomal disorders

	Per 1000 live births*
Trisomy 21	1.5
Trisomy 18	0.12
Trisomy 13	0.07
XXY (Klinefelter syndrome)	1.5
45,X (Turner syndrome)	0.4
XYY syndrome	1.5
XXX syndrome	0.65

*Births of appropriate sex only for sex chromosome abnormalities.

Table 4.3 Chromosome abnormalities in spontaneous abortions and stillbirths

	Percentage
All spontaneous abortions	50
Up to 12 weeks	60
12–20 weeks	20
Stillbirths	5

Table 4.4 Major types of chromosome abnormality in spontaneous abortions

	Percentage
Trisomies	52
45,X	18
Triploidy	17
Translocations	2–4

TRISOMIES

TRISOMY 21

Most cases of Down's syndrome, the most important chromosome disorder, result from free trisomy of chromosome 21, and the overall population incidence (in the absence of prenatal diagnosis) is around 1 in 650 live births. Early and rapid chromosome analysis is important in all clinically suspected cases, since the clinical diagnosis, though usually clear, is not always so and the risk of potential complications is considerable. There is a well recognized (but often misinterpreted) relationship of trisomy 21 with maternal age, as shown in Tables 4.5 and 4.6. Paternal age is of little significance, an observation that fits with the confirmation by molecular studies that over 90 per cent of cases of the major

Table 4.5 Risk of Down's syndrome in relation to maternal age (live births)

Maternal age at delivery (years)	Risk	Maternal age at delivery (years)	Risk
15	1:1580	33	1:575
16	1:1570	34	1:475
17	1:1565	35	1:385
18	1:1560	36	1:305
19	1:1540	37	1:240
20	1:1530	38	1:190
21	1:1510	39	1:145
22	1:1480	40	1:110
23	1:1450	41	1:85
24	1:1400	42	1:65
25	1:1350	43	1:49
26	1:1290	44	1:37
27	1:1210	45	1:28
28	1:1120	46	1:21
29	1:1020	47	1:15
30	1:901	48	1:11
31	1:795	49	1:8
32	1:680	50	1:6

Data from Cuckle HS et al. (1987), Br J Obstet Gynaecol **94**, 387–402 (combined from eight studies).

Table 4.6 Maternal age and chromosome abnormalities found at amniocentesis (rate per 1000)

Maternal age (years)	Trisomy 21	Trisomy 18	Trisomy 13	XXY	All chromosome anomalies
35	3.9	0.5	0.2	0.5	8.7
36	5.0	0.7	0.3	0.6	10.1
37	6.4	1.0	0.4	0.8	12.2
38	8.1	1.4	0.5	1.1	14.8
39	10.4	2.0	0.8	1.4	18.4
40	13.3	2.8	1.1	1.8	23.0
41	16.9	3.9	1.5	2.4	29.0
42	21.6	5.5	2.1	3.1	37.0
43	27.4	7.6		4.1	45.0
44	34.8			5.4	50.0
45	44.2			7.0	62.0
46	55.9			9.1	77.0
47	70.4			11.9	96.0

Based on Ferguson-Smith MA (1983), Br Med Bull **39**, 355–364.

trisomies are of maternal origin. Parental chromosome analysis is not necessary (though often requested) in an isolated and uncomplicated case of trisomy 21. It can be seen from the two tables that the risk estimate varies according to whether live-birth or amniocentesis data are used. Which is most appropriate will depend on the circumstances. In making a decision on whether or not to request amniocentesis in a relatively low-risk situation, Table 4.5 is usually most helpful. Where a decision has already been made in favour of testing, Table 4.6 may be more relevant. In any event, it should be made clear which criteria are being used. It is important to note the following points:

- The incidence in offspring of young women (25 years old and under) is very low (<1 in 1000); it may rise again slightly in the youngest mothers.
- The risk does not rise above that of the overall population risk until a maternal age of around 30 years.
- The risk of a Down's syndrome child reaches 1 per cent at a maternal age of about 40 years and rises steeply thereafter, with a slight fall possible in the few births to women in their late 40s. Increasing use of IVF procedures in older women points to the need for more accurate data for this group.

Recurrent trisomy 21

The risk of another affected child being born to a couple who have had one trisomic Down's syndrome child is increased over the normal risk, but the increase does not show a simple relation to maternal age. Confirmation of a low overall recurrence risk comes from combined amniocentesis data, which show a risk of 1 in 200 or 0.5 per cent for trisomic Down's syndrome and of 1 per cent for all chromosomal abnormalities in pregnancies where the indication was a previous child with trisomy 21. Because live birth and amniocentesis data are similar here, an appropriate risk for non-translocation Down's syndrome recurring is 1 in 200 under the age of 35 years. Above this age the risk appears to be little different from the general population age-specific risks given in Tables 4.5 and 4.6. There is no detectable increase in risk for second-degree or more distant relatives.

Risk for offspring of Down's syndrome patients

Risks would be expected to be high, but data are scanty since affected males or females rarely reproduce. A risk of around 1 in 3 for offspring of female patients seems likely. There is no satisfactory information for mosaics.

OTHER VIABLE AUTOSOMAL TRISOMIES (13, 18 AND 22)

Other trisomies are rare (as live births) in comparison with trisomy 21. Recurrence (except for translocation cases) is uncommon but data are few; most age-related recurrence risk will be for the more common Down's syndrome, for which the risks given above should be used. Maternal age is also a factor; Table 4.6 gives the age-specific risks for trisomies 18 and 13 at amniocentesis. The live-birth risks are considerably lower because of the frequency of spontaneous abortion, being around one-third the amnio-centesis rate for trisomy 18 and half that for trisomy 13. Since trisomy 13 can be due to a translocation, and both conditions may also be mimicked by non-chromosomal (often autosomal recessive) disorders, cytogenetic analysis is essential in any suspected case.

Non-viable autosomal trisomies are extremely common in spontaneous abortions and it is questionable whether amniocentesis in a subsequent pregnancy is warranted when such an abnormality is detected. How far risks for a future live-born child are increased by a previous chromosomally abnormal abortion is still uncertain; if the abnormality was a late abortion or stillbirth then it seems wise at present to use the same risk figures as for a live birth.

SEX CHROMOSOME ABNORMALITIES

Recurrence in a family is exceptional for any of the sex chromosome abnormalities (Table 4.7). Even among the offspring of affected fertile individuals, transmission is rare, for reasons not fully understood.

The 45,X (Turner) syndrome is frequently associated with aortic coarctation and almost invariably with streak gonads, primary amenorrhoea and short stature. It is commonly seen in spontaneous abortions. Mosaics or partial deletions of the X chromosome (see p. 30) may show streak gonads without the full phenotypic features, as may iso-chromosomes (see p. 76).

Hypogonadism is likewise a primary feature of the XXY (Klinefelter) syndrome, but not of the XYY syndrome, where tall stature is the most conspicuous feature, the association with behavioural problems being much less strong and specific than originally believed.

Long-term information on individuals with sex chromosome abnormalities is becoming available from studies of infants detected at birth by population studies. In general

Table 4.7 The more common sex chromosome disorders: clinical features

Clinical features	Klinefelter syndrome	XYY syndrome	Turner syndrome	Triple X syndrome
Chromosome constitution	XXY	XYY	45,X	XXX
Phenotypic sex	Male	Male	Female	Female
Gonads	Atrophic testes	Normal	Streak ovaries	Often normal
Fertile	No	Yes	No	Yes
Intelligence	Normal/slightly reduced	Usually normal	Usually normal	Usually reduced
Behavioural problems	May occur	May occur	Minimal	May occur
Other features	Hypogonadal features	Tall; severe acne	Short; neck webbing; aortic coarctation	Few

the phenotypic effects in XXY, XYY and 45,X individuals are mild; in particular, serious mental retardation is exceptional, although there is a slight reduction in mean intelligence quotient (IQ), along with an increased incidence of learning disability, often correctable. This may be more marked in XXX individuals. It is important that parents of a newly diagnosed child, as well as couples in whom such a condition has been detected by amniocentesis, are given an accurate picture of the likely situation, rather than one biased by the more serious problems of the minority attending hospital clinics.

CHROMOSOME ABNORMALITIES IN RECURRENT ABORTION AND INFERTILITY

This topic is covered in Chapter 22.

CHROMOSOME TRANSLOCATIONS

TRANSLOCATION DOWN'S SYNDROME

The great majority of cases of Down's syndrome have 47 chromosomes due to trisomy 21, but in about 5 per cent of cases the chromosome number is normal (46) and the extra chromosomal material is translocated onto another chromosome. This type of rearrangement is known as a Robertsonian translocation. Most commonly, the second chromosome involved is chromosome 14, and less commonly chromosome 22, 13 or 15. Very occasionally two chromosomes 21 are translocated onto each other.

The genetic risks in such a situation depend entirely on whether there is an abnormality in the parental chromosomes. If the chromosomes are normal, as in 75 per cent of cases, the risk to further offspring is minimal, probably similar to that following a trisomic child at the same maternal age, and under 1 per cent in younger women. If one parent has an abnormal karyotype, the situation is entirely different.

The usual parental abnormality is a balanced Robertsonian translocation, in which the chromosome number is 45, but the total amount of chromosomal material is normal; one chromosome 21 will be absent, and an abnormal chromosome will be seen composed of the 21 and the chromosome onto which it has been translocated. Banding techniques will allow precise identification.

The possibilities for offspring of such a parent are shown in Figure 4.3. In theory, one might expect all the categories to occur in equal proportions, but since trisomy 14 or the absence of one chromosome 14 or 21 (monosomy) is lethal and rarely results in an identified pregnancy, the risk of a child with translocation Down's syndrome should be 1 in 3. In fact, it is considerably lower, particularly when the father is carrying the balanced translocation. Table 4.8 summarizes the risks.

Two cautions should be given regarding these risks: first, the risk of an abnormality detected at amniocentesis is higher than given in Table 4.8 for live births, probably around 1 in 8 for pregnancies of a woman who is a balanced 14/21 translocation carrier;

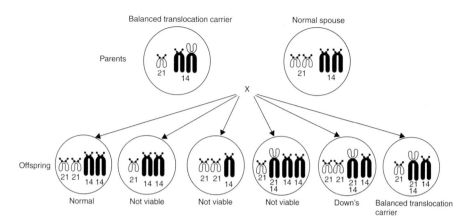

Figure 4.3 Possibilities for offspring in families with translocation Down's syndrome.

Table 4.8 Possibilities for offspring in families with translocation Down's syndrome

Type of translocation	Parent carrying balanced translocation	Risk to offspring (%)
14/21	Mother	10
	Father	2.5
	Neither parent	<1
21/22	One parent	Data scanty, risks probably as for 14/21 translocation
	Neither parent	Low (probability <1)
21/21	One parent (either sex)	100
	Neither parent	Low (probablity <1)

and secondly, data have been obtained principally from women who have already had an abnormal child – where the balanced chromosomal abnormality is detected incidentally, the risk may well be lower.

Data for the rarer 21/22 translocation are much less extensive than for 14/21, but risks are similar. However, in the case of the very rare 21/21 balanced translocation all pregnancies will be abnormal because the only alternatives are the unbalanced translocation Down's syndrome and the lethal monosomy.

Once a case of translocation Down's syndrome has been identified, it is essential to test the parents; if one of them proves chromosomally abnormal, other relatives should also be offered testing in order to identify unsuspected balanced translocation carriers (of either sex), who can then be offered prenatal diagnosis in any future pregnancy. It is rare now for a case of Down's syndrome not to be karyotyped, but clearly this is especially important in the infants of younger mothers, in whom trisomy is less frequent (although it is much more common than translocation at all ages). A register of both translocations and trisomies will often save unnecessary amniocentesis in relatives at a later date.

Table 4.9 Figures for the approximate likelihood of a chromosomally unstudied Down's patient representing an inherited translocation

Age of mother (years)	Likelihood of being inherited translocation (%)	Risk for offspring of a healthy sib (%)	
		Female	Male
<20	2.8	0.14	0.035
20–24	2.7	0.135	0.03
25–29	1.8	0.09	0.02
30–34	1.3	0.065	0.015
35–39	0.4	0.02	0.005
40–44	0.1	0.005	0.001
45–49	0.04	0.002	0.0005
<30	2.3	0.12	0.03
>30	0.5	0.025	0.006
Total	1.2	0.06	0.15

Based on the data of Albright GG, Hook EB (1980), *J Med Genet* **17**, 273–276.

Data are available on the likelihood of an unstudied case of Down's syndrome being the result of an inherited translocation at various maternal ages (Table 4.9). It can be seen that risks for offspring of healthy relatives are extremely small and rarely warrant amniocentesis.

RECIPROCAL TRANSLOCATIONS

Down's syndrome is not the only disorder that may result from autosomal translocations. Some may be responsible for other multiple malformation syndromes, or parental abnormalities may be discovered as a result of chromosomal studies for recurrent abortion or infertility (see Chapter 22). The principal form of rearrangement is a reciprocal translocation, where there is an exchange of chromosome material between chromosomes but no change in total chromosome number. It can be appreciated that such changes, especially if small, may be difficult to recognize; it may occasionally also be difficult to be sure if the rearrangement is balanced or unbalanced. FISH techniques may be helpful in such situations. The risk to offspring will depend on whether and how the rearrangement interferes with the normal process of meiosis. The individual situation will need careful study, and it is possible to work out the specific risks from the breakpoints or from diagrams of meiosis involving the abnormal segments, as shown by Gardner and Sutherland and by Young (see 'Further reading'). It is wise to consult closely with the cytogenetics laboratory, but the following general points can be made:

- The recurrence risk of an abnormality is very low if neither parent is a balanced carrier for the translocation.
- If the rearrangement in the affected individual appears balanced, it should be questioned whether it is related to the condition concerned or coincidental. Study of

the family may help by showing healthy members with the same chromosome 'abnormality'.

- Reciprocal translocations involving certain chromosomal segments, e.g. the short arm of chromosome 9 and the distal part of the short arms of chromosomes 4 and 5, have a high risk of an unbalanced defect (possibly as high as 30 per cent). Otherwise, recurrence risks where one parent is a carrier are approximately 20 per cent (those given in Table 4.8 for 14/21 translocation Down's syndrome).
- X-autosome translocations may impair fertility as well as resulting in unbalanced abnormalities in offspring. If the rearrangement has disrupted a specific gene, it may result in a female balanced X-autosome translocation carrier showing an X-linked disease, such as Duchenne dystrophy.
- Balanced Robertsonian translocations of chromosomes other than 21 (most often 13 and 14) are usually phenotypically normal despite the overall chromosome number being 45; they are relatively common, and are not usually associated with unbalanced chromosome defects in the offspring.

INVERSIONS

Rearrangement of genetic material within a chromosome is increasingly recognized by chromosome banding techniques. When the rearrangement is confined to one arm of a chromosome (paracentric inversion), the risk of abnormality in the offspring is small and possibly due to ascertainment bias (3 per cent has been suggested); however, if the centromere is involved (pericentric inversion) in an autosome, this may cause problems in pairing of chromosomes at meiosis, and gametes with an unbalanced chromosome complement may be formed. This may be discovered in a parent after a child with an unbalanced chromosome abnormality has been born, or it may be an incidental finding. Once again, figures are scanty as to the risks of abnormality: where an abnormal child has been born and the inversion is familial, the risk is probably comparable to that seen for translocations and amniocentesis is advisable in future pregnancies; where it is an incidental discovery, it is much less certain whether there is a significant increase in risk. The situation should be discussed carefully with the cytogenetics laboratory. Pericentric inversion of chromosome 9 is common and is a normal variant.

MOSAICISM

A chromosomal mosaic is an individual whose organs contain more than one chromosomally distinct line of cells. When one of the cell lines is normal (e.g. 45,X/46,XX Turner mosaicism), the phenotype of the individual will usually be intermediate between the full disorder and normal. Some chromosome disorders are only known in mosaic form (e.g. mosaic trisomy 8), the full condition probably being lethal.

Mosaicism may be undetected in blood chromosome preparations, and skin biopsy should be performed for culture if it is seriously suspected. Mosaicism in placental tissue (as studied in chorionic villus samples) may occur when the fetus is normal (see p. 120). Accurate risk figures for the offspring of patients showing chromosomal mosaicism are

Table 4.10 Some distinctive cytogenetic syndromes

Chromosome anomaly	Syndrome	Features
4p–	Wolf–Hirschhorn	Characteristic facies, frontal bossing, microcephaly, hypospadias
5p–	Cri-du-chat	Hypertelorism, characteristic cry
Trisomy 8 mosaicism		Craniofacial dysmorphism, everted lower lip, marked plantar furrows
12p tetrasomy	Pallister–Killian	Characteristic facies
18p–		Round facies, micrognathia, dental defect
18q–		Depressed mid-face, bulbous fingertips, genital anomalies
22q + dic(22)	Cat eye	Coloboma, anorectal atresia

not available, but prenatal diagnosis for their pregnancies should be offered, even though likely risks of abnormality are small.

Chromosomal mosaicism has recently been recognized to underlie some cases of malformation syndrome characterized by striped or whorled skin lesions; the increasing recognition by molecular techniques of mosaicism in single gene disorders has already been described in Chapter 2.

Mosaicism should be distinguished from chimaerism, where an individual is composed of cell lines from more than one zygote, which may rarely occur in a twin pregnancy.

DELETIONS

Deletions involve visible loss of a part of a chromosome. Phenotypic features may be less severe than when an entire chromosome is lost, so they are seen involving chromosomes where complete loss or trisomy is incompatible with a full-term pregnancy. Some of the increasing number of abnormalities that give relatively specific clinical features are included in Table 4.10. Risks of recurrence will be minimal in the absence of a rearrangement in a parent. Where chromosome studies are normal despite a distinctive phenotype, it is worth considering molecular studies, including in-situ hybridization; such studies have shown deletions in a number of previously undetected cases.

Ring chromosomes are essentially deletions in which the deleted ends of the abnormal chromosome have joined together. Parental chromosomes should be checked, but recurrence is rare if these are normal.

MICRODELETION SYNDROMES

New banding techniques, together with studies on chromosomes in a relatively elongated phase, have shown minor but consistent changes in several disorders not previously associated with visible chromosome defects, some of which follow mendelian inheritance. These

Table 4.11 Genetic disorders associated with chromosome microdeletions

Chromosome involved	Disorder
7q	Williams syndrome
8q	Langer–Giedion syndrome
11p	Wilm's tumour, aniridia and associated anomalies
13q	Retinoblastoma
15q	Prader–Willi/Angelman syndrome (see text)
16p	Rubinstein–Taybi syndrome
17p	Smith–Magenis syndrome
17p	Miller–Dieker lissencephaly syndrome
20p	Alagille syndrome
22q	DiGeorge/Shprintzen syndrome (see Chapter 19)

have been confirmed and extended by molecular studies. Table 4.11 lists some of these; it is important to recognize that not all patients with the clinical disorder show the abnormality, and to ensure that the laboratory knows that it is one of these small and difficult to detect abnormalities that is under suspicion. DNA probes from the specific region are becoming diagnostically useful in these disorders, as is FISH. These techniques should be used, if possible, when one of these disorders is strongly suspected. Deletions of 22q are proving to be frequent in specific forms of congenital heart disease, as discussed in Chapter 19. In Prader–Willi and Angelman syndromes, the same region of chromosome 15 is involved, but because of genomic imprinting, a different phenotype will result, depending on which parented region is lost, the loss being paternal in Prader–Willi and maternal in Angelman.

For all chromosome microdeletion syndromes, the recurrence risk in sibs will be low if parents are clinically normal and do not show the chromosomal or molecular defect present in the affected child.

UNIPARENTAL DISOMY

It is a fundamental fact of genetics that a child receives one copy of every autosome from each parent, but occasionally this does not happen – when both copies originate from one parent, this is termed **uniparental disomy**. This may have no harmful effects, in which case it will be unrecognized, but problems may arise if either of the following are true:

- the transmitted copies both carry a mutated gene present in heterozygous state in the parent (this has occurred in rare cases of cystic fibrosis)
- part of the chromosome shows 'genetic imprinting' (see Chapter 2), so that two inactivated chromosome regions are transmitted.

Prader–Willi and Angelman syndromes provide the clearest examples of uniparental disomy in conjunction with imprinting, although this is less common than microdeletions. Recurrence is very unlikely with any form of uniparental disomy.

Now that specific genes have been identified in the critical region of chromosome 15, it is becoming possible to determine which are responsible for the phenotype of the two disorders, and to find specific mutations in the minority of cases where no deletion is present.

ISOCHROMOSOMES

Isochromosomes are most commonly seen for the X chromosome; the majority result from breakage in the short or long arm so that a symmetrical chromosome consisting of either two long arms, or rarely two short arms, is formed. Patients show varying degrees of the Turner phenotype.

HEREDITARY FRAGILE SITES

Fragile sites occur on several chromosomes, giving the appearance of breakage at a specific point. On the autosomes they are entirely harmless, being seen usually only in the heterozygous state. On the X chromosome, the occurrence of a fragile site near the end of the long arm is generally associated in males with a syndrome of X-linked mental retardation and macro-orchidism, the fragile-X syndrome. This is discussed in more detail in Chapter 12. Fragile sites may be of considerable importance in relation to translocation sites, and to the somatic genetic changes involved in neoplasia, but there is no evidence that carriers of autosomal fragile sites are especially prone to cancer or to other diseases.

NORMAL VARIATIONS

Human chromosomes vary considerably in their morphology and clinicians may be concerned by a report of a minor variant and uncertain of its significance. Since for the most part it is people with a disorder who have their chromosomes examined, these variations are frequently reported in association with clinical problems which later prove unrelated. Studies of the rest of the family may resolve the issue by showing the variant in healthy members; close discussion with the laboratory should avoid problems in most instances. Relatively frequent changes of this kind are especially seen in the heterochromatic regions of chromosomes 1, 9 and 16, and variable length of the long arm of the Y chromosome.

FURTHER READING

Gardner RJM, Sutherland GR (2003). *Chromosome Abnormalities and Genetic Counselling*. Oxford, Oxford University Press – a clear and detailed source of recurrence risks and underlying mechanisms in chromosome disorders.

ISCN (1995). *An International System for Human Cytogenetic Nomenclature*. Basel, Karger.

Rooney DE, Czepulkowski BH (eds) (2001). *Human Cytogenetics. A Practical Approach*, 2nd edn. Oxford, IRL Press.

Schinzel A (2001). *Catalogue of Unbalanced Chromosome Aberrations in Man*. Berlin, De Gruyter.

Young ID (2000). *Introduction to Risk Calculation in Genetic Counselling*, 2nd edn. Oxford, Oxford University Press.

Molecular genetics and genetic counselling

The possibility of analysing individual genes and detecting specific defects responsible for human genetic disorders has now reached the point where molecular genetics is an integral part of medical genetics services; increasingly it is also becoming part of wider diagnosis and medical practice.

Genetic counselling has been affected profoundly by these molecular advances. Not only have they resulted in valuable specific tests that allow carrier detection and prenatal diagnosis where these were previously unreliable or impossible, but we are also gaining insight into the basis of the variability in expression that is characteristic of so many genetic disorders, and which provides some of the most difficult problems of genetic counselling. At an operational level, the establishment of molecular diagnostic services alongside cytogenetics laboratories, and their increasing interrelationship, means that molecular techniques are now an essential part of the way in which we manage the problems of families with genetic disorders.

This chapter touches on some of the more important aspects of molecular genetics relating to genetic counselling, the current status of molecular genetic services and also some of the issues arising in genetic testing.

LABORATORY ASPECTS

It is not essential for those involved in genetic counselling to have a detailed knowledge of laboratory methods of DNA analysis, particularly since techniques used are changing rapidly, but it is helpful for the clinician to have a brief outline of the principal approaches. The book of Strachan and Read (see 'Further reading') gives an excellent and clear account of the field. Anyone involved regularly in genetic counselling should develop close links with their local molecular genetics laboratory.

ISOLATING DNA FROM HUMAN CELLS

It is surprisingly easy to isolate pure DNA from human cells: DNA is much more stable than enzymes or most other large molecules, and a series of fairly simple steps allows it to be isolated from any cell type that has a nucleus, including white blood cells, buccal cells, amniotic cells, chorionic tissue and skin fibroblasts. The DNA will be essentially the same whatever its tissue of origin, a considerable advantage over most proteins, which are tissue-specific. A sample of only 20 mL of whole blood (often less) gives ample DNA for multiple diagnostic procedures; what is more, it is very stable and can be stored for years if necessary. Techniques of DNA amplification, such as the polymerase chain reaction (PCR), can utilize and amplify minute quantities of DNA, allowing material such as mouthwashes, stored filter-paper screening blood samples and hair roots to be used for the detection of specific mutations, although blood remains the choice for most testing.

POLYMERASE CHAIN REACTION AND THE DETECTION OF POINT MUTATIONS

Although in some disorders (e.g. Duchenne dystrophy) a high proportion of mutations are the result of large deletions in DNA detectable by Southern blotting, this is the exception and for many conditions the majority of gene defects are the result of point mutations. These can be recognized, once discovered, by constructing DNA primers to cover the short stretch of sequence affected by the mutation; however, obtaining sufficient copies for analysis represented a problem until the PCR was devised, which utilizes thermal cycling to produce amplification of the sequence. This has revolutionized the detection of mutations by giving a highly sensitive method that can be used on very small samples. Often a 'multiplex' system (detecting a number of possible mutations at once) can be used.

DNA HYBRIDIZATION (SOUTHERN BLOTTING)

The types of molecular abnormality detected by this approach are principally those altering the length of a DNA fragment, whether by deletion, duplication, or by altering the point on which a restriction enzyme works. The band corresponding to a fragment may be absent, or its size (as shown by its position) may be altered. Most point mutations in a gene will not be detected. Most useful is the ability of DNA hybridization to detect normal inherited variations (polymorphisms) within or around the gene, which can be used to track a disease gene within a family even though no specific molecular defect may be detectable. This abundance of stable genetic variation in DNA not only has proved to be of great value in clinical application, but has been the basis of the development of the human gene map (see below). With the development of other techniques, Southern blotting is now relatively rarely needed.

DIRECT DNA SEQUENCING

Automated techniques of DNA sequencing have allowed this approach to become part of molecular diagnostic practice, as well as forming the current basis of the human genome project. Sequencing approaches are particularly suitable for smaller genes, and for situations where the precise mutation in a family may not already be known. Against this, however, must be set the possibility that a change in sequence detected might not be causative for the particular disorder. As with all techniques, it requires careful interpretation in an individual context.

THE HUMAN GENOME PROJECT

The sequencing of the human genome, essentially completed in 2003, represents both an epic chapter in the understanding of human biology and the foundation for practical applications in relation to human genetic disorders. In some ways, though, it represents the starting point rather than the end; we still do not understand how most genes work in either health or disease, but we have the information to begin exploring these questions.

The sequencing of the genome was preceded by an important phase of **gene mapping**, allowing the 'positional cloning' of many important disease genes (e.g. cystic fibrosis, Huntington's disease), as well as giving direct practical applications in the form of gene markers linked to important inherited disorders. Now that all the genes have been specifically identified (around 35 000), it is possible to note some of the aspects that are of most immediate relevance to genetic counselling and genetic testing:

- *Genetic heterogeneity* – this has proved to be the rule rather than the exception, with more than one locus responsible for a clinical disorder in most instances (e.g. adult polycystic kidney disease). Sometimes clinical and other differences can be recognized once it is possible to separate the different genetic forms.
- *Multiple phenotypes from a single locus* – this has been a more surprising finding, with some widely different disorders proving to result from mutations in the same gene (e.g. *RET* oncogene mutations in both multiple endocrine neoplasia and Hirschsprung's disease.
- *Extensive homology of genes and mutations across different species*, even those far apart – this has been of immense importance in allowing the use of model organisms in research and in understanding developmental processes and defects (see Chapter 6), which show a particularly high degree of sharing across all species.
- *Recognition of subsets of common disorders* following mendelian inheritance within a much larger 'multifactorial' group (see Chapter 3).
- *With a few exceptions, human genetic diseases seem to be rather randomly scattered* around the different chromosomes, with genes involving similar pathways or diseases often widely separated. However, there has been considerable conservation during evolution, so that areas of the mouse genome, for example, can be shown to correspond to specific human regions. This is proving important in showing homology between human disorders and the numerous well-studied mouse mutants. The X chromosome shows the highest degree of homology between species.

THE MOLECULAR BASIS OF MUTATION IN GENETIC DISEASES

The different types of mutation that may produce genetic disorders have already been mentioned briefly; many of these mechanisms were already known from experimental studies on *Drosophila* and other experimental organisms and from work on well understood molecules such as human haemoglobin. Now that information is becoming available on numerous human genes and diseases, the wide variety of mutations is apparent. In some disorders, such as cystic fibrosis, a single common mutation may predominate, while in others, dozens or hundreds of mutations may occur with a relatively even frequency. There may be particular `hot spots' in the gene where most mutations occur, as in Duchenne dystrophy; while the actual form of the mutation may range from deletions of varying sizes, duplications or insertions of DNA, to point mutations, in different parts of the gene. The phenotypic effect of the mutation may depend more on its site than on its size, particularly on whether it interrupts the 'reading frame' and hence radically alters the amino acid sequence of the protein produced. For most genetic disorders, we are only just beginning to gain a clear picture of the correlation (if any) between the type, extent and site of a mutation and its clinical effects, but already this is beginning to be useful in giving an approximate guide to likely prognosis, as in myotonic dystrophy, Gaucher's disease and cystic fibrosis. Computer-based mutation databases (see 'Further reading') can help to synthesize this information.

THE CLINICAL APPLICATIONS OF MOLECULAR GENETICS

Most regional medical genetics centres now have molecular genetic diagnostic laboratories alongside cytogenetic laboratories and clinical genetic services. While the scope and organization of these vary, the close links, formal and informal, between laboratories and clinical geneticists around the world mean that it is usually possible for molecular genetic testing to be carried out for a family, once the basic research stage has been validated. At the very least, DNA can be isolated and stored for future analysis. Thus the onus is now very much on clinicians to be sure that families under their care are aware of what can and cannot be done in terms of molecular prediction, to keep in close touch with their local genetic service, and to ensure that DNA is banked on those patients with a genetic disorder where information from DNA analysis may be essential in allowing an accurate prediction for relatives in the future.

Previous editions of this book listed those diseases for which molecular analysis was possible, but the rapid advances of the past few years have so increased this list that it is now better to assume that molecular analysis is potentially possible for any single-gene disorder, to be aware of the minority where it is still not possible, and to check whether recent advances may have altered the situation. There can be few fields of medicine where what is possible is changing so rapidly. The computer databases and internet sites given in the 'Further reading' section and Appendix (p. 380) are probably the best way for anyone to learn the current situation.

Unfortunately, there is a growing gap between what has been discovered and what is available in service; once initial research interest has faded, the disorder may be 'dropped' as research workers move on to other fields, while for rare disorders, it may prove difficult to set up systematic service funding. There is an urgent need for a systematic network that will cover a wide range of less common genetic disorders on a national or international basis. In the UK this is now being addressed through the UK genetic testing network, and there are comparable initiatives for Europe as a whole and for North America (see the Appendix for website addresses).

MUTATION ANALYSIS

Whether the defect detected is a deletion or a point mutation, its discovery allows a specific test to be applied to relatives at risk, regardless of pedigree structure. This is particularly helpful in the isolated case, where linked markers often cannot be used. This emphasizes the point already made (but all too often ignored) that DNA should be isolated and stored from such cases (with appropriate consent), to allow future mutational tests that can help family members.

If mutations can be detected in most or all affected individuals, this raises the possibility of the test being used as part of primary diagnosis, rather than within established families. This may be extremely helpful in clinically variable disorders (e.g. myotonic dystrophy, where detection of the specific expansion can confirm or exclude the diagnosis), or where a particular genetic disorder is part of a range of possible diagnoses. However, it must be borne in mind that the genetic possibilities may not have been explained to patients and relatives (see below).

A further note of caution in interpreting the finding of an apparently specific mutation is the need for firm proof of cause and effect, already mentioned in connection with DNA sequencing. In the early stages of research after a gene is isolated, it may be far from clear whether a particular change is a causative mutation or a harmless normal variation unrelated to the disease state. This emphasizes the need for a clear body of peer-reviewed evidence before a test is accepted as the basis for service molecular diagnosis.

A final point to be emphasized is that the detection of a mutation in a person at risk does not make a diagnosis of a clinical disorder. Many mutations are proving to have much lower penetrance than was initially thought likely; while the mutation will of course show a mendelian pattern in a family, this does not necessarily mean that the related disorder will. This obvious point is often overlooked and many healthy individuals with a predisposing mutation are falsely (and harmfully) labelled as having a 'disease' as a consequence (see 'Presymptomatic testing' below).

LINKED DNA POLYMORPHISMS

There remain many conditions that have been mapped but where the gene itself remains unknown, or where it may be impossible to identify a specific mutation. In this situation, linked DNA markers may be the only possible approach to prediction and may be extremely valuable, especially now that highly polymorphic microsatellite markers have been developed. However, their use raises numerous possibilities for error and misinterpretation, some of which are considered below. While linked markers will usually be replaced by gene-specific tests when available, the process is being balanced by the discovery of linked markers for previously unmapped diseases. It is thus important that the use and limitations of linked markers are not forgotten. The main issues are as follows:

- *What is the recombination rate between marker and disease?* This will represent the minimal error rate. Bear in mind that until data are abundant, this figure may have wide confidence limits, and that it may vary between male and female meioses. Now that most markers used are within the gene itself, these error rates are normally very low.
- *Is there evidence for genetic heterogeneity in terms of more than one locus?* Since most families seen for counselling are relatively small, this is a particularly important point; again, the answer may not be clear until much information has been collected, as seen in disorders such as adult polycystic kidney disease and tuberous sclerosis, where two loci for each exist, with overlapping phenotypes.
- *Is the family structure suitable for linkage prediction?* This requires consideration before tests are offered; where parents or affected members are dead or unavailable, it may be impossible to make a prediction. Even when a missing person's genotype can be inferred, this gives extra scope for error.
- *Is the 'phase' known?* This term may be unfamiliar so an explanation is given as an example in Figure 5.1. In Figure 5.1(*a*) it is clear which marker allele has been passed on with the disease gene – the 'phase' is known; in Figure 5.1(*b*), by contrast, this is not known because the grandparents are dead; the potential error in prediction will be greater than the recombination rate.
- *Is the family completely or partially informative?* This is illustrated in Figure 5.2; it can be seen that in Figure 5.2(*a*) a prediction can be made whatever the genotype of the

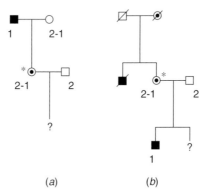

(*a*)   (*b*)

Figure 5.1 The importance of linkage 'phase' in DNA prediction; two families with Becker X-linked muscular dystrophy. (*a*) It is clear that the individual marked with an asterisk has received the disease gene from her father along with allele 1, i.e. the linkage phase is known. Transmission of allele 1 to a pregnancy would indicate the fetus was affected unless recombination had occurred. (*b*) Since the grandparents are dead, it is not known whether the disease gene has been passed on with allele 1 or 2, i.e. the phase is unknown. No prediction would have been possible for the first pregnancy. Knowing that the affected son has received allele 1 makes it likely that allele 1 and the disease gene are together on the same chromosome, but this could be due to recombination, increasing the error rate for prediction in a future pregnancy.

offspring, while in Figure 5.2(*b*) only those 50 per cent of offspring who are homozygous can be predicted as normal or abnormal, no prediction being possible for those who are heterozygous. It is essential to know this in advance if prenatal diagnosis is being considered.

- *Do flanking markers exist?* If two close marker loci on either side of a disease can be shown not to have recombined, it will be most unlikely that error from recombination will have occurred in relation to the disease.

Risk estimation using linked markers may thus be extremely difficult, even in an apparently simple pedigree. When it is realized that one may also have to incorporate risk data from other tests and more distant pedigree information, it should be clear that the procedure should not be embarked on lightly. Computer programs exist which are helpful and accurate, although they should not be used blindly.

CARRIER DETECTION

Molecular techniques have revolutionized carrier detection for many genetic disorders, as described in more detail in Chapter 7. DNA abnormalities and polymorphisms do not show dominance or recessiveness and are thus readily detectable in the heterozygous state. This has its greatest advantage in X-linked disorders, because one avoids the problems produced by X-chromosome inactivation, a process that has made all other attempts at carrier detection in these disorders fraught with uncertainty. Now that accurate molecular approaches are available, we at last have reliable carrier detection for such disorders as the haemophilias and muscular dystrophies, although previous carrier test results should not be ignored.

PRENATAL DIAGNOSIS

DNA does not usually alter during embryonic development (with the possible exception of unstable trinucleotide repeat mutations), so a further advantage of the molecular

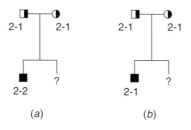

(a)   (b)

Figure 5.2 DNA prediction in cystic fibrosis. (*a*) A 'fully informative' pedigree. The affected child has received allele 2 from the father and from the mother. Only genotype 2-2 in a subsequent pregnancy would be predicted to be affected. (*b*) A partially informative family. It is not certain which parent contributed allele 1 and which allele 2. In a subsequent pregnancy only homozygotes (1-1 or 2-2) could be predicted as unaffected, while those typing 2-1 would have a 50 per cent chance of being affected. **NB**: Most predictions for cystic fibrosis would now use specific mutation detection.

approach is that it can be used in early prenatal diagnosis (see Chapter 8), in particular in first-trimester material from chorion biopsy.

There has already been widespread application of molecular prenatal diagnosis, now normally based on direct mutational detection; the range of disorders involved includes most serious mendelian disorders where the gene has been isolated or accurately mapped. Chapter 8 gives further details.

Chorion villus sampling provides a sample which can be analysed directly without the need for cell culture, and DNA yield of which is generally superior to that of amniocentesis. Since the risk of an affected pregnancy in prenatal diagnosis of mendelian disorders is usually high, the possible extra miscarriage rate is not usually such a critical factor as it may be in low-risk cytogenetic indications. The potential use of molecular techniques in pre-implantation diagnosis, together with the need for caution, is also discussed in Chapter 8.

PRESYMPTOMATIC TESTING

The fact that tests based on DNA are essentially independent of disease onset and other phenotypic features makes it possible to use them in a wide variety of late-onset disorders where clinical features of the condition may not be detectable for many years. Although this has obvious advantages where earlier treatment or preventive measures are possible, such situations are few at present. Even where there are such options, as in some of the familial cancers, important issues are raised that need detailed discussion before testing is done. Depending on the individual disorder, a variable proportion of individuals at risk will decline the offer of testing when fully informed. This proportion ranges from around 10 per cent in familial polyposis, where effective surgical treatment exists, through around 50 per cent in familial breast cancer, where outcome of early treatment is much less clear, to more than 80 per cent in Huntington's disease, where no effective therapy exists and where the reasons for people wishing to be tested relate more to relief of uncertainty and to reproductive decisions than to medical measures.

There is a general consensus that presymptomatic testing should not be considered as a purely laboratory activity, but that it should be closely linked to genetic counselling, so that fully informed consent can be based on a proper foundation of information, preparation and support. Precisely how this can be ensured will vary according to the disorder; its complexity will reflect the difficulties inherent in the condition and there is no need for an identical model to be applied universally. There is, however, a range of issues that are common to most disorders of late onset, and some to all genetic disorders. These include the implications of an abnormal result for future employment and insurance; family and reproductive issues, including the genetic implications to relatives; strategies for coping with an abnormal result and likely support from family and friends; and the more general issue of whether the consequences of all these aspects should lead to a decision to proceed with testing or to decide against it. Chapter 28 discusses some of these wider issues.

Most experience so far has come from Huntington's disease (see Chapter 12), which represents an extreme situation on account of its severity and lack of therapy. A 'two-stage' approach has been generally adopted here and found to be necessary, both to allow the complex issues to be fully discussed and to give a 'pause for reflection' that permits individuals to withdraw from the testing process should they so wish. Testing protocols for other neurological degenerations have followed a comparable line, as has genetic testing for familial breast cancer. It is probably fair to say that as other specialities begin to appreciate the complexity of the issues, this two-stage approach will prove to be the norm, rather than the exception. It has the additional advantage of allowing two separate samples to be analysed.

DIAGNOSTIC GENETIC TESTING

The term 'diagnostic' is often used rather loosely and inaccurately in relation to genetic testing. While it is reasonable to use the term molecular diagnostics for this whole field, it must be remembered that most of the analyses relate to determination of genotype, which may or may not provide a definite diagnosis, while many of the individuals tested are healthy individuals, rather than 'patients' with symptoms requiring a diagnosis. This distinction may seem pedantic, but there are very real differences in the approach needed to symptomatic and to healthy individuals, which influence greatly any associated genetic counselling.

Increasingly, with specific mutation testing feasible, true molecular genetic diagnosis is now possible when a patient is being investigated whose clinical features suggest a particular genetic disorder. Such testing may make unnecessary other more invasive (or more expensive) tests such as biopsies or electrophysiology, or the different approaches may be used in conjunction or sequentially. In this diagnostic situation, detailed genetic counselling, as practised in relation to presymptomatic testing, may often not be necessary, and a simpler explanation is frequently adequate. Likewise, diagnostic genetic testing is something increasingly requested by a wide range of clinicians as part of their practice, without involvement of a specialist clinical genetics service; again, this is in contrast to presymptomatic testing, where such specialist involvement is usually important.

Before it is concluded, though, that diagnostic genetic testing can be handled just as any other medical test, several important points need to be considered. First (but often omitted) is the need to inform the patient that a genetic disorder is under consideration, and that an abnormal result may have a major impact on the wider family. This is especially relevant for those disorders with a small genetic subset (e.g. prion dementias), where the individual and family concerned may have no perception that the disorder could be inherited. Secondly, it is essential that any symptoms are related to the disorder being tested for; this is especially so if a family history has been recognized. Thus, to take the example of Huntington's disease given in Chapter 12, genetic testing for an individual whose complaint is headache (unrelated to the disorder) would really be presymptomatic, not diagnostic, testing and should be handled accordingly. As the practice of genetic testing becomes more widespread, many clinicians requesting such tests may not have thought about these important issues.

GENETIC TESTING – THE WIDER PROCESS

The above paragraphs on the applications of genetic testing have illustrated how important it is for this to be regarded not purely as a laboratory activity (although laboratory quality issues are vital) but as part of a more general process. In some cases the associated aspects are relatively simple and can readily be handled by whoever is initiating the test. In others, however, notably in presymptomatic testing for serious late-onset disorders, the issues can be exceedingly complex and may need the time and skills of a specialist in this area. Chapter 28 discusses some of these aspects further. Deciding what the particular situation needs is going to be an increasingly important skill in the training of clinicians and others involved, with implications just as great as deciding on criteria for specialist referral and complex interventions in other fields of medicine.

FURTHER READING

Advisory Committee on Genetic Testing (1998). *Genetic Testing for Late Onset Disorders*. London, HMSO.

Bridge PJ (1997). *The Calculation of Genetic Risks: Worked Examples in DNA Diagnostics*. Baltimore, Johns Hopkins University Press.

Cooper DN, Krawczak M (1993). *Human Gene Mutation*. Oxford, Bios.

European Directory of DNA Diagnostic Laboratories – *http://www.eddnal.com*

GeneTests (International Directory of Genetic Laboratories) – *http://www.genetests.org*

Harper PS (1997). What do we mean by genetic testing? *J Med Genet* **34**, 749–752.

Holtzman NA, Watson MS (1997). *Promoting Safe and Effective Genetic Testing in the United States*. Washington, DC, National Institutes of Health.

Jameson LJ (ed.) (1998). *Principles of Molecular Medicine*. New Jersey, Humana.

McKusick VA, Amberger JS (2002). The morbid anatomy of the human genome. In: Rimoin DL, Connor JM, Pyeritz RE, eds. *Emery and Rimoin's Principles and Practice of Medical Genetics*. Edinburgh, Churchill Livingstone, pp. 137–234 – this continually updated list of mapped and cloned disease genes can also be accessed through McKusick's *Mendelian Inheritance in Man* and OMIM (*http://www.ncbi.nlm.nih.gov/omim*).

Scriver CR, Beaudet AL, Sly WS, Valle D (2001). *Metabolic and Molecular Bases of Inherited Disease*. New York, McGraw Hill (and updated CD Rom and online versions – *http://genetics.accessmedicine.com*) – contains molecular details on many specific disorders.

Strachan T, Read AP (2003). *Human Molecular Genetics*. Oxford, Bios.

Trent RJ (1997). *Molecular Medicine: an Introductory Text*. Edinburgh, Churchill Livingstone.

Mutation databases

Human Gene Mutation Database – *http://www.hgmd.org* – a valuable general database of the range and types of mutation found in genetic disorders based on the book by Cooper and Krawczak (see above).

Locus-specific mutation databases – these are increasing in number and often also contain helpful general information; they can be accessed through the Human Gene Mutation Database (see above). Two valuable examples are Phenylalanine Hydroxylase Mutation Database (for PKU) and Cystic Fibrosis Mutation Database.

Dysmorphology and genetic syndromes

Congenital malformations represent one of the most frequent and important reasons for seeking genetic counselling, with 2–3 per cent of births in most populations affected by a condition that falls into this category. Until very recently, clinicians have had to rely almost entirely on their own skills and experience to make an accurate diagnosis, with laboratory studies helping in only a minority of cases. This is now changing rapidly, and the underlying basis of congenital malformations is one of the most exciting and practically relevant fields of science and medicine.

A range of different laboratory approaches can be used to help genetic counselling (see Table 6.1), but the most rapidly growing area is the study of the metabolic and molecular pathways underlying normal development, along with the corresponding gene defects that produce congenital malformations. Advances in this field, including the use of mouse and other models, have now reached the point where a series of developmental pathways can be traced, and defects grouped in families according to the specific type of molecular abnormality.

The situation is now comparable to that reached some years ago for inborn errors of metabolism. Garrod himself foresaw this a century ago and the currently available

Table 6.1 Laboratory investigations in diagnosis of congenital malformations

Autopsy (including radiology)
Cytogenetics (including FISH and microdeletion studies, where appropriate)
Biochemistry (e.g. peroxisomal disorders)
Molecular analysis:
    known genes
    developmental pathways

information has now been brought together in a book, *Inborn Errors of Development* (see 'Further reading'), that will undoubtedly become the key reference source for the scientific analysis of congenital malformations.

In case any reader should think that these scientific developments make clinical skills redundant, it should be emphasized that the reverse is the case. It is only possible to use the new laboratory approaches effectively if they are clinically guided and targeted, and this relies entirely on a careful and sensitive clinical approach.

The clinical geneticist has a special advantage in the clinical diagnosis of malformation syndromes, partly as the result of providing a service for a large population – often a million or more – enabling considerable experience to be gained of even the rarest disorders, which a paediatrician or obstetrician may encounter only a few times during a professional career. The 'genetic approach' of emphasis on accurate and specific diagnosis, and of keeping long-term records and registers that allow comparison of old material with new cases, and the dysmorphology groups that have grown up to discuss difficult cases and exchange information have all placed the clinical geneticist at the centre of this field; but it is others who will be involved first, and who will have to make the principal decisions concerning management.

DEFINITIONS

Confusion of terminology abounds in the study of congenital malformations. The very term 'dysmorphology' is disliked by some, but has the advantage of clearly identifying the field as the study of disordered development, without specifying the causes or limiting the subject to genetic influences. In general, the field covers what are broadly known as congenital abnormalities or birth defects, i.e. abnormalities that are apparent at or before the time of birth and where there are recognizable structural anomalies. Thus, most inborn errors of metabolism do not fall into this area, except for those few where visible defects are present at birth, such as maternal phenylketonuria and some of the peroxisomal defects. Likewise, many other progressive mendelian disorders are excluded, such as Duchenne muscular dystrophy and Tay–Sachs disease, even though histological or biochemical study may show clear changes before birth.

The term 'malformation' is now generally restricted to a specific primary abnormality of development, e.g. a congenital heart or neural tube defect. A malformation syndrome is the occurrence together as an entity of several such defects as primary events, the cause being unknown in many but clear-cut in some, e.g. the occurrence of central nervous system defects, congenital heart disease and cleft palate due to trisomy 13. A malformation sequence occurs when a primary malformation itself determines additional defects, such as foot deformity and hydrocephalus secondary to spina bifida. Some defects in organs already normally developed can be clearly identified as the result of compression, constriction or immobility; such abnormalities are best termed 'deformities', while the term 'disruption' is used when there is major destruction of a structure already formed, e.g. amputation due to amniotic bands.

Such distinctions of nomenclature may seem pedantic, but agreement and consistency are essential if confusion is to be avoided. These basic groupings also largely determine our thoughts and investigations into the causes of such defects, as well as being important for estimation of genetic risks and for the prognosis and management of the affected individual.

Unfortunately, not all syndrome names are based on a scientific approach. It is not uncommon to be faced with referral of a family with a syndrome that one has never heard of, only to find that the diagnosis is really something quite familiar masquerading under a strange name. A book is included in the 'Further reading' section (Jablonski) which is useful for this 'decoding' process.

THE DIAGNOSTIC APPROACH TO THE DYSMORPHIC CHILD

Although many aspects of the diagnostic approach to the dysmorphic child are similar to those already outlined more generally for genetic disorders, there are differences of emphasis. Pregnancy history is of crucial importance, because it may reveal a specific non-genetic cause, such as teratogenic infection or drug-related, a mechanical uterine factor causing deformation or disruption (increasingly identifiable with widespread early use of ultrasound), or features such as hydramnios or lack of fetal movements that may be a clue to the cause of abnormalities only apparent after delivery.

A full pedigree and information on relevant members is essential, as in any other situation where genetic counselling will be needed, and may show a clear genetic cause in a group where recurrence risk would otherwise be low, e.g. congenital contractures. In examination of the affected infant, careful measurements are essential, while vague terms should be avoided. Precise measurement not only avoids confusion as to whether the characteristic is really abnormal (adequate reference ranges are now available; see 'Further reading'), but also allows serial evaluations to be made. As in any clinical situation, the extent and direction of the examination will be influenced by pointers given in the history and pedigree. Thus, if a syndrome known regularly to involve the eye is suspected, then a full ophthalmic assessment may need to be undertaken, even in the absence of any obvious eye defect.

A special note should be made of the importance of photography in the investigation of the dysmorphic infant. Not only does it supply an accurate means of documenting structural defects, but it also allows evaluation of serial changes much better than reported descriptions or even measurements can. Most valuable of all is the ability of a good photograph to convey an overall impression of a defect to a group of people who may never have seen the patient. Despite this, photography is unfortunately often still regarded as a hobby rather than a serious medical investigation. One should be aware of the sensitivity that patients and families may feel about photography but, as with most procedures, people are usually willing to help provided that the trouble is taken to explain why photographs are important and that full consent is obtained and recorded.

Radiography is another technique that is too often neglected, especially in the abnormal stillbirth or fetus. It is remarkable how an investigation with potentially harmful effects on the living is so seldom performed on the dead, to whom it can do no harm, but where a specific diagnosis may be immediately apparent. Lethal bone dysplasias and osteogenesis imperfecta are particular examples, but the value of a normal skeletal X-ray of a stillbirth should not be underestimated in excluding particular disorders.

Cytogenetic studies should be undertaken in all dysmorphic infants with multiple defects; skin culture will frequently yield results postmortem and has the further advantage of detecting mosaicism. High-resolution studies detecting small deletions may be appropriate where certain combinations of defect are present; a close link between clinical and laboratory staff will help in determining when such additional studies are needed.

Although biochemical studies currently prove helpful in only a small proportion of dysmorphic infants (e.g. peroxisomal disorders such as Zellweger syndrome, and some lysosomal storage diseases), consideration should also be given to storing tissue for future analysis. Cultured fibroblasts may be saved after cytogenetic analysis, while in fatal cases, skin and liver tissue can be deep-frozen.

Molecular analysis is now of major importance in the diagnosis of malformation syndromes and is increasing rapidly in its applications. The progressive understanding of the molecular basis of malformation syndromes is probably the most exciting area of dysmorphology and is considered later in the chapter. A sample of DNA or tissue from which it can be isolated should be kept for future analysis.

Autopsy by an experienced paediatric pathologist is valuable in any infant death or pregnancy loss associated with malformation. It may show unsuspected internal defects, e.g. renal abnormalities, that are related to the dysmorphic features. However, a careful external examination with photographic and radiological records can still be of great value, even if autopsy is not permitted.

Finally, careful literature search, discussion with and presentation to colleagues, and the use of computer databases are all important diagnostic measures, as mentioned later. In particular, the recognition of relatively unusual diagnostic features may provide a useful 'handle' that can distinguish a syndrome from other related conditions.

SYNDROME DIAGNOSIS AND CLINICAL MANAGEMENT

The accurate diagnosis of malformations is sometimes disparaged by clinicians as an exercise in classification that contributes little to the welfare of the affected child. Nothing could be further from the truth, yet it is surprising how often clinical geneticists have to point out to their paediatric and obstetric colleagues the existence of some major complication, the possibility of which they were unaware of because a precise diagnosis had not been made. Quite apart from affecting the risks of recurrence on which genetic counselling is based, management of the individual case may be critically affected. A few examples among many encountered by the author are given below:

- *Holt–Oram syndrome* – an atrial septal defect in an infant with limb defect was missed because the possibility of cardiac involvement was not considered.
- *Thrombocytopenia–absent radius (TAR) syndrome* – lack of awareness of this disorder led to a diagnosis of Fanconi anaemia, with a prediction of probable mental retardation and high risk for malignancy (both of which are absent in TAR).
- *Exomphalos* – prenatal detection by ultrasound led to caesarean section; the infant had multiple other defects due to a major chromosome anomaly; if recognized antenatally, active management would probably not have been undertaken.

Now that highly sophisticated (and often successful) neonatal intensive care and surgery are available, it is all the more important that a full and accurate diagnosis of any genetic syndrome is made rapidly, even prenatally if possible. While laboratory tests, in particular chromosome analysis, are often a vital part of this, the diagnostic skill of a clinical geneticist experienced in dysmorphology may be of even greater value in ensuring the appropriate management of many of these difficult problems.

THE AETIOLOGICAL BASIS OF MALFORMATION SYNDROMES

Many of the important syndromes are described in the individual chapters of Part II of this book and can be located using the index. Here an outline is given of some of the aetiological groups that are increasingly becoming defined. Not only is it important to establish aetiology, where possible, for practical reasons of genetic counselling, but some of these disorders are proving to be of great importance in basic research, particularly where specific genes are involved. As the techniques of molecular genetics are applied to dysmorphology, many more syndromes will prove useful as models for disordered developmental processes that can be analysed at the molecular level.

CHROMOSOMAL SYNDROMES

While the major chromosomal disorders (see Chapter 4) have been recognized for many years (e.g. trisomy 21, trisomy 13), the past few years have delineated many others which involve parts of specific chromosomes (e.g. Wolf–Hirschhorn syndrome, 4p-), or mosaicism for entire chromosomes (e.g. mosaic trisomy 8). Syndromes of this type involving an autosome are usually accompanied by mental retardation, but in many cases the combination of physical abnormalities is sufficiently specific to allow a presumptive diagnosis before the chromosome constitution is known. While most cases are sporadic, it is important to recognize the small proportion where one parent is a balanced carrier.

MICRODELETION SYNDROMES

In the microdeletion syndromes, the individual components may be the result of deletion of contiguous genes, and the combination of clinical features is a most valuable clue to the localization and relative ordering of the loci involved. The deletions involved may be visible, especially if high-resolution cytogenetic analysis is used, but in some cases may only be detectable by use of molecular techniques; FISH (see Chapter 4) can be valuable where small chromosome rearrangements have occurred. Some members of this group are listed on p. 75; examples of particular importance are those involving chromosome 11p and giving various combinations of Wilms' tumour, aniridia, genital defects and mental retardation (the WAGR complex), and the complementary paternal and maternal deletions of 15q resulting in Prader–Willi and Angelman syndromes, respectively. Since some cases of these two syndromes have no detectable deletion, they may result from the dysfunction of specific genes in this region rather than from multiple contiguous gene deletion. A development of considerable importance is the recognition that a significant proportion of cases of congenital heart disease result from microdeletions of 22q, with a considerably broader and often more subtle range of features by comparison with the originally recognized categories of DiGeorge syndrome and velocardiofacial syndrome (see Chapter 19). Since the phenotype in some microdeletions can be relatively mild and compatible with reproduction, study of parents (clinical as well as chromosomal) is of particular importance.

TERATOGENIC SYNDROMES

In teratogenic syndromes (see Chapter 26), the factor may be infective (e.g. rubella), drug-related (e.g. anticonvulsants) or metabolic (e.g. maternal phenylketonuria). The number of well documented and specific syndromes in the group remains small (e.g. maternal warfarin). Some may closely mimic genetic syndromes, so it is important not to assume a teratogenic cause without good evidence.

SYNDROMES DUE TO DISORDERED FUNCTION OF SPECIFIC GENES IN DEVELOPMENT

The possibility of identifying the specific genes responsible for individual malformation syndromes has become one of the most important and rapidly evolving fields of medical genetics, and has immediate practical consequences. It clearly reinforces the need for an accurate clinical classification of dysmorphic syndromes, as well as providing the possibility of early prenatal diagnosis for families. Two main types of advance are in progress: the identification of disease loci by gene mapping and positional cloning, along the lines described in Chapter 5; and the search for defects in specific developmental genes.

The first approach has provided valuable information on the mapping of a number of important malformation syndromes, leading to identification of the gene itself in some cases.

The second approach is more recent, and has resulted from the isolation of important genes involved in developmental processes of such experimental species as the mouse, *Drosophila* and even simpler organisms such as the nematode *C. elegans* and yeast. Notable examples include a series of segmentation (homeotic) genes and various genes involved in cell signalling, allowing the concept of 'inborn errors of development' to become firmly established, as discussed earlier in this chapter.

Many of these genes are strongly conserved between species, so that the human counterparts can be isolated and tested for abnormalities in various syndromes. In addition, at a more clinical level, clear homologies exist between a number of mouse mutants and human malformations, so that if a molecular defect is found in the mouse model, it is likely to be relevant also to the human condition. Table 6.2 gives a selection of examples; others will be found in the specific chapters. Interestingly, some of the genes involved in developmental defects are proving to be involved in neoplasia as well (e.g. the *RET* oncogene in both Hirschsprung's disease and multiple endocrine neoplasia type 2).

Table 6.2 The molecular basis of congenital malformations (specific examples)

Disorder	Gene
Apert syndrome	Fibroblast growth factor (*FGFR 2*)
Campomelic dysplasia	*SOX 9* (SRY related developmental gene)
Hirschsprung's disease	*RET* oncogene (also involved in MEN 2)
Holt–Oram syndrome	Specific gene, 12q (transcription factor)
Opitz syndrome (X-linked)	*MID 1* (mid-line developmental gene)
Rubinstein–Taybi syndrome	*CREB* binding protein (16p)
Saethre–Chotzen craniosynostosis	*TWIST* (*Drosophila* homologue)
Thanatophoric dysplasia	Fibroblast growth factor (*FGFR 3*)
Treacher–Collins syndrome	Specific gene 5q (function unknown)
Waardenburg syndrome	*PAX 3* (mouse homologue)

These exciting developments offer the possibility of matching human developmental defects with the individual genetic steps in embryonic development. The possibility of constructing transgenic mouse models in addition to those occurring naturally further strengthens this approach. Malformation syndromes can now be seen as the equivalent of inborn errors of metabolism, specific defects that will eventually tell us as much about normal embryonic development as rare inborn errors have told us about metabolic pathways. The recent publication of Epstein *et al.*'s *Inborn Errors of Development* (see 'Further reading') gives an authoritative source for defects in different developmental pathways, although rapid change will undoubtedly occur.

GENETIC RECURRENCE RISKS IN MALFORMATION SYNDROMES

For many of the more common disorders, empiric recurrence risks exist and are mentioned in the appropriate chapter in Part II of this book. Frequently, however, such data are inadequate or non-existent, and the clinician is faced with giving genetic counselling without a secure basis on which to estimate the risk of recurrence. The greatest potential for error in such a situation lies in mistaking a disorder following mendelian (particularly autosomal recessive) inheritance for a similar but non-genetic or polygenic condition. In the absence of a positive family history, and especially if full documentation is not available, such a mistake is all too easy. For this reason, lists are given in Tables 6.3–6.5 of some of the disorders where mendelian inheritance is probable. While the potential for recurrence in sibs is greatest for the autosomal recessives (Table 6.3) and X-linked disorders (Table 6.5), variability of expression can be a trap with autosomal dominant inheritance, and this group is listed in Table 6.4. As a counterbalance, a list is given of disorders where (for reasons usually unknown) recurrence is rare (Table 6.6, page 96). It must be borne in mind that an increasing range of malformations with specific developmental molecular defects are proving to be new and genetically lethal dominant mutations. Chromosomal disorders, craniofacial syndromes and skeletal dysplasias are considered in the relevant chapters.

Table 6.3 Malformation syndromes following autosomal recessive inheritance

Bardet–Biedl syndrome
Campomelic dysplasia
Cerebro-oculofacioskeletal (Pena–Shokeir) syndrome (some families)
Chondrodysplasia punctata (rhizomelic type)
Cockayne syndrome
Cohen syndrome
Cryptophthalmos (Fraser) syndrome
Dubowitz syndrome
Ellis–van Creveld syndrome
Fanconi pancytopenia
Fryns syndrome
Holoprosencephaly (some families)
Hydrolethalus syndrome
Jarcho–Levin syndrome
Johanson–Blizzard syndrome
Leprechaunism (Donohue syndrome)
Marden–Walker syndrome
Meckel syndrome
Multiple pterygium syndrome
Neu–Laxova syndrome
Orofaciodigital syndrome type II (Mohr syndrome)
Roberts syndrome
Rothmund–Thompson syndrome
Seckel syndrome
Seip lipodystrophy syndrome
Smith–Lemli–Opitz syndrome
Thrombocytopenia–absent radius (TAR) syndrome

COMPUTERIZED DATABASES

The recognition and delineation of new syndromes has benefited immensely from the development of computerized databases of known and unknown disorders. Several systems are now available which are regularly updated and are becoming essential tools of the clinical geneticist and others involved with dysmorphic children. These systems not only provide help to the non-expert, but give a framework by which new entities can be worked out. By including information published or presented all over the world, they are especially helpful in rare or atypical disorders; by suggesting various alternative diagnoses and giving key references, they also stimulate the clinician to think in new directions. Molecular details and available tests are now becoming part of these databases.

Two main systems currently exist: the London Dysmorphology Database and POSSUM. Both have illustrations of patients and are regularly updated. It must be emphasized that

Table 6.4 Malformation syndromes following autosomal dominant inheritance

Beckwith–Wiedemann syndrome (some families)* (maternally transmitted)
Craniosynostoses (including Crouzon's disease and Saethre–Chotzen syndrome)
EEC syndrome (ectrodactyly, ectodermal dysplasia, clefting)
Freeman–Sheldon (whistling face) syndrome*
Greig cephalopolysyndactyly
Holt–Oram syndrome
Larsen syndrome
Mandibulofacial dysostosis (Treacher Collins syndrome)*
Multiple lentigines–deafness (LEOPARD) syndrome
Nail–patella syndrome
Noonan syndrome (some families)*
Oculodentodigital syndrome
Opitz hypertelorism–hypospadias (G) syndrome (some families)
Popliteal pterygium syndrome (some families)
Rieger syndrome
Robinow (fetal face) syndrome
Stickler syndrome*
Townes–Brocks syndrome
Trichorhinophalangeal syndrome (type I)
Van der Woude syndrome
Waardenburg syndrome

* Expression variable and sometimes minimal.

Table 6.5 Malformation syndromes following X-linked inheritance

Aarskog syndrome (faciogenital dysplasia)
Börjeson–Forssman–Lehmann syndrome
Coffin–Lowry syndrome
Corpus callosum agenesis with retinal defects (Aicardi syndrome)
(dominant, lethal in male)
Ectodermal dysplasia, hypohidrotic
FG syndrome (Opitz)
Focal dermal hypoplasia (dominant, lethal in male)
Lenz microphthalmos syndrome
Menkes syndrome
Orofaciodigital syndrome, type I (dominant, lethal in male)
Otopalatodigital syndrome
X-linked alpha-thalassaemia mental retardation (ATRX) syndrome

they do not normally make the diagnosis for you, and they require practice and knowledge for their optimal use.

An additional database of more general information available on the internet is that provided by the National Organization for Rare Disorders (NORD) (see Appendix).

Table 6.6 Malformation syndromes in which recurrence in sibs is rare (this does not necessarily exclude a genetic basis)

Amniotic bands syndrome
CHARGE association
Goldenhar syndrome
Hemifacial microsomia
Klippel–Feil syndrome
Klippel–Trenaunay–Weber syndrome
de Lange syndrome (see Chapter 14)
McCune–Albright (fibrous dysplasia) syndrome (probably somatic mutations)
Moebius syndrome
Poland syndrome
Proteus syndrome
Rubinstein–Taybi syndrome (microdeletions or new mutations at 16p13)
Russell–Silver syndrome
Sacral agenesis (caudal regression syndrome)
Septo-optic dysplasia
Sotos syndrome
Sturge–Weber syndrome
VATER association
Weaver syndrome

FURTHER READING

Aase JM (1990). *Diagnostic Dysmorphology*. New York, Plenum.

Cohen MM (1997). *The Child with Multiple Birth Defects*. New York, Oxford University Press.

Donnai D, Winter R (1995). *Congenital Malformation Syndromes*. London, Prentice-Hall.

Epstein CJ, Erickson RP, Wynshaw-Boris A (2003). *Inborn Errors of Development*. New York, Oxford University Press – a landmark in the field both practically and scientifically.

Gilbert SF (1997). *Developmental Biology*. Sunderland, MA, Sinauer – a beautifully illustrated guide to basic embryology.

Gorlin RJ, Cohen MM, Hennekam RCM (2001). *Syndromes of the Head and Neck*. Oxford, Oxford University Press – a comprehensive account of malformation syndromes covering a much wider range than the title implies.

Graham JM (1988). *Smith's Recognizable Patterns of Deformation*, 2nd edn. Philadelphia, WB Saunders.

Hall JG, Froster-Iskenius VG, Allanson JE (1989). *Handbook of Normal Physical Measurements*. Oxford, Oxford University Press.

Harper PS (1997). The naming of genetic syndromes and unethical activities. In: Harper PS, Clarke AJ, eds. *Genetics, Society and Clinical Practice*. Oxford, Bios, pp. 221–225.

Jablonski S (1991). *Jablonski's Dictionary of Syndromes and Eponymous Diseases*. Malabar, FL, Krieger – useful when faced with a strange syndrome name but not recommended for other purposes.

Jones KL (1997). *Smith's Recognisable Patterns of Human Malformation*, 5th edn. Philadelphia, Saunders

National Organization for Rare Disorders (NORD). PO Box 8923, New Fairfield, CT 06812, USA – *http://www.rarediseases.org*

POSSUM (version 5.0, 1998) (Pictures of Standard Syndromes and Undiagnosed Malformations). CD-Rom. Melbourne, Murdoch Institute for Research into Birth Defects.

Stevenson RE, Hall JG, Goodman RM (1993). *Human Malformations and Related Anomalies*. Oxford, Oxford University Press.

Wiedemann H-R, Kunze J (1997). *Clinical Syndromes*, 3rd edn. St Louis, Mosby.

Wilkie AOM, Amberger JS, McKusick VA (1994). A gene map of congenital malformations. *J Med Genet* **31**, 507–517.

Winter R (1996). Analyzing human developmental abnormalities. *Bioessays* **18**, 965–971.

Winter RM, Baraitser M (1991). *Multiple Congenital Anomalies*. London, Chapman & Hall – a valuable written companion to the London Dysmorphology Database.

Winter RM, Baraitser M (2002). *The London Dysmorphology Database*. Oxford, Oxford University Press.

CHAPTER 7

Carrier testing and genetic prediction

One of the major tasks in genetic counselling is to identify those individuals who, while apparently healthy themselves, have a high risk of transmitting a genetic disorder. Recognition of a particular mode of inheritance will often allow the risk to be estimated and, in some cases, excluded, but where the risk is high, it may often be impossible to tell with certainty on clinical grounds alone whether or not a particular family member possesses the abnormal gene. For this reason, tests that will identify the correct genotype of a person are of great importance and in many instances form an integral part of the overall process of genetic counselling. This chapter explores the range and limitations of tests of carrier detection and attempts to show how the information can be used in conjunction with other genetic and clinical data to make as accurate a prediction as possible.

WHAT DO WE MEAN BY 'CARRIER'?

The term 'carrier' is widely used in medicine, and is often applied to those harbouring an infective agent, quite apart from its use in medical genetics. The term may be used by different people with entirely different connotations, and a precise definition is important if confusion is not to arise. A working definition of the carrier state in inherited disease is as follows:

> A carrier is an individual who possesses in heterozygous state the gene determining an inherited disorder, and who is essentially healthy at the time of study.

From this definition, several important points follow:

- A carrier is a heterozygote; thus the term can only be applied satisfactorily to mendelian disorders determined by a single locus. It is logical to talk of a carrier for cystic fibrosis,

Table 7.1 Genetic risks for carriers of mendelian disorders

Inheritance	Risk to offspring of carrier
Autosomal recessive	Very low unless the disorder is extremely common, consanguinity is present or the same disorder is in the spouse's family
Autosomal dominant	50% (risk of overt disease will vary with disorder)
X-linked recessive	50% of male offspring affected; variable expression of disorder possible in female offspring

but not of a carrier for spina bifida, where the genetic determination is poorly understood and non-mendelian. The definition can, however, be stretched to individuals with a balanced chromosomal abnormality such as a translocation, where the inheritance is essentially mendelian (see Chapter 4), and to asymptomatic individuals with a mitochondrial mutation.

- Although a carrier is heterozygous, this does not necessarily imply that the affected individual must be homozygous. This will only be the case in autosomal recessive disorders; in autosomal dominant disorders, almost all individuals with the abnormal gene, whether affected or carriers, will be heterozygous.
- Although the risk of a carrier transmitting the abnormal gene is high (normally 50 per cent), it does not always follow that there is a high risk of having an affected child. The risk may in fact be extremely low and will depend on the mode of inheritance (Table 7.1).
- The fact that a carrier is 'essentially healthy' at the time of study does not mean that minor clinical features may not be distinguishable, nor does it mean that the individual will necessarily remain healthy. Those carrying the mutation for Huntington's disease provide an example of the latter point.

It is clear from these considerations that carrier detection has to be approached in the light of the natural history of the particular genetic disorder and its mode of inheritance.

OBLIGATORY AND POSSIBLE CARRIERS

When the testing of carriers is being considered, it is often not recognized that in addition to individuals at a higher or lower risk of being a carrier, there are those who, on genetic grounds, must be carriers (Figure 7.1). Recognition of these 'obligatory' carriers is important for several reasons: it may save complex and unnecessary testing procedures, it allows much more definite genetic counselling to be given, and it also provides a reference population against which any new or improved carrier test can be evaluated.

Obligatory carriers for autosomal recessive disorders include all children and parents of an affected individual (mutation as an alternative is too rare to be a practical problem). In X-linked recessive inheritance, all daughters of an affected male will be obligatory carriers, while in autosomal dominant inheritance, obligatory carriers are people who have both a parent and a child affected but who show (or showed when alive) no abnormalities

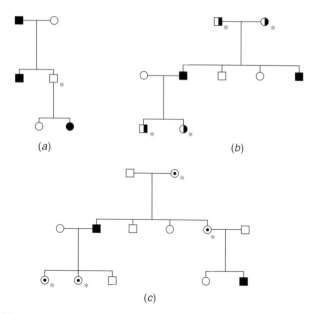

Figure 7.1 Obligatory carriers in mendelian inheritance. Obligatory carriers for the three major modes of inheritance are marked with an asterisk. By convention, carriers for autosomal recessive disorders are half shaded, and those for X-linked disorders dotted. (*a*) Autosomal dominant inheritance: any individual having both an affected parent and affected offspring must be a carrier. (*b*) Autosomal recessive inheritance: both parents and all offspring of an affected individual are obligatory carriers. (*c*) X-linked recessive inheritance: obligatory carriers include all daughters of an affected male and all women who have an affected son and at least one other affected male relative.

themselves. This situation is commonly seen in Huntington's disease and other late-onset disorders when an individual has died young of an unrelated cause but is later shown to have transmitted the disorder.

CARRIER DETECTION IN AUTOSOMAL RECESSIVE DISEASE

Autosomal recessive disorders provide by far the largest number of carriers numerically, but are by no means the most important in genetic counselling. We are all likely to be carriers for at least one serious recessive disorder and several lethal ones, quite apart from numerous polymorphisms such as blood groups where heterozygosity is normal and may have been beneficial in the past, if not now.

From the standpoint of genetic counselling there are three main situations that are encountered:

- an individual is or is likely to be a carrier for a rare autosomal recessive disorder
- an individual is or is likely to be a carrier for a common autosomal recessive disorder

- the situation is complicated by consanguinity or by marriage to an individual whose family may be affected by the same disorder.

The importance or lack of importance of the carrier state in these three situations is directly related to the principles of autosomal recessive inheritance, which have been discussed in Chapter 2.

RARE AUTOSOMAL RECESSIVE DISORDERS

Rare autosomal recessive disorders are the ones about which advice is most commonly sought, and family members may be greatly worried and alarmed by having been told they may be carriers. Such worry (usually induced by doctors in the first place) is entirely unnecessary, but is often extremely difficult to allay. Some individuals may believe that being a carrier means they have the disease in a mild form, or are in some way not entirely healthy. Others believe that, even though they are healthy themselves, their children will inevitably be affected.

Neither situation is, of course, the case. Heterozygotes for autosomal recessive disorders are almost always entirely healthy and will remain so, even when minor distinguishing features can be found. Likewise, even though the chance of the sibs of affected individuals (who are those most commonly seeking advice) being carriers is two-thirds, the risk of such carriers having affected children is exceptionally low, as shown in Table 7.2, and for all rare autosomal recessive disorders a confident reassurance can be given that this is the case. Some family members may request carrier testing for themselves and their spouses, if this is feasible, 'just to be sure'. In general, the author discourages this, because for most rare inborn errors of metabolism where testing is possible, it is likely

Table 7.2 Carrier detection in some common or important autosomal recessive disorders

Disorder	Test
Alpha-1-antitrypsin deficiency	Alpha-1-antitrypsin electrophoretic typing; DNA analysis
Combined immunodeficiency (one type)	Adenosine deaminase electrophoresis
Congenital adrenal hyperplasia	DNA analysis
Cystic fibrosis	DNA analysis
Galactosaemia	Galactose-1-phosphate uridyl transferase (red cells); DNA analysis
Mucopolysaccharidosis type I (Hurler)	Alpha-iduronidase (white cells); DNA analysis
Phenylketonuria	Phenylalanine load; phenylalanine tyrosine serum ratio; DNA analysis
Pseudocholinesterase deficiency	Pseudocholinesterase level; dibucaine number
Tay–Sachs disease	Hexosaminidase A (white cells); DNA analysis
Thalassaemias and other haemoglobinopathies	Red cell morphology, haemoglobin electrophoresis, DNA analysis

that the margin of error of the test makes misclassification a real possibility in a situation of low prior risk. Prenatal diagnosis is similarly rarely justified.

The advent of molecular testing for many rare autosomal recessive disorders has increased the likelihood of inappropriate carrier testing. Often it is possible to distinguish the heterozygous carrier within a family having such a disorder, but impossible to do so in the population as a whole. The unsatisfactory situation can thus be created where worry is increased by a sib being shown to be a carrier, without it being possible to resolve the situation by testing the unrelated partner. Even if a specific mutation has been detected in the family, there is no guarantee that a carrier partner would have the same mutation, so that an extensive search for all possible mutations may be needed if one has embarked on this course, often leaving the situation inconclusive.

COMMON AUTOSOMAL RECESSIVE DISORDERS

The common autosomal recessive disorders provide a much more important indication for carrier detection (Table 7.2), although the disorders have to be extremely common to present a significant risk to individual couples. Even for a disorder as relatively common as phenylketonuria (1 in 10 000 births), the risk for offspring of a healthy sib is only 1 in 300. Very few of the classic enzyme deficiencies for which carrier testing is available are as common as this, except for special concentrations such as Tay–Sachs disease in Ashkenazi Jewish populations. The haemoglobinopathies and thalassaemias provide the most important group on a worldwide basis, and carrier detection is fortunately feasible in most of these; population screening for the carrier state in these disorders is now widespread and is discussed on page 363. Particular countries (e.g. Finland, Quebec) or isolated populations may have high frequencies of other disorders, making carrier detection important for them. Laboratories and clinical genetic services both need to ensure that ethnic origins and the pattern of genetic disorders and mutations are taken into account in the analyses and risk estimates undertaken.

When carrier testing for one of the common autosomal recessive disorders is being undertaken, it is logical to test both the family member at risk and the spouse (or prospective partner) at the same time, since if only one proves to be a carrier, the couple can confidently be reassured; if population testing (and thus testing of an unrelated partner) is not possible, this should be pointed out before any testing is embarked upon, as it may make the whole exercise meaningless. Where an individual affected with an autosomal recessive disorder is concerned, only the partner need be tested, unless there is a particular need to characterize the mutation in the affected person.

Table 7.2 summarizes the state of carrier detection for some major autosomal recessive disorders. Cystic fibrosis is a good example of a disorder where all phenotypic tests for the carrier state proved unreliable but where testing for mutations now allows determination of which close relatives are carriers. This is made easier by the predominance of one common mutation (delta F508) in most north European populations; excluding the carrier state in an unrelated partner may require testing for a much wider range of less frequent mutations. The implications of this for population screening in cystic fibrosis are discussed in Chapter 27.

Consanguinity (see also Chapter 9) may occasionally produce the need for carrier testing in a rare autosomal recessive disorder where the risks would otherwise be negligible;

even more rarely, the same disorder may be present in the families of two unrelated partners. The heterozygote can be distinguished in the case of numerous rare inborn errors of metabolism, but it should be noted that there is often considerable overlap between the normal and heterozygote ranges, so that a clear indication of the likely margin of error should be obtained from the laboratory involved. Molecular testing is often easier when consanguinity is present, since if mutation analysis is being used, one is looking for the same mutation in both partners.

To conclude, it can be seen that for most autosomal recessive disorders, especially those that are rare, the time and energy of the person involved in genetic counselling should normally be employed to give a clear explanation of the (usually very low) risks and the lack of importance to one's health of being a carrier, rather than in indiscriminately recommending difficult, expensive and generally unnecessary tests of carrier detection. The limitations and inaccuracy of any testing situation should be clearly understood and explained, and testing only carried out when these aspects have been, as far as is possible, resolved.

CARRIER DETECTION IN AUTOSOMAL DOMINANT DISEASE

For practical purposes all individuals with a dominantly inherited disease are heterozygotes, so the carrier state can only exist where the disorder is mild, variable or late in onset. One cannot be a carrier for achondroplasia – either one has it or one does not (gonadal mosaicism can provide occasional exceptions to this; see p. 29). Thus, the number of dominantly inherited disorders where carrier detection is applicable is very small compared with autosomal recessive inheritance, but the importance in terms of risks to offspring is much greater.

Table 7.3 lists some of the major autosomal dominant disorders where carrier detection is feasible using clinical or biochemical approaches. These disorders fall into three principal categories. The first are disorders that frequently remain asymptomatic and which under normal circumstances might hardly be considered diseases; the acute porphyrias and malignant hyperpyrexia, both drug-aggravated disorders, are examples. The second group consists of those difficult disorders which show variable penetrance and expression, and which are especially important in genetic counselling because of this variability; tuberous sclerosis, osteogenesis imperfecta and myotonic dystrophy all fall into this class. The final group consists of diseases that sooner or later follow regular dominant inheritance, but where the true state of affairs may not be clear at the time individuals at risk wish to have children. Huntington's disease (see Chapter 12) is the most important and most difficult disorder in this group, but some of the other progressive neurological degenerations are comparable. In this group, tests of carrier detection are essentially tests of presymptomatic diagnosis.

Molecular testing is proving to have a major impact on carrier testing for autosomal dominant conditions, including most of those listed in Table 7.3. It has already found a place alongside more conventional approaches and, in some cases, is replacing them, especially where they are invasive or of limited accuracy. The lack of age dependence in molecular analysis is a considerable advantage, though equally a danger in terms of

Table 7.3 Carrier detection in variable autosomal dominant disorders: clinical and biochemical approaches

Disorder	Clinical or biochemical feature
Angioedema, hereditary	C1 esterase inhibitor levels
Hereditary spherocytosis	Red cell morphology, osmotic fragility
Holt–Oram syndrome	Minor digital abnormalities
Hypercholesterolaemia, familial	Lipoprotein and LDL cholesterol assays
Malignant hyperpyrexia	Elevated creatine kinase, muscle biopsy
Multiple epiphyseal dysplasia	Short stature, premature osteoarthritis
Muscular dystrophy (facioscapulohumeral)	Minimal weakness
Myotonic dystrophy	Minimal weakness, electromyography; lens opacities
Neurofibromatosis	Skin lesions, Lisch nodules
Osteogenesis imperfecta	Dental changes, deafness, blue sclerae
Polycystic kidney disease (adult)	Renal ultrasound
Porphyrias (acute intermittent, variegate, coproporphyria)	Specific enzyme assays
Tuberous sclerosis	Skin lesions (UV light), CT scan, dental pits
Van der Woude syndrome	Lip pits
Von Hippel–Lindau syndrome	Retinal lesions
Waardenburg syndrome	White forelock, hypertelorism

inappropriate childhood testing (see p. 370). The ease of the procedure from the individual's viewpoint, with only a blood sample required, is likewise a double-edged sword, with the danger that samples may arrive in the laboratory without appropriate genetic counselling having been performed.

The rapidity of advance in gene mapping and isolation makes it inappropriate to list those dominant disorders for which molecular carrier detection can be undertaken, since they are now in the majority. It can be assumed that carrier testing is at least potentially feasible for any such disorder whose gene has been mapped or isolated. Whether it is actually possible will depend on the range of mutations, whether there is genetic heterogeneity and, if linked markers rather than mutation analysis are being used, the structure of the particular family pedigree.

In contrast to autosomal recessive disorders, the risk of the offspring of a carrier for an autosomal dominant condition having overt disease at some stage of their life is high. Although in a few cases (e.g. the myopathy underlying malignant hyperpyrexia) the disorder remains constantly subclinical in successive generations, it is common to find more severely affected offspring born to asymptomatic parents. This in part reflects the natural variability of these disorders, but also results from the fact that the carrier parents form the mildest extreme of a range of variability, so that in 'reverting to the mean' the children are more likely to be clinically affected. In some instances, as with myotonic dystrophy, there may be maternal effects producing severe disease in the offspring of an asymptomatic mother, as well as special factors producing anticipation (see pp. 27 and 166).

Autosomal dominant disorders of late onset also produce a special difficulty in carrier detection because, in contrast to those with a static course and those with recessively inherited disease, the carrier is not just at risk of transmitting the disease but of developing it. Thus to identify an individual as a carrier of Huntington's disease (apart from those individuals with a subclinical mutation – see Chapter 12) is inevitably to mark out that person as being destined to develop the disease at some time in the future. The whole field of presymptomatic detection for late-onset disorders carries serious ethical and practical consequences (see Chapters 5 and 28). We now have considerable information on the effects of this in Huntington's disease (see p. 174), which is likely to provide a general model for other late-onset disorders, including the familial cancers, although these differ importantly from Huntington's disease in having preventable and treatable aspects.

CARRIER DETECTION IN X-LINKED DISEASE

A relatively small number of X-linked recessive disorders provide the most important of all applications of carrier detection. The reason for this is simple: the carriers are generally healthy and so will be likely to reproduce, but in contrast to autosomal recessive inheritance, they will be at risk of having affected male offspring regardless of whom they marry. In such a situation, the availability of carrier detection for women at high risk is a major contribution, and forms such an integral part of genetic counselling that it is often unwise to give a definitive risk estimate until information from testing is available.

The haemophilias and X-linked muscular dystrophies (principally Duchenne dystrophy) are overwhelmingly the most important disorders that have to be considered in this group, and the approaches to carrier detection and the problems of interpretation are remarkably similar in each. For this reason, although details are given with the individual disorders, they will be used here as examples of carrier detection in X-linked recessive disease. Table 7.4 summarizes some of the features. Fragile-X syndrome is also a frequent reason for carrier detection, but its unusual genetic features, with normal transmitting males, make it different from most other X-linked disorders in terms of carrier detection.

In both haemophilia and Duchenne dystrophy, a few carriers may be detectable clinically, probably as the result of X-chromosome inactivation having randomly resulted in a higher than expected proportion of those X chromosomes bearing the abnormal gene functioning in the particular tissue of importance. Unfortunately, this process will also result in the opposite – namely carriers in whom, principally, the normal X chromosome is functioning, and who will thus be difficult or impossible to detect even by the most sensitive tests. This variability of X-linked carriers is characteristic and must always be borne in mind. Tests based on DNA are not affected by X inactivation, and this property is one of the most important reasons for their use in X-linked heterozygote detection.

In some disorders, the problem of X-chromosome inactivation can be overcome by cloning cultured cells to separate out two populations, one of which will behave normally, the other abnormally, but it is a complex procedure. Molecular tests based on the differential methylation of the active and inactive X have proved useful in the X-linked immune deficiencies.

The phenotypic test generally used for Duchenne dystrophy, the elevation of serum creatine kinase levels, is considerably further removed from the basic molecular defect than the assays for factor VIII in haemophilia, with consequently less precision in detecting carriers. In both disorders, however, there is a considerable overlap between normal and

Table 7.4 Carrier detection in Duchenne muscular dystrophy and haemophilia A

	Duchenne muscular dystrophy	**Haemophilia A**
Clinical abnormalities (when present)	Minor weakness, often asymmetrical	Slight to moderate bleeding tendency
DNA testing approach	Deletions common; point mutations numerous, not always detectable; family analysis using intragenic probes still sometimes needed	Deletions infrequent; mutation analysis feasible in most cases; family analysis using intragenic and linked probes required in some cases
Main phenotypic test	Serum creatine kinase	Serum factor VIII assays (immunological and functional)
Proportion of definite carriers showing phenotypic test results outside the normal range	Two-thirds	Around 80%

carrier ranges, which makes it impossible to classify most individuals as 'normal' or 'abnormal'. Instead, a series of likelihood ratios must be used which will give odds for or against the carrier state for any particular result of a carrier test. By using these odds, one can arrive at a much more precise separation of carriers and non-carriers than would otherwise be possible, especially if the results are integrated with other genetic information, as described in Chapter 2. Although phenotypic tests in these and other X-linked disorders are being progressively replaced by molecular analysis, they remain valuable in both Duchenne dystrophy and the haemophilias. In particular, a clearly abnormal result will rarely be outweighed or contradicted by molecular evidence.

The isolated case of an X-linked disorder presents major problems in carrier detection. There is considerable uncertainty as to the proportion of such cases likely to represent new mutations and, correspondingly, the proportion of mothers who are carriers. It is likely that this may vary from one disorder to another, even when affected males do not reproduce. The prior risk of such a mother being a carrier will be somewhere between 50 and 100 per cent, depending on the relative mutation rates in the two sexes, and the interpretation of carrier testing will clearly be influenced by this figure. Even the recognition of gene deletion in such an isolated case does not always allow exclusion of the carrier state, because some mothers show gonadal mosaicism. This may be a further factor in apparent lack of phenotypic features in carrier women, and seems to be especially frequent in Duchenne dystrophy.

All daughters of a man with an X-linked recessive disease must be carriers, and so tests of carrier detection are irrelevant for such people. Despite this, they are often referred for 'genetic counselling and carrier detection' under the misapprehension that a normal result will somehow make a definite carrier less definite! False reassurance is a real danger in such a situation.

Table 7.5 shows some of the X-linked recessive disorders where carrier detection is helpful. The range of approaches is wide and may be morphological, functional, biochemical or molecular. The last of these approaches is rapidly becoming the definitive one. Taken as a

Table 7.5 Phenotypic changes in carrier detection for X-linked disorders

Disorder	Abnormality in carrier
Adrenal leucodystrophy	Long-chain fatty acid synthesis
Alport syndrome	Microscopic haematuria
Amelogenesis imperfecta	Patchy enamel hypoplasia (heterogeneous)
Anhidrotic ectodermal dysplasia	Reduced sweat pores, dental defects
Becker muscular dystrophy	Serum creatine kinase (less effective than in Duchenne)
Centronuclear myopathy (lethal type)	Muscle biopsy changes
Choroideraemia	Pigmentary retinal changes
Chronic granulomatous disease	Partial NADPH oxidase deficiency; discoid lupus-like skin lesions
Duchenne muscular dystrophy	Serum creatine kinase
Fabry's disease	Skin lesions; α-galactosidase assay
Fragile-X mental retardation	Variable mental retardation; may show chromosomal fragile site
Glucose-6-phosphate dehydrogenase deficiency	Quantitative enzyme assay and electrophoresis
Haemophilia A	Factor VIII assays
Haemophilia B	Factor IX assay
Hunter syndrome (MPS II)	Enzyme assay on hair bulbs and serum (variable)
Hypogammaglobinaemia (Bruton type)	Reduced IgG (some individuals only)
Immune deficiency (SCID)	X-inactivation analysis
Lesch–Nyhan syndrome	HGPRT assay on hair bulbs
Lowe syndrome	Amino aciduria, lens opacities
Ocular albinism	Patchy fundal depigmentation
Retinoschisis	Cystic retinal changes
Vitamin D-resistant rickets	Serum phosphate (may be clinical features)
Wiskott–Aldrich syndrome	X-inactivation studies; IgA levels
X-linked congenital cataract	Lens opacities
X-linked ichthyosis	Corneal opacities, reduced steroid sulphatase
X-linked mental retardation	Various non-fragile-X forms; carrier detection rarely feasible
X-linked retinitis pigmentosa	Pigmentary changes; abnormality of electroretinogram, more than one locus

group, X-linked disorders are probably the most satisfactory in terms of our ability to detect the carrier state and its applicability in preventing recurrence of the disease within families.

METHODS OF CARRIER DETECTION

The techniques available for detecting the carrier state vary greatly according to the nature of the particular disease and our understanding of its metabolic basis. It is impossible to give all the details here, and available approaches are mentioned as far as possible with individual disorders, but it is worth considering the broad forms of approach and some of the limitations that exist.

Molecular analysis (see Chapter 5 for details)

This is now the approach of choice where the gene has been isolated. Deletions or point mutations may be recognized, or intragenic polymorphisms used. In the immune deficiencies, the inactivated X chromosome may be distinguishable by its methylated status. Where linked markers at a distance from the gene are used, the risk of error from recombination must be considered. In addition, as already discussed, there may be problems with DNA carrier prediction if the affected individual is dead, there is uncertain paternity, genetic heterogeneity, or if results depend on inferring genotypes of missing relatives.

Measurement of the primary enzyme or other defect

This is a very satisfactory approach, where available, and is feasible for numerous inborn errors of metabolism, mostly following autosomal recessive inheritance, as well as for non-enzymatic defects such as haemophilias and various haemoglobinopathies. Even in this group, however, the range of results in heterozygotes may show considerable overlap with the normal range, and less commonly with that of the abnormal homozygotes. The appropriate tissue to use will also vary. Serum may be adequate, but more often red or white blood cells or cultured fibroblasts are required and the techniques may be difficult and specialized. X-linked disorders are particularly variable, as already discussed.

Secondary biochemical changes

The value of these will, in general, be related to how close the abnormality is to the primary defect. Important examples are the use of creatine kinase measurement in Duchenne muscular dystrophy, elevation of haemoglobin A levels in beta-thalassaemia, and abnormalities of porphyrin excretion in the acute porphyrias. As our knowledge increases, such tests will tend to be superseded or used as preliminary screening tests. Even when a disorder is thoroughly understood in enzymatic terms, a secondary test may be the most useful; thus in phenylketonuria the enzyme is confined to the liver, and until the gene was isolated carrier detection was usually achieved by studying the blood phenylalanine–tyrosine ratio under standardized conditions, or by performing a phenylalanine loading test.

Cytogenetic studies

These are of obvious importance in families with a balanced translocation, but new techniques are showing applications in disorders not previously considered chromosomal, as discussed in Chapter 4. Where a small deletion or translocation is involved (see Table 4.10), the presence or absence of any anomaly in a relative is likely to determine whether the risk is high or low. In the important case of fragile-X mental retardation, molecular analysis for the mutation is proving to be of greater value than cytogenetic study in the identification of asymptomatic gene carriers, whether these are females or normal transmitting males (see Chapter 13).

Physiological tests

These are of particular use in those autosomal dominant conditions where we have little biochemical understanding. Examples include the use of electroretinography in detecting the carriers of X-linked retinitis pigmentosa and nerve conduction in Charcot–Marie–Tooth disease. Many are now being superseded by molecular tests (e.g. slit-lamp eye examination and electromyography in myotonic dystrophy).

Microscopic techniques

These may rely on biopsy, as in Duchenne muscular dystrophy; blood film examination, as with sickle-cell anaemia or thalassaemias; or biomicroscopy, as in slit-lamp examination for the lens opacities of myotonic dystrophy or the Lisch nodules of neurofibromatosis.

Radiology

This may show minor skeletal abnormalities in such disorders as osteogenesis imperfecta, while internal defects may be visible, e.g. cerebral calcification in tuberous sclerosis and renal abnormalities in polycystic kidney disease.

Clinical observation

Many carriers may exhibit clinical features that show their genotype and, although the absence of such evidence rarely excludes an individual being a carrier, their presence provides a strong positive indication. Ophthalmic disorders (e.g. choroideraemia and retinitis pigmentosa) are particularly susceptible to carrier detection in this way, as are skin disorders. Female carriers of an X-linked recessive disorder may show a 'patchy' appearance, as already noted; again, this is particularly evident in skin, dental and eye disorders where the tissue concerned is open to inspection.

FURTHER READING

Scriver CR, Beaudet A, Sly WS, Valle D (1996). *The Metabolic and Molecular Bases of Inherited Disease*. New York, McGraw-Hill – gives details of carrier detection for many specific disorders.
Young ID (2000). *Introduction to Risk Calculation in Genetic Counselling*. Oxford, Oxford University Press – general approaches to risk estimation are clearly described.

CHAPTER 8

Prenatal diagnosis and related reproductive aspects

The development of techniques for diagnosing genetic disorders *in utero* has proved to be a major advance in medical genetics, and has so altered the outlook for families at risk of having affected children that it has become one of the main options open to those receiving genetic counselling, especially where there is a high risk of a serious and untreatable disorder. Prenatal diagnostic procedures have frequently been developed by, or in close association with, those actively involved in genetic counselling, and, perhaps as a result of this, have in general been used appropriately and responsibly. The increasingly widespread use and diversified nature of the techniques, notably the use of ultrasound, have more recently tended to result in prenatal diagnostic procedures being applied as a substitute for genetic counselling, in isolation from the estimation of genetic risks and other relevant factors supporting it. The author believes strongly that this is an unfortunate and potentially harmful trend, and that prenatal diagnosis, like other clinical and laboratory techniques, must be seen in the context of the entire situation: the risk of a pregnancy being genetically affected, the other measures such as carrier detection which may define that risk more precisely, the potential for treatment of the disorder in question and, most importantly, the attitude and wishes of the couple concerned.

Such an approach means that, wherever possible, a prenatal diagnosis must be considered, discussed and planned before a pregnancy occurs. To begin this process during pregnancy is highly undesirable (although sometimes inevitable), because not only may procedures have to be hurried, but most pregnant women (and their partners) are not in a state where an objective assessment of the factors for or against prenatal diagnosis and possible termination of pregnancy can easily be undertaken. It is likely that much of the emotional trauma sometimes associated with prenatal diagnosis results from an absence of careful prior planning. The availability of chorion villus sampling (CVS) in the first trimester makes it even more important that the situation is planned carefully in advance of pregnancy.

Most genetic counselling in relation to prenatal diagnosis will inevitably, and rightly, be carried out by obstetricians and those involved in primary care, with specialists in medical genetics responsible for those cases where the genetic aspects are complex. A welcome development has been the growth of interdisciplinary fetal medicine groups, where obstetrician, radiologist, medical geneticist and other colleagues can meet regularly to discuss specific cases, but there remain too many instances where skilled genetic advice has been sought too late, or not at all.

The widespread use of screening tests in pregnancy now means that most prenatal diagnosis is undertaken where there is no previous risk or expectation of a genetic disorder. The population aspects of this are considered in Chapter 27, but the very real implications that this has for individual families are dealt with later in this chapter.

THE CRITERIA AND INDICATIONS FOR PRENATAL DIAGNOSIS

When prenatal diagnosis is being considered in genetic counselling, several basic factors must be examined (see Table 8.1), but the most important is whether the couple concerned actively wish for prenatal diagnosis; all too often it is suggested simply because it may be technically feasible and without adequate information.

Because most prenatal diagnostic procedures involve a large amount of worry (and a small amount of discomfort) to the mother, and a significant morbidity and mortality to the fetus (with 100 per cent mortality if the test proves abnormal and termination is requested), prenatal diagnosis should normally only be carried out if the general criteria summarized in Table 8.1 are fulfilled. These are self-evident, but as in most clinical situations, cases of real doubt may occur.

Severity of disorder

This is beyond doubt in most of the disorders for which prenatal diagnosis is employed, including Down's syndrome and other autosomal trisomies, open neural tube defects and the rare neurodegenerative metabolic disorders. Other conditions may be more

Table 8.1 Criteria for prenatal diagnosis

Is the disorder sufficiently severe to warrant termination of the pregnancy?
Is treatment absent or unsatisfactory?
Is termination of an affected pregnancy acceptable to the couple concerned?
Is an accurate prenatal diagnostic test available?
Is there a significant genetic risk to the pregnancy?

questionable, especially those where physical abnormalities (e.g. limb defects, cleft lip and palate) are likely to be accompanied by normal intellect and life expectancy. Albinism, which has few general health implications in northern climates, may, because of the likelihood of skin cancer, be a fatal disorder in tropical countries. Such variable categories may be expected to increase and to present difficult decisions, the outcome of which will vary from family to family, and between different societies. Relatively minor but visible defects may be considered unacceptable in some cultures, whereas serious internal disorders may be accepted. Some of the more general problems posed for society by these new developments are discussed in Chapter 27.

Treatment availability

Treatment may be clear-cut and satisfactory in some disorders which might otherwise be considered for prenatal diagnosis. Thus, in phenylketonuria, now detectable prenatally by molecular analysis, most children treated from birth have near normal health and intelligence, at least in countries where dietary treatment is available; by contrast, in galactosaemia, liver damage is occasionally present at birth and the long-term outlook for the infant is less clear. Whether prenatal diagnosis is undertaken here will probably depend on the attitudes and previous experience of the parents. In congenital adrenal hyperplasia (see Chapter 22), the outlook with treatment for a second child is much better than for the first-born, in whom delayed diagnosis commonly results in death or serious morbidity, while treatment *in utero* is also a possibility.

Acceptability of termination

The acceptability of termination of pregnancy to a couple must be determined before any prenatal procedures are contemplated. In some cases it is unacceptable on religious grounds or because of the prevailing attitude of the community; in others, it is a more personal ethical view. Acceptability may be a relative phenomenon. Thus many couples find fetal sexing by amniocentesis – with late termination of a male pregnancy which may be normal – unacceptable, whereas these same individuals may accept first-trimester termination following CVS, or alternatively late termination of a definitely affected male pregnancy. It is essential to know the attitude of a couple before pregnancy occurs because this may well affect their decision whether or not to have further children.

Unacceptability of termination should not be considered as automatically ruling out prenatal diagnosis. In rare instances, parents may feel that they will gain by being able to prepare for an affected child, although this is exceptional, especially when the finite risk of prenatal procedures is pointed out. Serious potential ethical problems arise if prenatal diagnosis is undertaken for a late-onset disorder and the pregnancy continues (see Chapter 28).

Feasibility of prenatal diagnosis

The feasibility of diagnosis is something that may well change rapidly with scientific advances, so it cannot be too strongly stressed that the clinician giving genetic counselling must obtain accurate information on this point before suggesting the possibility to a couple, and must be satisfied that the technique is applicable as a service rather than as a research procedure. Failure to do this is as reprehensible as submitting a patient to some new surgical procedure without enquiring as to its benefit and mortality. This is especially relevant when using new molecular advances, where the boundary between research discovery and established techniques can be hard to define, especially for very rare disorders, or those where the gene has been recently isolated.

Genetic risk

The final point to be emphasized is that the risk of the disorder occurring in a particular pregnancy must be estimated accurately before prenatal diagnosis is considered – in other words, the consideration of prenatal diagnosis must be an integral part of genetic counselling. All too often the author has seen patients referred for prenatal diagnosis when the risk to the pregnancy has not been properly evaluated, and where the risk frequently proves to be so low as to make prenatal procedures unwarranted. Even if prenatal diagnosis were free of risk (which it is not), such a slipshod approach cannot be justified. If the clinician involved cannot accurately evaluate the risk (which will not be the case after reading this book, it is hoped), then the advice of a colleague who can do so should be sought.

AMNIOCENTESIS

A variety of techniques exist by which a prenatal diagnosis may be achieved for different disorders. At present, amniocentesis, the procedure by which a sample of amniotic fluid and its cells is obtained from the pregnant uterus, is still the technique with the widest application, especially for cytogenetic studies on lower-risk pregnancies. It is important, however, not to forget that other approaches exist (Table 8.2), which are rapidly increasing in importance.

Table 8.2 Approaches to prenatal diagnosis

Amniocentesis
Chromosomal disorders (especially where risk is low)
Open neural tube defects

Chorion villus sampling
DNA and enzyme analysis
Chromosomal disorders (especially when risk is high)

Ultrasound scan
Placental localization, gestational dating and exclusion of twins
Structural malformations, including limb, neural tube, cardiac and other internal defects
Nuchal thickening and related measurements

Fetal blood and tissue sampling
Thalassaemias and related disorders (when DNA analysis not feasible)
Other severe haematological and metabolic disorders detectable from fetal blood

Maternal blood biochemical screening
AFP (neural tube defects and Down's syndrome)
β-hCG, oestriol and other biochemical markers (Down's syndrome)

The information that can be obtained from amniocentesis is illustrated in Figure 8.1. The sample should consist of clear fluid, in which are suspended the cells (fetal in origin) that can be cultured for chromosomal, biochemical or molecular studies, or in some situations analysed directly. A bloodstained sample usually indicates damage to the placenta; a discoloured fluid may indicate impending or actual fetal death, and is an important factor to note because the subsequent inevitable abortion might otherwise be attributed to the amniocentesis itself. Both these findings reduce the chance of a successful cell culture.

Once obtained, the sample is usually spun immediately and duplicate cell cultures set up. The supernatant fluid can be used for alpha-fetoprotein (AFP) estimation and, less frequently, for metabolic studies. Most diagnostic studies, however, whether chromosomal or biochemical, require cultured amniotic fluid cells, and depending on the number required, it may be 8 days to 3 weeks before sufficient are available. It is important that cultures are checked regularly to ensure that satisfactory cell growth is occurring; if not,

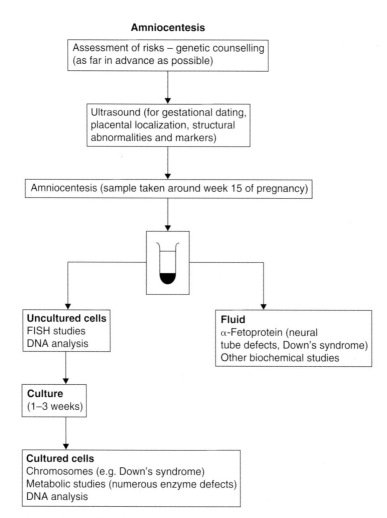

Figure 8.1 Amniocentesis – the main steps.

it may be preferable to repeat amniocentesis soon, rather than to wait until it is certain that growth will not occur, by which time it may be too late.

PRACTICAL ASPECTS

It is important that clinicians referring patients for amniocentesis or suggesting its application should realize what is involved and how best to utilize the service that is provided. The need for proper assessment and genetic counselling before a pregnancy is undertaken has already been stressed, but several points are often overlooked.

Timing

The earliest time that a satisfactory sample can reliably be obtained is at 15–16 weeks' gestation, so the couple must be prepared to accept a termination as late as 18 weeks. It is not uncommon for a patient's attitude to change during pregnancy, particularly once fetal movement has occurred. Early amniocentesis (at 12–14 weeks) has been introduced in some centres to allow an earlier result to be given, but preliminary results suggest a higher risk of pregnancy loss than conventional amniocentesis and it is unlikely to be generally adopted.

Who performs the procedure?

There is no doubt that the risks are increased if amniocentesis is done by an 'occasional operator' and there is much to be said for a centralized service in which skilled amniocentesis, accurate genetic counselling and appropriate laboratory facilities can all be combined.

The procedure itself

Some patients expect amniocentesis to be a painful procedure, but this is not the case. Direct needling, after ultrasound scan has localized the placenta and confirmed the correct gestation, can be done under local anaesthesia without need for hospital admission, although rest afterwards is advisable. It is surprising how many women are referred without a clear picture having been given of what amniocentesis entails, something that is clearly the responsibility of the obstetrician and referring clinician. In many centres, as noted earlier, a fetal medicine group has been set up, with the clinicians involved meeting weekly. This allows unexpected findings to be discussed, along with the likely genetic risks and possible diagnosis, something that is especially important in interpreting the findings of ultrasonography in pregnancies not known previously to be at risk.

Results and follow-up

The couple must be warned that a definitive result may take 10 days to 3 weeks (sometimes longer for biochemical and DNA studies) and that there is a possibility that a repeat sample may be needed. Results of rapid trisomy testing on uncultured cells should still be regarded as provisional. The possibility of abnormality unrelated to that primarily being looked for should be mentioned (e.g. a sex chromosome anomaly in a pregnancy at risk for Down's syndrome), and a clear policy must be defined in the event of no definite answer being reached because of culture failure or other reasons. Follow-up after delivery is important not only to check the correctness of the prediction, but also because the outcome may affect the genetic risk to subsequent pregnancies.

THE RISKS OF AMNIOCENTESIS

Amniocentesis is not without risk to the pregnancy. Approximate figures that can be used in discussion with families, based on a number of large studies, are as follows:

- *Abortion* – the added risk is around 0.5 per cent, but repeat amniocentesis carries a much higher risk (5–10 per cent), as does the performance of the procedure by an inexperienced person. Each centre should audit its own figures.
- *Perinatal problems* – these are not significant; an increase in postural orthopaedic deformities was suggested in one early UK study, but this has not been confirmed.
- *Maternal risks* – these are minimal, apart from a possibility of rhesus sensitization (Rh-negative mothers should receive anti-D antibody).

In general, amniocentesis has proved to be a safe and reliable procedure, but it is essential that it is used selectively and appropriately, and that the risks are carefully explained to couples who may be considering it. Each centre should monitor and make available its own risks and failure rate.

CHORION VILLUS SAMPLING

Prenatal diagnosis in the first trimester using fetal tissue obtained from chorionic villi has proved to be a major advance, especially for molecular diagnosis, but has not superseded amniocentesis for low-risk cytogenetic indications.

Currently, samples are obtained either transabdominally or transcervically at 10–11 weeks' gestation under ultrasound guidance; at this stage chorionic tissue has not yet become localized into a placenta. It is difficult to obtain tissue transcervically after 12 weeks, although transabdominal placental sampling is feasible at a later stage. Maternal tissue is dissected away microscopically, and the remaining villi consist of pure fetal tissue which can be used for a variety of diagnostic approaches, including the following:

- *Molecular studies.* Uncultured chorionic villi are much the most satisfactory sample for these and can provide a rapid and accurate prenatal diagnosis for any disorder for which mutation analysis or DNA markers are available. There is no evidence that the DNA of this tissue gives significantly different results from other fetal samples.
- *Enzyme studies.* The normal ranges in this material may differ considerably from amniotic fluid cells, while in X-linked diseases, differential X inactivation may give very low levels in a female heterozygote.

Experience with CVS is now extensive. It is likely that the rate of miscarriage is higher than in amniocentesis (2–3 per cent extra, compared with 1 per cent, and considerably more in inexperienced hands). Reports of an excess of limb defects possibly related to the procedure, especially in biopsies taken at 9 weeks or earlier, have not been confirmed at 10 weeks or later, but in general, amniocentesis remains the primary approach for pregnancies at lower risk, with CVS used in higher-risk situations and notably for molecular analyses.

CHROMOSOMAL DISORDERS

The recurrence risks for the major types of chromosome disorder have been discussed in Chapter 4, and the strength of indication for prenatal diagnosis will depend on the magnitude of this risk as well as on the nature of the disorder and the attitude and experience of the couple concerned in relation to it. The relative risks of amniocentesis and CVS will need careful consideration, especially where the risk of abnormality in the pregnancy is low. The main chromosomal indications for prenatal diagnosis are considered individually below (see also Table 8.3).

ADVANCED MATERNAL AGE

The risk with advanced maternal age is primarily for Down's syndrome, with a lesser risk of other trisomies. The difference in risk of having a live-born child with an abnormality and that for an abnormality found at amniocentesis has already been emphasized (see Tables 4.5 and 4.6, p. 67), but there is general agreement that this risk is sufficient that all women aged 35 years or over should be informed of the risks of Down's syndrome and offered amniocentesis. Although the uptake of amniocentesis varies greatly between countries and regions, this often reflects a failure of obstetricians and others to give adequate information, together with geographical variability in the services provided. The pattern of amniocentesis has been considerably affected by the development of biochemical screening tests for Down's syndrome in the second trimester, usually a combination of AFP, human chorionic gonadotrophin (hCG) and oestriol assessment (discussed further below and in Chapter 27). As a result of this, it is becoming possible to modify the age-specific risks so that some older women whose risk is considerably reduced will no longer opt for amniocentesis.

Table 8.3 Principal chromosomal indications for prenatal diagnosis (see Chapter 4 for detailed risk figures)

One parent carrier of a balanced autosomal translocation
Advanced maternal age
Abnormal Down's screening test
Ultrasound findings suggestive of Down's syndrome or other chromosome disorder
Previous child with autosomal trisomy or similar abnormality
Parent mosaic for chromosomal abnormality
Chromosomal instability syndromes

TRANSLOCATION DOWN'S SYNDROME

The rare, but high-risk, group with translocation Down's syndrome comprises only 5 per cent of all cases of Down's syndrome. The risks for the offspring of balanced carriers of the various forms of translocation have been discussed in Chapter 4 and are given in Table 4.8 (p. 71). It is clearly vital that the precise type be established from study of the index case, and that relatives at risk should be investigated using blood before a pregnancy occurs. CVS may be preferred to amniocentesis in a high-risk situation. If the individual is a chromosomally normal sib or more distant relative, there is no indication for prenatal tests. Where the parents of a child with translocation Down's syndrome are both chromosomally normal, the risk of a further affected child is also low, probably similar to that for trisomic Down's (see below). Although it may be reasonable to offer prenatal diagnosis to such couples in a subsequent pregnancy, it should not be undertaken under the false assumption that the risk of Down's syndrome is high.

TRISOMIC DOWN'S SYNDROME AND OTHER AUTOSOMAL TRISOMIES

All studies agree that the recurrence risk for trisomic syndromes is low, with the exception of very rare families in which there appears to be some special factor causing clustering of chromosomal abnormalities, possibly by predisposing to non-disjunction or gonadal mosaicism. It is important that the chromosomes of the child, or of both parents if the child is dead, be studied before another pregnancy is considered, and that the age of the mother is considered in estimating the recurrence risk (see Chapter 4).

In practice, most couples who have had an affected child do elect for prenatal diagnosis in a subsequent pregnancy, even in full knowledge of the risk from the procedure and the low probability that the abnormality will recur. Provided that they have the full facts, this seems reasonable.

For other relatives of a child with isolated trisomic Down's syndrome, there is no evidence of an increased risk in their offspring, and this should be made clear at the time of diagnosis of the index case to avoid unnecessary worry. Where the index case is no longer living and no definite chromosomal status has been recognized, it is preferable to undertake an urgent blood karyotype of the at-risk relative rather than perform an unnecessary amniocentesis. Unfortunately, there is still no test – chromosomal or molecular – that will distinguish, prior to conception, the couple particularly likely to have a trisomic child.

PROBLEMS WITH CHROMOSOMAL PRENATAL DIAGNOSIS

The following problems may complicate prenatal chromosomal diagnosis.

Faulty diagnosis in the index case

Down's syndrome said to affect an older relative may prove to be an entirely different disorder, and the records (or the affected individual, if available) should be checked wherever possible. A cytogenetic register of all known cases of Down's syndrome in a region is helpful.

Chromosomal abnormality unrelated to clinical abnormality

This is seen particularly in cases of mental retardation, where chromosome studies are commonly performed. It should be particularly suspected if healthy family members show the same chromosomal pattern.

Normal variants

These may be mistakenly considered to be the cause of the problem in the index case, as mentioned above, or they may be discovered in the amniotic cells of the fetus at amniocentesis. In most cases, there should be little doubt as to whether they are pathological; again, help may come from finding the same pattern in a healthy parent. The findings should always be discussed with the cytogenetic laboratory that has actually performed the analysis.

Unrelated or unexpected abnormalities

These may be chromosomal (e.g. sex chromosome anomalies or a balanced translocation), or a raised AFP level may suggest a neural tube defect in a pregnancy studied primarily for a chromosomal indication. Such findings may lead to a difficult dilemma, and in general one has to discuss the facts with the couple and respect their decision. It is always easier if the possibility of such a situation arising has been explained prior to the amniocentesis.

Mosaicism

Interpreting this is often difficult, not only the likely consequences and severity in the child, but also whether it is a genuine reflection of the chromosome state of the fetus. This is especially the case in CVS samples, where mosaicism is often confined to the placenta; amniocentesis may be needed to check this, but close liaison with the laboratory is wise.

STRUCTURAL MALFORMATIONS

NEURAL TUBE DEFECTS

A series of factors have combined to reduce the birth frequency of neural tube defects in most populations where these have previously had a high incidence. This is a major achievement which, like rhesus isoimmunization, is in danger of being overlooked now that major defects of this type no longer represent such an important cause of serious abnormality, disability and death in childhood. The principal factors include:

- a natural decline in incidence, especially in high-risk populations, probably related to maternal nutritional status
- primary prevention in high-risk pregnancies and the wider population by use of folic acid, taken preconceptually and as a food supplement
- increasing resolution of prenatal ultrasonography
- maternal serum AFP screening.

The first of these steps was the discovery that pregnancies ending in an open neural tube defect had elevated amniotic fluid levels of AFP, which provided an accurate prenatal test for pregnancies known to be at high risk. The subsequent development of ultrasonography provided a means of both confirming the diagnosis and detecting most closed lesions. As ultrasound scanning has become more sensitive and is used more routinely, this has allowed detection in pregnancies not known to be at risk. The first true screening approach came from maternal serum AFP analysis. In areas of high incidence, this remains the main screening test, in conjunction with an ultrasound scan. In areas where the incidence is low, high-resolution ultrasonography alone is often preferred, as the proportion of false-positive raised AFP samples will be higher in these areas.

Amniocentesis is now often not performed where a clearly abnormal pregnancy is detected, since delay will inevitably result. Where there are doubts, this test should be undertaken, together with chromosome analysis on the amniotic fluid if there is any suspicion of a complex malformation syndrome.

In general, these methods of prenatal diagnosis of neural tube defects have proved reliable and free from major problems. However, several points need to be borne in mind:

- There are a number of other causes of a raised serum AFP level (Table 8.4), including normal twin pregnancy. These can often be distinguished by the level of acetylcholinesterase in amniotic fluid, which is specifically raised in neural tube defects.
- Routine obstetric ultrasound scanning is an inadequate substitute for high-resolution ultrasonography performed by an expert, at the optimal gestation (usually around 18 weeks).

Table 8.4 Abnormalities other than neural tube defects that may cause a raised amniotic fluid alpha-fetoprotein level

Spontaneous intrauterine death
Omphalocele and gastroschisis
Bowel and oesophageal atresias
Turner syndrome
Congenital nephrosis (Finnish type)
Sacrococcygeal teratoma
Bladder exstrophy
Focal dermal hypoplasia and other skin defects
Meckel syndrome

- High-risk pregnancies must be considered separately from general population screening and the risks estimated appropriately.
- Any pregnancy terminated should have an expert fetal autopsy, since numerous syndromes associated with neural tube defects exist, some mendelian, others chromosomal (see Chapter 12).

OTHER STRUCTURAL ABNORMALITIES: ULTRASOUND SCANNING IN PRENATAL DIAGNOSIS

Ultrasonography is now a sensitive, valuable and widely available approach to prenatal diagnosis. Table 8.5 summarizes some of the main applications, but a few general points must be made:

- There is an immense difference between the results of expert units specializing in detection of malformations and the results of radiologists, radiographers and obstetricians using ultrasound as a more general tool. This applies to both false positives and false negatives and to the interpretation of any possibly abnormal results. The rapid spread of ultrasonography outside specialist centres can be actively harmful unless there is a comparable spread of expertise, which is often still not the case. Most genetics centres are aware of pregnancies that were terminated because of supposed ultrasonographic abnormality and where the fetus proved to be entirely normal.

Table 8.5 Ultrasound in prenatal diagnosis of structural malformations

General applications
Accurate gestational dating
Multiple pregnancy
Placental localization before amniocentesis or chorion biopsy
Central nervous system abnormalities
Anencephaly
Spina bifida (in conjunction with other approaches)
Hydrocephalus and hydranencephaly
Microcephaly (see Chapter 12 for limitations)
Skeletal defects
Severe neonatal bone dysplasia (e.g. achondrogenesis)
Osteogenesis imperfecta (severe congenital forms only)
Limb defects (especially of digits)
Internal abnormalities
Severe congenital heart defects
Renal agenesis
Infantile polycystic kidney disease
Severe obstructive uropathy
Omphalocele and gastroschisis
Fetal tumours

- Although ultrasound is itself apparently risk-free, one must also consider the risks of any attendant or consequent investigations resulting from apparently abnormal or uncertain findings. These may be considerable.
- In investigating genetic abnormalities, the prior risk of the situation must be taken into consideration. Ability to detect or exclude an abnormality in the face of a high genetic risk is quite different from doing so when the risk is low or when ultrasound scanning is used as a screening procedure. This obvious fact is still ignored by many of those using the technique.
- Many ultrasonographic 'abnormalities' or 'soft markers' may be transient and physiological rather than pathological in nature. Others may indicate abnormality in only a proportion of cases (e.g. nuchal oedema in trisomy 21; choroid plexus cysts in trisomy 18).
- The best results from ultrasound scanning are likely to be when it is used in conjunction with other appropriate investigations. The balance of value of the various tests will change, but they should be considered together for each particular problem. Likewise, the interpretation of puzzling findings is best carried out in conjunction with other specialities, preferably as part of a fetal medicine group, as mentioned earlier.

The diagnosis of congenital heart disease by ultrasonography provides a good example of how uncertain is the role of the technique. Although severe lesions can be detected in the middle trimester of pregnancy, currently available information still does not allow one to decide how accurately less severe defects can be recognized or excluded, or whether this is a suitable investigation for families with the more common forms of congenital heart defect, especially where the recurrence risk is low.

MATERNAL SERUM SCREENING FOR DOWN'S SYNDROME

Although population maternal serum screening was originally started for neural tube defects in areas of high incidence, as indicated above, the finding that AFP levels were frequently reduced in Down's syndrome has led to its use in screening antenatally for this disorder, especially since the additional measurement of levels of β-hCG, oestriol and pregnancy-associated plasma protein-A (PAPP-A) has given a greater discrimination than AFP assessment alone. An additional screening technique for Down's syndrome is the fetal nuchal fold thickness as measured by ultrasound scan; this still requires further evaluation.

The value of this approach is that (in theory at least) the number of invasive tests, i.e. amniocentesis, can be kept constant or even reduced, while the proportion of tests with abnormal results is raised. In practical terms, this can allow mothers of all ages to be offered amniocentesis if the screening test passes an agreed threshold of risk (often 1 in 250), while other women can avoid amniocentesis if their risk following serum screening is reduced to below this level.

In practice, the situation is often less simple. Older women may be reluctant to forego a definitive test (and their obstetricians may fear the legal consequences). The greater completeness of coverage may itself increase the amniocentesis rate, overloading the cytogenetics laboratory, while many women (and often their doctors) may be worried by being given a specific risk estimate, however small it is, and request amniocentesis. An additional problem, as with all screening, is that an abnormal screening result produces severe distress and anxiety in women who have not perceived themselves to be at high risk, and who may have been given inadequate information about the test. Many genetic clinics have found themselves having to attempt to resolve such traumatic situations, an almost impossible task. There can be no doubt that for these women at least, screening has caused more harm then good.

The overall issues of population screening are debated in Chapter 27; for maternal serum Down's syndrome screening, the evidence currently suggests that it will allow the avoidance of Down's syndrome in a considerably greater proportion (60–70 per cent) of pregnancies than age-related screening alone. How this can be weighed against any adverse effects on women being screened is an open question, for which more evidence, social as well as scientific, is urgently needed as such screening becomes more widespread. What is clear is that good practice necessitates the full provision of information to allow informed choices by women and their partners.

X-LINKED DISORDERS

Where a pregnancy is at high risk for an X-linked disorder, fetal sexing offers the possibility of determining whether the fetus is indeed at risk. However, in most disorders, direct molecular prenatal diagnosis of an affected male is now possible, and even where it is not, linked DNA markers can often be used. First-trimester fetal sexing using both DNA and cytogenetic methods is now feasible with CVS, and should always accompany metabolic studies, which may give variable and misleading results in X-linked conditions.

Where a woman is only a possible carrier, not a definite one, it is vital to estimate the risk before fetal sexing is undertaken and to use methods of carrier detection where applicable (see Chapter 7). The most successful approach to prenatal diagnosis is where no prenatal procedure is required at all, because the carrier state has been excluded. As with any prenatal diagnostic investigation, this should be approached as a planned procedure with the issues for and against resolved, as far as possible, beforehand.

Occasionally, in haemophilia or Becker muscular dystrophy for example, fetal sexing may be requested for a pregnancy with an affected father, with a view to termination of a female fetus, which would inevitably be a carrier. The author has serious misgivings about the wisdom of this, because such daughters would almost always be healthy, and because advances within the next generation are likely to allow them the option of direct prenatal diagnosis in their own future children, even for disorders where this is not possible at present. The situation is less clear-cut for disorders where heterozygous females frequently show some clinical effects, such as ornithine transcarbamylase deficiency and fragile-X mental retardation.

Prenatal sex selection (usually by ultrasound and sometimes by amniocentesis), solely for parental choice, is currently illegal in most countries, including the UK. However, it is being grossly abused in some parts of the world, notably India, almost always in favour of a male pregnancy. Developments in sperm sorting, ineffective until very recently, have raised the issue of whether this should be permitted for non-medical reasons. A recent UK report has recommended against this at present.

INBORN ERRORS OF METABOLISM

The development of prenatal diagnostic techniques for a variety of inherited metabolic disorders has been one of the major achievements of human genetics, even if the number of families at risk for such disorders is small in comparison with chromosomal disorders such as Down's syndrome. So many serious inborn errors are now prenatally detectable that this aspect is one of the first to be raised by any couple who have had an affected child.

Chapter 23 covers some of the more important disorders and virtually all of them are now diagnosable prenatally, by either biochemical or DNA analysis, or a combination of both.

The following points need to be borne in mind when prenatal diagnosis of a metabolic disorder is being considered:

- The great majority of these disorders follow autosomal recessive inheritance, so that only sibs of affected patients are at high (1 in 4) risk. Risks for other relatives are rarely high enough to warrant undertaking prenatal diagnosis.
- Most disorders require chorionic villi or cultured amniotic fluid cells for their diagnosis; in general, if a particular enzyme defect can be detected in the cultured skin fibroblast, it can also be detected in cultured amniotic fluid cells or villus material, but normal ranges may differ considerably.
- Large numbers of cells are often required, making direct analysis of chorionic villi especially suitable; the need for cell culture with amniocentesis may add delay and uncertainty, which should be explained beforehand. A late termination may be unacceptable to a couple who would accept termination in early pregnancy.
- Many of the enzymatic techniques are exceptionally specialized and can only be undertaken by a few laboratories. Careful advance planning is essential because cells may have to be sent long distances. Fortunately, a remarkable degree of cooperation exists between laboratories involved in this work, although careful distinction is needed between a centre that is interested in a disorder and one that has proven experience in its prenatal diagnosis. DNA analysis also requires great familiarity with the probes concerned, but there is a higher degree of 'common technology' between the different disorders.
- Wherever possible, samples from the affected individual should be studied alongside those at risk. If the affected child is likely to die, every effort should be made to reach a precise enzymatic or molecular diagnosis beforehand, and to arrange for storage of DNA, cultured cells or postmortem material to be used at a later date. Failure to do this may result in serious problems in relation to a future pregnancy.

A few inherited metabolic diseases can be diagnosed directly from amniotic fluid itself, although the use of cultured cells is usually desirable as a back-up. These include the organic acidurias (propionic and methylmalonic aciduria), mucopolysaccharidoses, the 21-hydroxylase form of congenital adrenal hyperplasia, and congenital nephrosis (diagnosed by elevated amniotic AFP levels).

MOLECULAR PRENATAL DIAGNOSIS

The impact of molecular genetics has been felt in the area of prenatal diagnosis more than in most other branches of medical genetics. There are many reasons for this, including the independence of the techniques from gestational timing and tissue specificity, the lack of variability in heterozygotes, and the suitability of first-trimester samples. Most of all, molecular analysis has extended the possibility of prenatal diagnosis to numerous serious disorders, often dominantly inherited, where lack of specific biochemical knowledge previously precluded any attempts at prenatal diagnosis. In any inherited disorder for which the specific gene has been isolated, it can be assumed that prenatal diagnosis is potentially feasible.

The range of molecular approaches available is the same as already indicated in Chapter 5, and also outlined in relation to carrier detection in Chapter 7. Where a mutation has been identified in an affected relative, search for this will avoid the necessity for additional tests. Where this is not possible, a wider search for mutations may be needed and this may have limitations. If linked genetic markers are being used, intragenic markers will be reliable provided that other family members can be typed; for recessive disorders a previous affected child is usually the critical sample. The importance of storing a sample from such key individuals for the future must yet again be emphasized.

If linked DNA markers outside the gene are used, the risk of error due to recombination must be carefully estimated and discussed before embarking on prenatal testing.

FETAL BLOOD AND TISSUE SAMPLING

Direct umbilical cord sampling under ultrasonographic control has superseded placental aspiration as a method of obtaining pure fetal blood, but DNA techniques render it unnecessary in many situations where it was used before – notably in the haemoglobinopathies and haemophilias.

Fetal skin biopsy has proved both reliable and safe for a variety of severe conditions, including lethal and dystrophic epidermolysis bullosa, ichthyosiform erythroderma, Sjogren–Larsson syndrome and severe oculocutaneous albinism; there is usually no visible scar. As with fetal blood sampling, molecular analysis using DNA from a chorion villus sample is progressively replacing this approach.

PRE-IMPLANTATION DIAGNOSIS

For many couples at high risk of transmitting a serious genetic disorder, this could offer the possibility of avoiding termination of an established pregnancy. It is now possible to undertake molecular analysis of cells from an early embryo produced by *in vitro* fertilization, and to implant only those embryos shown to have an unaffected genotype.

In principle this should allow pre-implantation diagnosis to be offered for any disorder where a specific molecular or chromosomal defect can be identified. In practice, there are major reservations, which mean that pre-implantation diagnosis must still be considered as a research procedure in most situations until much more evidence is available. These include:

- inadequate numbers studied to give meaningful rates of error or failure to obtain a result
- absence of long-term data on potential harmful effects of the procedure
- lack of prior experience in identifying the defect for most individual disorders
- limited success rate for IVF in general.

In view of these serious limitations, it is most unfortunate that some centres offer pre-implantation diagnosis without making it clear to referring clinicians or families what prior experience they have had with individual disorders, what preparatory research they have undertaken, or whether what they are offering is research or service. Even more disturbing is the fact that pre-implantation diagnosis is not always being offered in the context of full genetic counselling. Given the complex genetic situations commonly involved, expert information on the wider genetic aspects is essential if families are to make an informed choice between the possible options open to them. There is a clear need for effective regulation in this field if this promising and important development is not to be discredited by premature applications.

FETAL CELL ANALYSIS OF MATERNAL BLOOD

This is another field that remains a research procedure. It has long been known that a small number of fetal cells are present in maternal blood; the development of techniques to separate and identify these gives the possibility of DNA analysis or fluorescence in-situ hybridization to provide a non-invasive approach to prenatal diagnosis. Current research is concentrating on the use of this technique as part of a primary screening test for Down's syndrome. At present, it seems unlikely that it will prove reliable enough to be applied as a service.

TWINS AND PRENATAL DIAGNOSIS

The discovery of a twin pregnancy poses obvious practical problems in undertaking amniocentesis, but it also alters the genetic risk figures that would normally be given for a singleton pregnancy. The problems involved in estimating the modified risks are summarized in Table 8.6. It is assumed here that a third of twin pairs are monozygous.

In general, the risks are considerably higher than for a singleton pregnancy, and they are altered if information is available on one twin from amniocentesis. The figures do not include the increased risk of malformations known to be associated with monozygotic

Table 8.6 Genetic risks in twin pregnancies

	Chromosome abnormality	Neural tube defect	X-linked (fetal sexing only)	X-linked (specific diagnostic test)	Autosomal recessive
Before amniocentesis					
Risk for singleton pregnancy	Y*	1/25	1/2	1/4	1/4
Risk of at least one twin being affected	5/3 Y	2/25	2/3	3/8	3/8
Risk of both twins being affected	≃1/3 Y	<1/100	1/3	1/8	1/8
Twin A normal; risk of twin B being abnormal	2/3 Y	1/25	1/3	1/6	1/6
After amniocentesis (one sac successfully tested)					
Twin A abnormal; risk of twin B being normal	2/3 − 2/3 Y	9/10	1/3	1/2	1/2
Twin A abnormal; risk of twin B being abnormal	1/3 + 2/3 Y	1/10	2/3	1/2	1/2

*Risk (Y) will vary with maternal age, etc.
After Hunter AGW, Cox DM (1985), *Clin Genet* **16**, 34–42.

twin pregnancies (see p. 142). Clearly the couple concerned should be informed of these altered risks, and the same is true even when prenatal diagnosis is not being considered.

A further point to be noted is that the normal range of maternal serum AFP concentrations is raised in twin pregnancies. Twin percentiles are now available for assessing AFP levels; it should be noted that all twin pregnancies ending in a neural tube defect had a serum AFP concentration at least 75 times the normal singleton median value.

Techniques of selective abortion are possible when only one of a twin pair is found to be abnormal, but twin pregnancies remain a difficult field of management. Multiple births are also increasingly seen following IVF procedures.

MATERNAL ASPECTS OF GENETIC COUNSELLING IN PREGNANCY

Although prenatal diagnosis is principally concerned with the fetus, genetic counselling in pregnancy also needs to look at the maternal aspects. In many dominantly inherited disorders, the mother will be affected by the disorder, which may pose direct risks to her health in pregnancy or give obstetric complications. Prognosis of an affected parent is a further relevant point in relation to any decisions.

Examples of the range of problems needing consideration are given in Table 8.7.

Table 8.7 Genetic disorders in pregnancy and maternal health

Maternal health adversely affected by pregnancy
Cystic fibrosis (respiratory decompensation)
Homocystinuria, sickle-cell disease (thrombotic episodes)

Obstetric complications increased
Achondroplasia (pelvic disproportion, uterine myomas)
Ehlers–Danlos syndrome (premature rupture of membranes)
Myotonic dystrophy (postpartum haemorrhage, anaesthetic problems)
Steroid sulphatase deficiency (delayed labour, increased risk of stillbirth)

FURTHER READING

Abramsky L, Chapple J (2003). *Prenatal Diagnosis. The Human Side*, 2nd edn. London, Chapman & Hall.

Brock DJH, Rodeck CH, Ferguson-Smith MA (eds) (1992). *Prenatal Diagnosis and Screening.* Edinburgh, Churchill Livingstone.

Clarke A (1997). Prenatal genetic screening. Paradigms and perspectives. In: Harper PS, Clarke A, eds. *Genetics, Society and Clinical Practice.* Oxford, BIOS, pp. 119–140.

De Crespigny L, Dredge R (1991). *Which Tests for my Unborn Baby?* Oxford, Oxford University Press – a clearly written guide for the educated and articulate parent-to-be.

Gardner RJM, Sutherland GR (2003). *Chromosome Abnormalities and Genetic Counselling.* Oxford, Oxford University Press – a valuable source for all aspects of chromosomal prenatal diagnosis.

Milunsky A (1998). *Genetic Disorders and the Fetus*, 4th edn. Baltimore, Johns Hopkins University Press.

Prenatal Diagnosis (Wiley InterScience) – this journal is a valuable source of recent advances.

Scriver CR, Beaudet AL, Sly WS, Valle D (2001). *The Metabolic and Molecular Bases of Inherited Disease.* New York, McGraw Hill.

Simpson JL, Golbus MS (1998). *Genetics in Obstetrics and Gynaecology.* Philadelphia, WB Saunders.

CHAPTER 9

Special issues in genetic counselling

CONSANGUINITY

Consanguinity, or marriage between close relatives, is a common and important issue in genetic counselling. Where an inherited disorder is present in the family, consanguinity may significantly influence the risks, while even without a known disorder, couples who are closely related may be concerned about the risks to their offspring.

There are three aspects of consanguinity that need to be considered in relation to genetic counselling:

- What is the exact relationship between the two individuals?
- How is the risk of a genetic disorder in the family influenced by the occurrence of consanguinity?
- How likely is it that any harmful gene might be handed by both members of the couple to a child, i.e. that the child is homozygous by descent for that gene?

An attempt is made here to answer these questions in simple terms, avoiding a complex mathematical approach. These same questions are of more general interest to population geneticists, and detailed accounts of the subject can be found in genetics textbooks (see 'Further reading', Chapter 1).

GENETIC RELATIONSHIPS

An accurate idea of how individuals are related is important in all genetic counselling, regardless of the presence or absence of consanguinity, but when a marriage between close relatives is being considered, it becomes essential. Table 9.1 summarizes the main categories of relationship, and it is always important to construct a precise pedigree pattern rather than relying on verbal descriptions, which may be confusing. Table 9.2 gives examples.

Table 9.1 Degrees of relationship

	Proportion of genes shared
First degree	
Sibs	
Dizygotic twins	1/2
Parents	
Children	
Second degree	
Half-sibs	
Uncles, aunts	1/4
Nephews, nieces	
Double first cousins	
Third degree	
First cousins	
Half-uncles, aunts	1/8
Half-nephews, nieces	

Table 9.2 Patterns of relationship

Relationship (between shaded individuals)		Degree of relationship	Proportion of genes shared	Chance of homozygosity by descent (F)
	Monozygotic twins	–	1	–
	Dizygotic twins	First	1/2	1/4
	Sibs	First	1/2	1/4
	Parent-child	First	1/2	–
	Uncle (aunt)-(niece) nephew	Second	1/4	1/8
	Half-sibs	Second	1/4	1/8
	Double first cousins	Second	1/4	1/8

Table 9.2 (cont.)

Relationship (between shaded individuals)	Degree of relationship	Proportion of genes shared	Chance of homozygosity by descent (F)
First cousins	Third	1/8	1/16
Half-uncle–niece (or similar combination)	Third	1/8	1/16
First cousins once removed	Fourth	1/16	1/32
Second cousins	Fifth	1/32	1/64
Second cousins once removed		1/64	1/128
Third cousins		1/128	1/256

Marriage between first-degree relatives is almost universally prohibited by law and social custom, but incestuous relationships, usually between father and daughter or between sibs, are more common than is generally recognized, and give rise to particular problems discussed below. Marriage between second-degree relatives is also legally barred in many countries, although uncle–niece marriage is frequent in some Asian communities.

First cousin marriages are the most common reason for couples seeking genetic advice; these are legal in many Western countries, but may be the subject of religious or social restrictions. In many Asian communities they are actively encouraged. The less common half-uncle–niece marriage shown in Table 9.2 is, in genetic terms, identical to a first cousin marriage.

Table 9.3 Legal restrictions on marriage (UK and USA)

Marriage	UK	USA
Full sibs	Illegal	Illegal (all states)
Parent–child	Illegal	Illegal
Grandparent–grandchild	Illegal	Illegal
Half-sibs	Illegal	Illegal in 42 states
Uncle (aunt)–niece (nephew)	Illegal	Illegal
Half-uncle–niece (or half-aunt–nephew)	Illegal	Illegal in 18 states
First cousins	Legal	Illegal in 30 states
First cousins once removed	Legal	Illegal in 7 states
Double first cousin	Legal	Illegal in N. Carolina

Among the more distant relationships, the problem of terminology may cause confusion. The term 'removed' refers to a difference in generations between the individuals – thus the son of one's first cousin is a first cousin once removed, while the children of one's parents' first cousins are one's second cousins.

It should be noted that the 'degrees' of relationship shown in Table 9.1 are those used in genetic terminology, and also in English canon and common law, but not in civil law, where a different approach is used. Thus, uncle and niece, who would generally be considered second-degree relatives, would be termed 'third-degree relatives' in civil law.

Some of the legal aspects of consanguineous marriages are given in Table 9.3. It is helpful in genetic counselling to be aware of these because many couples have unspoken fears about the legality of a relationship as well as the genetic risks. Clearly the situation will vary between countries, and in the USA between individual states. The situation in the USA, provides some remarkable inconsistencies, although some have been amended: thus first cousin marriages are illegal in over half the states, while half-niece or half-nephew marriages are prohibited in only a quarter of states. Some states prohibit marriages between first cousins once removed. On the other hand, 11 states allow marriages between half-sibs. Some continental European countries have recently relaxed or removed restrictions on marriage between even the most closely related individuals.

Quite apart from these complexities, there are a number of restrictions on marriages between unrelated individuals. Thus, the wife of an uncle may be considered as a legal aunt even though no genetic relationship exists. In addition, different religions may have specific prohibitions over and above the legal requirement.

Taking all these facts together, it can be seen that there are numerous legal as well as genetic pitfalls confronting those involved in genetic counselling for consanguineous marriages. If there is any doubt, the couple should obtain legal advice and this aspect should be clarified before the genetic risks are discussed in detail.

SOCIAL ASPECTS OF CONSANGUINITY

Working in the field of medical genetics, it is easy to regard consanguinity as a 'problem' and something to be discouraged. In fact, it is a preferred pattern of marriage over large parts of the world, something that would not have occurred without good reasons.

These are obvious to members of such populations, but need to be emphasized. Quite apart from legal and property rights, a consanguineous marriage often greatly strengthens the position of a woman, who is much less likely to be ill-treated if her husband's family are bound by ties of kinship. These considerations apply just as much to immigrant groups in Western countries, who are even more dependent on family links to survive and prosper. Thus consanguinity is a beneficial pattern for many millions of couples, though one with a genetic price to pay in terms of autosomal recessive disorders.

RISKS OF CONSANGUINITY WITH A SPECIFIC GENETIC DISORDER IN THE FAMILY

Where a specific genetic disorder occurs in a consanguineous marriage, this may have serious implications for the extended family, who will have to weigh up the social benefits against the genetic risks. It is thus clearly important that the extended family as well as the immediate family have information on the precise risks involved, as outlined below. Such risks decline rapidly with distance of relationship.

In general, consanguinity will have no effect on risks if the disorder is X-linked recessive or autosomal dominant, unless both partners of the couple actually have the condition or carry the gene concerned. Autosomal recessive inheritance provides the main problem; it is likely that risks are also increased for polygenic disorders, even though this is difficult to estimate.

The essential question to be asked for an autosomal recessive disorder is this: what is the chance that the harmful mutant gene will have passed down both sides of the family simultaneously and appear in homozygous state in the child? The situation is best illustrated by the example shown in Figure 9.1. Here, a man having a sister with a rare autosomal recessive disorder has married his first cousin. We can ignore the very small added risk of new mutation or the mutant gene being present by chance.

The chance of the husband carrying the mutant gene is 2 in 3 (not 2 in 4, as is commonly thought, because the homozygous affected category has been excluded). The chance of a child receiving the gene from him is thus 1 in 3.

The chance of the wife (first cousin) also being a carrier must now be estimated. Both parents of the husband must be carriers and one of the common paternal grandparents also must be, so the chance of their daughter being a carrier is 1 in 2 and for their

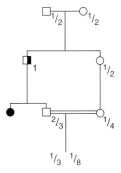

Final risk $^1/_{24}$

Figure 9.1 Genetic risks in a consanguineous marriage (see text for explanation).

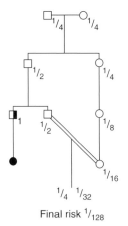

Figure 9.2 Genetic risks in a consanguineous marriage (first cousins once removed). The chance of a child being homozygous for (i.e. affected by) the rare autosomal recessive disorder present in the husband's niece is 1 in 128.

grand-daughter (the wife in the couple being considered) it is 1 in 4. The chance of the mutant gene being transmitted to her child will be 1 in 8. The risk of the child receiving the gene from both sides simultaneously, i.e. of having the disorder, is simply the product: $1/3 \times 1/8 = 1/24$.

A second example is given in Figure 9.2; it is a little more complex, but the approach is the same. Every generation added to the path diminishes the risk by one-half.

Figure 9.3 summarizes some of the general risks in this situation. This information could be important for genetic counsellors and others working in isolated areas with little access to specialist advice, as is the case in many parts of the world where consanguinity is the norm. Indeed, there is no reason why community or religious leaders should not use such a table for the commonest situations, since they are often involved when marriages are being arranged. A simple computer program, based on those already widely used in population genetics, could also be readily produced. The figures show clearly how substituting a more distant consanguineous marriage for a closer one could give an acceptably low risk, and thus allow the social benefits of consanguinity to be retained. If the situation is simply presented in terms of consanguinity being a problem, rather than of a graded risk, considerable social damage could result that might well outweigh the potential harm from a genetic disorder.

GENERAL RISKS OF CONSANGUINITY

Estimates of risk for the offspring of consanguineous marriages when no disorder is known in the family are based on two approaches:

- information on the probable number of deleterious recessive genes carried by healthy individuals in the population
- surveys of the outcome of pregnancies from consanguineous marriages.

Several studies have suggested that everyone carries at least one gene for a harmful recessive disorder, and probably at least two for lethal conditions that would result in a spontaneous abortion or stillbirth. Using this as a basis, risks can easily be estimated if one knows the relationship of the couple concerned.

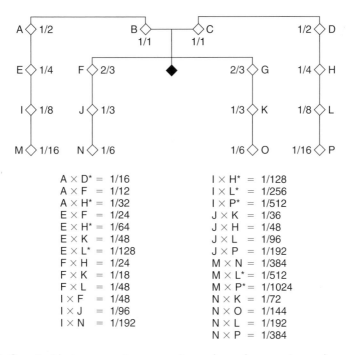

A × D* = 1/16		I × H* = 1/128	
A × F = 1/12		I × L* = 1/256	
A × H* = 1/32		I × P* = 1/512	
E × F = 1/24		J × K = 1/36	
E × H* = 1/64		J × H = 1/48	
E × K = 1/48		J × L = 1/96	
E × L* = 1/128		J × P = 1/192	
F × H = 1/24		M × N = 1/384	
F × K = 1/18		M × L* = 1/512	
F × L = 1/48		M × P* = 1/1024	
I × F = 1/48		N × K = 1/72	
I × J = 1/96		N × O = 1/144	
I × N = 1/192		N × L = 1/192	
		N × P = 1/384	

Figure 9.3 Genetic risks in consanguineous marriages where a known autosomal recessive disorder is present in the family (sex of individuals not specified for simplicity). The diagram indicates the main categories of marriage for which genetic risk estimates may be sought. In each case, the risk of the disorder will be 1/4 × the product of the two individual carrier risks: e.g. for E × L, the risk is 1/4 × 1/4 × 1/8 = 1/132. Selected examples are summarized above. **NB**: Some of the relationships are not consanguineous, even though genetic risks are increased. These are indicated by an asterisk.

The simplest approach is to trace the fate of such a harmful mutant gene from the common ancestor or ancestors to the offspring at risk, in a manner similar to that described in the previous section. Figure 9.4 shows this for a first cousin marriage, where it is clear that the risk of one harmful recessive gene reaching the offspring by both sides simultaneously is 1 in 64. Because the other common ancestor has to be considered as well, the total risk is 1 in 32. If the two lethal genes carried by each individual are considered in the same way, the risk is 1 in 16. This latter estimate is identical to the risk of any gene being homozygous by descent in the offspring, a figure known as the coefficient of consanguinity (F); this forms the generally used yardstick for measuring closeness of relationship between two individuals (see Table 9.1) and can also be used in connection with populations as well as individuals, as discussed below.

Studies of the actual empiric risks to the offspring of consanguineous marriages, summarized in Table 9.4, show considerable variation between populations.

It is also difficult to separate an increase in specific genetic disorders from problems with a large environmental contribution. Thus, in an extensive early study in Japan, the offspring of first cousin marriages followed over a 10-year period showed a 3 per cent increase in mortality over those with unrelated parents, but only a small increase in severe malformations (1.7 vs. 1.0 per cent). The offspring of marriages between first cousins once removed and between second cousins showed no increase in malformation rate. The data from different studies are well summarized in Vogel and Motulsky's book (see 'Further reading').

Studies of the offspring of incestuous matings have confirmed the high predicted risk to offspring, and show a risk of around 1 in 3 of childhood death or severe abnormality. In addition, there appears to be an increased risk of mental retardation without physical abnormality, so that only about half of the children may be fully normal. This poses a special problem because such children are commonly placed for adoption, and adoption agencies and potential adoptive parents will want to know how great is the risk of an undetected serious recessive disorder. It seems likely that around three-quarters of such disorders will express themselves in the first 6 months of life, so it is probably reasonable to wait until around this age before finalizing an adoption placement. It is also worth actively testing for the more common autosomal recessive disorders such as cystic fibrosis and phenylketonuria.

There is no clear evidence for a significant effect of consanguinity on intelligence in first cousin or more distantly related marriages.

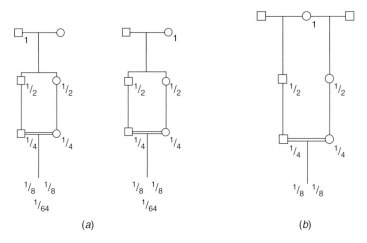

(a)   (b)

Figure 9.4 (a) First cousin marriage: the chance of a harmful gene in a common ancestor being homozygous by descent in the child is 1 in 64. Because there are two common ancestors, the risk will be twice this (total risk 1 in 32). (b) Marriage between half first cousins: the situation is as for full first cousins but there is only one common ancestor to be considered (total risk 1 in 64).

Table 9.4 Observed increase in severe abnormalities and mortality among offspring of consanguineous parents

Parental relationship	Increase (%)
Incestuous matings	30
First cousins	3
First cousins once removed and second cousins	1

Occasionally there may be a need to resolve uncertainty as to whether a child is indeed the offspring of an incestuous mating. In this situation, information can be obtained from the proportion of DNA polymorphisms for which the individual is homozygous.

In summary, consanguinity without known genetic disease in the family appears to cause an increase in mortality and malformation rate which is extremely marked in the children of incestuous matings, but which is of little significance when the relationship is more distant than that of first cousins. First cousin marriages, the most common counselling problem, seem to have an added risk of about 3 per cent, so that a total risk of 5 per cent for abnormality or death in early childhood, about double the general population risk, is a reasonable, though approximate, guide. It is possible but not certain that the risk is less for populations with a long tradition of cousin marriage; it is only recently that genetic disorders are being fully recognized and accurately diagnosed in these populations. By contrast, some immigrant groups of Asian origin in the UK show an unusually high frequency of recessively inherited disorders, some extremely rare. This may well reflect increased consanguinity due to isolation and restriction of marriage partners.

MULTIPLE CONSANGUINITY

Individuals may be related to each other in more than one way. This causes difficulty in drawing the pedigree as well as in calculating the precise degree of relationship. The simplest approach is to deal with each mode of relationship separately, work out the coefficient of consanguinity for each, and then add them.

More complex situations may need the help of a colleague expert in population genetics, but this method should be sufficient for most counselling situations. Figure 9.5 gives an example. The couple are first cousins by one set of parents, but also second cousins by the other set. Their coefficient of consanguinity (F) is thus that for first cousins (1/16) plus that for second cousins (1/64) giving a total of 5/64. The risk of a serious recessive disorder, assuming one harmful recessive gene per person, would be about half this, i.e. 5/128 or about 4 per cent.

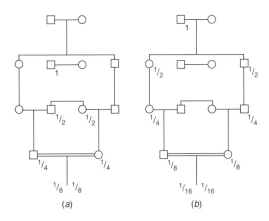

(a)   (b)

Figure 9.5 Estimation of risks with multiple consanguinity. One harmful recessive allele is assumed for each individual. (a) Risk is $2 \times 1/8 \times 1/8 = 1/32$. (b) Risk is $2 \times 1/16 \times 1/16 = 1/128$. Total risk is $1/32 + 1/128$ (about 4 per cent).

Alternatively, the route of a harmful gene can be plotted as in Figure 9.5, taking the 'inner loop' (first cousin) first and then the outer (second cousin) loop. The two pathways give risks of 1/32 and 1/128, respectively (each path must be gone over twice for the two common ancestors), giving a combined risk of 5/128, as did the first approach.

INBRED POPULATIONS

It is possible for a couple to be closely related simply because they are both members of an inbred population which has many of its genes in common. Such populations, particularly when isolated or derived from a small founding population, such as the Amish of North America, are often notable for the rare recessively inherited diseases occurring in them, and for many of them estimates of the coefficient of consanguinity (F) for the population as a whole are available. Even in the most inbred, the level of consanguinity rarely approaches the first cousin level.

In some cases, the frequency of carriers of a harmful gene in the population may be known, and this may be used in counselling. Thus, for a healthy man whose sister had Tay–Sachs disease, the risk of marrying a carrier would be 1 in 20 if he married someone of Ashkenazi Jewish descent, but only 1 in 400 if he married a non-Jewish person.

In the absence of such information, the risks are similar to those where the partners are known relatives with a particular coefficient of consanguinity. Thus a couple from the highly inbred Canadian Hutterite community ($F = 0.03$ or $1/67$) would be predicted to have a risk of recessively inherited disorders in the offspring similar to that of second cousins ($F = 1/64$). Practical proof of these risks is rarely available, however.

Where a known consanguineous marriage occurs in an already inbred population, the two contributions must be added. Thus the risk of homozygosity by descent (F) for a first cousin marriage in a Welsh gypsy population would be 1/16 (F for first cousin marriage) +1/50 (F for whole population) 1/12. The risk for a serious recessive disorder would be half this, i.e. 1/24 (as discussed above).

PATERNITY AND RELATIONSHIP TESTING

The uncertainty of paternity is a subject that has always concerned people, more for legal and social reasons than for any connections with genetic disease. Indeed, some societies in the past have not recognized the existence of paternity at all, while only in comparatively recent times has it been accepted that the paternal and maternal contributions to the child are approximately equal. The possibility of non-paternity must always be considered when trying to explain a puzzling pedigree pattern; non-maternity, by contrast, is an exceptionally rare problem – it is seen chiefly in possible confused identity of infants in maternity hospitals and in instances where a woman claims a kidnapped baby to be her own.

The testing of paternity depends almost entirely on the use of genetic polymorphisms detectable in the blood; clearly the more polymorphic a system is, the greater the chance of it distinguishing between two individuals, which is the object of the exercise. This is now possible using the technique of 'DNA fingerprinting', resulting from the discovery

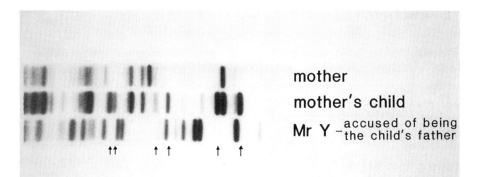

mother

mother's child

Mr Y $-$ accused of being the child's father

Figure 9.6 Use of the hypervariable mini-satellite DNA approach in paternity testing ('genetic fingerprinting'). The arrows indicate bands present in the child but not in the mother, which should thus be present in the biological father. The putative father can here be seen to lack these and is readily excluded. (Example kindly provided by Professor Alec Jeffreys, University of Leicester.)

by Jeffreys and colleagues of hypervariable mini-satellite DNA sequences giving a pattern unique to each individual (apart from identical twins) (see Figure 9.6).

The difference between individuals results from the existence of a variable number tandem repeat polymorphism (see Chapter 5), which can detect a considerable number of genetic loci, and which can be thought of as a large number of separate polymorphisms combined into a single test. The end result is a large number (30–40) of distinct bands, half of which come from the father, and half from the mother. Provided that one parent and the child are known, the bands inherited from the other parent can be determined and matched against any proposed candidate for paternity.

This technique is in widespread use for paternity testing (in animals as well as in humans), for immigration procedures involving kinship, and in forensic investigations such as rape and murder cases. The growth of forensic DNA databases has serious potential for abuse, however, particularly if disease-related or behavioural-related genotypes were to be used. Regulatory bodies need to monitor this area closely.

Modification of the techniques and development of locus-specific markers have increased stability and reliability, so that this is now an exceptionally powerful and legally acceptable tool for use in a wide variety of medicolegal situations. Nevertheless, it is not infallible, like any technique, and can be misinterpreted and misused. Practical and ethical guidelines for paternity testing are provided by the report given in the 'Further reading' section. There are important issues of consent involved. The same approach can also be used, though with less certainty, in establishing or excluding less close relationships.

TWINS

Studies of twins have played an important part in human genetics, but most of the available data are neither suitable nor relevant to genetic counselling. Only a few of the more important areas are discussed here; some further reading is given at the end of this chapter. Twinning in relation to prenatal diagnosis is discussed in Chapter 8.

DETERMINATION OF ZYGOSITY

Determination of zygosity may be simple, e.g. twins of unlike sex must be dizygotic. Triplets and other multiple pregnancies resulting from fertility drugs are likewise usually not monozygotic. In a like-sex twin pair, the most reliable clinical information comes from whether the twins consider themselves identical and are confused by others. This has been shown to correspond closely with detailed genotyping. Placentation is not a reliable guide. DNA fingerprinting now gives a definitive method of confirming zygosity.

RISKS OF MONOZYGOTIC TWIN PAIRS

For a fully penetrant mendelian disease, there should be complete concordance, i.e. both twins should either have or not have the disorder. There is often remarkable similarity in clinical features and age at onset.

For dominantly inherited disorders, an affected pair of monozygotic twins with normal parents is compatible with a new mutation (unlike dizygotic twins) and there is no increased risk of the disease in subsequent children of the normal parents.

For non-mendelian disorders, the risk to a co-twin will vary with the degree of genetic causation of the disease, being very high where genetic factors are predominant (as seen also in normal facial features and dermatoglyphics).

RISKS OF DIZYGOTIC TWIN PAIRS

Since dizygotic twins are genetically no more alike than sibs, risks for mendelian disorders are essentially the same as for sibs. For non-mendelian conditions, the shared intrauterine (and to some extent postnatal) environment gives a somewhat higher risk than that seen in sibs, but few accurate figures are available. In some instances concordance may be less than expected – thus in neural tube defects, affected co-twins are exceptional and it is possible that such pregnancies are lost, a point of relevance when one twin is found to be abnormal in prenatal diagnosis.

TWINNING IN FAMILIES

Monozygotic twins are rarely familial and have a rather constant incidence of around 4 in 1000 pregnancies. Dizygotic twinning, by contrast, shows marked geographical variation and frequently is around 6 in 1000 in European and white American populations, but it occurs in about 1 per cent of pregnancies in American blacks, and up to 4 per cent of pregnancies in parts of Nigeria. The recurrence risk for dizygotic twins is about 1.7 per cent for Europeans.

MALFORMATIONS IN TWINS

Monozygotic (but not dizygotic) twins have an increased overall malformation rate of around 5 per cent, twice that for a singleton pregnancy, a fact of considerably greater importance in genetic counselling than the twinning itself. The increase is for a variety of structural malformations, including neural tube defects and congenital heart disease.

CONJOINED TWINS

The phenomenon of conjoined twins can be regarded as an extreme example of mono-zygotic twinning and is most unlikely to recur in a family. Ultrasonography should now be able to give early warning of the problem. A partially developed co-twin may cause confusion on ultrasound scan.

TWIN RISKS IN COMMON DISORDERS

Twins have played an important role in determining the relative importance of heredity and environment in common non-mendelian disorders. The critical point is not the absolute concordance in twins but the difference between monozygotic and dizygotic twin concordance rates. Unaffected monozygotic co-twins are of special importance; thus the demonstration that the increased risk of schizophrenia in the children of such co-twins is similar to that in the children of the affected monozygotic twins provides strong evidence for a primary genetic basis of the disorder.

Estimates for the risk of monozygotic co-twins are available for a number of common disorders and are mentioned in the relevant chapters; however, it is not always certain that these data are representative.

A final point of caution concerning monozygotic twins relates to DNA testing. Should such a twin request presymptomatic testing (e.g. for Huntington's disease), the result would automatically apply also to the co-twin. Obviously testing in such a situation needs handling with the greatest care.

LEGAL PROBLEMS IN MEDICAL GENETICS

Few areas of medical practice can avoid serious consideration of the legal aspects; medical genetics, involving many controversial and relatively new situations, might be expected to be especially vulnerable. Yet it is surprising (in the UK anyway) how rarely serious medicolegal problems do arise. The author suspects that this probably speaks more for the tolerance and goodwill of our patients than for the skills of the medical profession. The fact that we spend a great deal of time with our patients may also be relevant, as may the practice of providing families with a written letter.

Obviously there are areas which are bound to be difficult in legal terms, such as artificial insemination and *in vitro* fertilization (discussed in Chapter 10), the identification of relatively mild disorders such as sex chromosome defects in pregnancy, and the demand for fetal sexing for non-medical reasons. However, these are not the issues likely to involve the clinician with the law. Recent discussions with the various medical defence unions in Britain leave no doubt that the main problem is that of 'negligence', as in other areas of medical practice.

Negligence in this respect is not likely to mean giving an imprecise recurrence risk in genetic counselling, but rather giving no information at all when it could have been given, by a colleague if not by oneself. Thus the obstetrician or other clinician who fails to give genetic counselling, or to inform the patient that particular tests are available, is indeed likely to be held negligent if this is felt to fall short of what might reasonably be expected from a person in that position, while a specialist in medical genetics might be expected to have provided information of greater detail and accuracy. The laboratory is more likely to face problems from misidentification of samples than from the misinterpretation of results, though both are important.

In the USA the situation is probably not radically different, although the climate is much more litigious.

Among the broader legal issues that need consideration, most link closely with the social and ethical problems discussed in the final section of this book. Few are unique to genetics, but genetic situations often highlight them or bring them up in new form.

CONSENT

This is probably the most important general issue. It arises when genetic testing is being undertaken, especially in the case of children and others unable to consent fully, in the scope and nature of research studies on genetic disorders, the long-term storage of samples and in the use and transfer of laboratory or clinical information for third parties, such as insurance companies or employers. Since genetic information is often relevant and necessary for family members, particular issues arise as to how far consent is necessary within the context of genetic counselling for family members. This and related areas raise both ethical and legal issues. In general, there is little legal precedent, so that it is unlikely that a person following ethical guidelines and accepted standards of good practice will be exposed to unexpected legal challenges. However, recent episodes arising outside medical genetics in which good practice has not been followed have resulted in a sharp change of attitudes, making it essential that practice in all areas involving consent is clarified.

FURTHER READING

Baird PA, McGillivray R (1982). Children of incest. *Pediatrics* **101**, 854–857.

Bittles AH (2003). Consanguineous marriage and childhood health. *Dev Med Child Neurol* **45**, 571–576.

Krawczak M, Schmidtke J (1994). *DNA Fingerprinting*. Oxford. BIOS.

McGillivray R, Campbell DM, Thompson B (1988). *Twinning and Twins*. New York, Wiley.

Milunsky A, Annas GJ (1985). *Genetics and the Law III*. New York, Plenum.

Modell B, Darr A (2002). Genetic counselling and customary consanguineous marriage. *Nat Rev Genet* **3**, 225–229.

Vogel F, Motulsky AG (1996). Diagnosis of zygosity. In: *Human Genetics. Problems and Approaches*, Appendix 5. Berlin, Springer.

The genetic counselling clinic

A primary aim of this book is to encourage clinicians to regard genetic counselling as an integral part of the management of patients and their families, and to dispel the view that all genetic problems must of necessity be referred to a specialist clinic. Nevertheless, the organizational aspects of genetic counselling require careful consideration, whoever is doing it, and the following notes are intended to cover some of the practical aspects which need close attention if a satisfactory and efficient service is to be provided for patients.

Adequate time is essential if genetic counselling is to be at all worthwhile, and it may be argued that the main advantage of a patient being seen in a specialist genetic clinic is the greater amount of time that a medical geneticist is likely to be able to devote to the problem, compared with a busy clinician. All too often patients complain not that their doctor advised them incorrectly, but that he or she was too busy to answer their questions adequately or even to appreciate that the problem existed.

Clearly the first duty of any doctor interested in a patient's genetic problems is to ensure that this time is provided. The author finds an hour to be the usual time required to establish what are the main issues, take full pedigree details, undertake examination of the patient and discuss the genetic risks and possible measures of support. A follow-up visit is frequently required to interpret the results of investigations or records that have been obtained on relatives, and half an hour is usually allowed for this. Investigation of an extended family may take considerably longer and it is wise to attempt this in stages. The arrival of a complete kindred of people can create consternation in a clinic, while the conflicting views of several branches of a family are also best dealt with separately.

SETTING

The necessity of adequate time usually means that a specific session is best set aside for genetic counselling, whether this be in a family doctor's office or surgery, or in a hospital clinician's outpatient department. Whatever the precise location, several needs must be borne in mind. Quiet and freedom from disturbance are essential. The design of many hospital outpatient departments makes this almost impossible, while the rumpus associated with most children's clinics is also a distraction. The absence of a telephone is an advantage (they can now usually be unplugged), and the coming and going of well-meaning nurses must be discouraged. The author, until he was fortunate enough to have his own genetic counselling area, found it necessary to place a sign on the door, reading 'Genetic Counselling: Do Not Disturb'.

The number of people present must be small if patients are not to be inhibited in discussing personal details – usually not more than one medical colleague and a genetic counsellor or other co-worker. A single student could perhaps be added, but pressure to accommodate large student or postgraduate groups should be resisted. One-way screens are sometimes advocated to avoid this problem, but the author dislikes them.

If the clinic is held in a paediatric setting, there must be facilities for examining adults as well; the unexpected emergence of a large, undressed adult in the midst of a paediatric clinic may cause anxiety. Legal requirements now exist in the UK regarding clinical facilities for children.

EQUIPMENT

Very little equipment is needed. It is a pleasure in these days of expensive technology and centralization to be able to provide a high-class service to people in relatively remote areas without the need for cumbersome equipment or excessive cost to the community (or to the patient). A full set of examination equipment is essential, for many patients sent for counselling will prove to be really in need of diagnosis. Facilities for taking blood and for radiography (especially skeletal X-rays) are essential, as is a good camera or access to a medical illustration department; samples for most laboratory tests, including cytogenetic, biochemical and DNA studies, can be taken at a distance if necessary, and brought back or even mailed to the central laboratory for analysis.

PEDIGREES AND RECORDS

The number of families seen increases with a remarkable rapidity, and unless a clear and simple system is decided on from the outset, the clinician will soon be unable to find relevant information. The keeping of systematic records is also the basis for much of the research on inherited disorders, and should allow for follow-up and long-term preventive measures, where appropriate.

A clear and detailed pedigree is the foundation of good genetic counselling and a simple lined sheet is useful to keep it neat and orderly. The temptation to construct a rough pedigree for later improvement should be resisted – time and energy are rarely enough for this to happen and with practice a clear pedigree can be produced quickly using the method and symbols described in Chapter 1. Relevant information can be recorded at the foot of the page using letters to identify the particular individuals; Figure 1.2 on page 7 shows typical examples on the author's pedigree chart.

Other medical details will also need recording and in the author's clinic the policy has always been to write these, or put a copy, in the regular hospital case-record, where a copy of all correspondence is also placed, unless it contains details that might adversely affect other individuals. A copy of all notes and letters, along with the pedigree, is kept in the medical genetics department, where it is immediately available for consultation, in contrast to the main hospital case-record, which may be in use elsewhere or missing.

An easily workable index system is vital, especially in regions like Wales where many unrelated people share the same few surnames. It can be embarrassing to discover that the Mrs Davies whom one thought had a child with Duchenne dystrophy is, in fact, a different Mrs Davies who is at risk for Huntington's disease. Computerized systems are now almost universal in medical genetics clinic and other medical records, as well as for specific disorders. Some of these allow integration of clinical genetics records with molecular and cytogenetic laboratory information. A clear diagnostic index system is also essential.

THE GENETIC COUNSELLING SERVICE

Much genetic counselling, especially for common disorders, will be provided by clinicians who are not specialists in medical genetics. There will always be patients who require a specialist referral, however, and at present the awareness of genetic problems and consequent need for genetic counselling is growing faster than the ability of general clinicians to provide it. Many countries, including the UK, have evolved a system of regional genetic counselling centres to provide a specialist service and, since resources are limited and potential demand very large, it is important to consider how these are best utilized by doctors and other referring personnel.

In the UK, there is now a genetic counselling and clinical genetics centre in every health care region, usually based in the medical teaching centre of the region concerned and commonly staffed by, or closely associated with, an academic medical genetics unit. There is usually a close link with cytogenetic, molecular and other laboratory services. Hospital regions in Britain commonly serve a population of two to five million people, and vary in the size of the area. The service of the author and his colleagues covers Wales, a country which functions as equivalent in size to a single region within the UK National Health Service (NHS), with a population of three million and a maximum distance of 300 kilometres from the teaching centre. Here, as in some other parts of the UK, a service of regular district-based clinics has been set up to serve more distant parts of the region, which are serviced from the main unit in the medical teaching centre, originally on a 'hub and spoke' basis, but now with two sub-centres. In addition to this service, a number of specialist clinics have been set up in the main centre, often jointly with relevant clinicians to deal with particular problems, e.g. Marfan syndrome, muscular dystrophies and neurogenetic disorders.

The genetic counselling service in the UK has evolved historically within the framework of the NHS and thus differs in many ways from the pattern seen in much of continental Europe and the USA. It may well prove to be one of the major and (hopefully) lasting achievements of the NHS that the development of medical genetics has been able to take place relatively painlessly inside the service, without the necessity for charging of fees to patients or relatives. This applies equally to the provision of cytogenetic, molecular and prenatal diagnostic services. Whether the existing structure of services will prove adequate to cope with the steady increase in demand remains to be seen, and will depend partly on how clinical geneticists, genetic counsellors and clinicians in hospital practice and primary care can develop appropriate mutual roles in providing genetic services, as well as on whether the government is prepared to support the service by adequate funding. The pressure from the former government in Britain to commercialize services and to disband or fragment regional services and planning mechanisms seriously harmed the development of medical genetics services and similar problems have occurred in other countries. While the UK outlook is now more encouraging, considerable support and commitment from those planning and administering health services are needed to restore the situation.

Most clinical genetics services around the world are led by medically qualified staff with specialist training in genetics. Many countries, including the USA and Britain, have a carefully constructed and monitored programme of training and accreditation for those specializing in the field. The rapid development of such allied areas as prenatal diagnosis, screening and early therapy, together with the delineation of numerous clinically recognizable syndromes, has added to the importance of a medical training, even though much of the underlying research responsible for these advances has been made by non-medical scientists.

The author believes strongly that most genetic counselling should preferably be undertaken by people who are medically trained, largely for the reason that it is often quite impossible to separate the actual counselling from the associated aspects of clinical diagnosis. On numerous occasions, what is referred as an apparently straightforward problem of risk estimation and counselling produces a completely unexpected diagnostic problem, which a non-medical person would not only be unable to solve, but might well fail to recognize. Thus, in planning for the future, the author is in no doubt that training in both medicine and genetics is desirable for those intending to devote all or much of their time to genetic counselling. It may be argued that to train such individuals is expensive; this is true, but it is preferable to have a relatively small number of well trained people and for them to be used selectively. This view returns to the underlying theme of this book, that most genetic counselling is and will continue to be done by regular clinicians as a part of the overall management of patients under their care, while the medical geneticist is principally involved in those families where the situation is less simple, and in educating clinical colleagues.

This view should not be taken as implying that non-medically trained staff are not important in genetic counselling – quite the opposite is the case. Any well-developed clinical genetics service needs to rely heavily on members of its team who are non-medical, and this trend will undoubtedly increase. Provided that training of such staff is thorough, that their remit is clear and that links and support within the team are satisfactory, this mixed structure of a clinical genetics service should add to its quality and effectiveness, as has been the experience in many other fields of medicine. An increasing number of referrals for genetic counselling are proving able to be satisfactorily handled by genetic counsellors without the direct involvement of a medically trained clinical geneticist.

At present, non-medical co-workers in genetic counselling tend to follow two main streams. The first, most common in America, is the 'genetic counsellor' model, with extensive graduate training in basic genetics and in psychological aspects. In the second, the 'genetics nurse specialist', training in genetics and genetic counselling follows a more general nursing background. In both cases there are important roles that can complement that of the medically trained clinical geneticist. In the UK, there has been rapid development of specific training programmes, career structures and professional bodies.

A home visit prior to the clinic appointment can be most valuable, although geography and resources may not always mean this is feasible. This will frequently clarify and reassure those referred as to the purpose of the clinic; it is surprising how often this will not have been explained and they may have fears and concerns about it. A home visit will usually dispel these and will often also identify sensitive issues that might have been difficult to raise for the first time in a hospital setting, or might have resulted in non-attendance. Likewise, such a visit may uncover the true needs and concerns, which may not be those stated in a referral letter.

A further valuable role of a home visit (though this can also often be achieved by an unhurried phone call) is to determine which records or family details are needed before a clinic appointment is scheduled. Advance preparation of this kind can avoid much wasted time subsequently. Construction of a pedigree is often done at this time, although in the author's view, this also forms an important part of the actual genetic counselling process and is something that should not always be delegated. Taking the family details gives a valuable opportunity to 'break the ice' and form a relationship with a family being seen for the first time. Much can be learned about their fears and worries, their general attitude to the disorder in the family, how well they are likely to understand risk figures, and whether there are disagreements and tensions within the family. On several occasions it has become clear during this preliminary process that someone coming primarily for counselling is affected by the disorder. Huntington's disease is an example of such a condition, where a period of quiet observation during history-taking may give much more information than a formal examination.

Non-medical staff have further valuable roles to play in the genetic counselling clinic. A trained genetics nurse or counsellor, involved with the family from the point of first referral, will often be able to detect problems that family members have not spoken about, and ensure that they have actually understood what the person giving genetic counselling thinks they have; the two often prove surprisingly different. In many instances, practical support may need to be arranged; this may prove as valuable as the genetic counselling itself.

The help of such staff is also invaluable in contacting the extended family at home, taking samples from relatives, and obtaining additional information left incomplete at the time of a clinic visit. It is difficult to provide more than a very limited genetic counselling service without the availability of such non-medical personnel, and the author has been especially fortunate in having such colleagues working with him.

COUNSELLING AFTER STILLBIRTH AND TERMINATION OF PREGNANCY

The need for parental support and for the natural process of grieving to occur after neonatal death or stillbirth is well recognized, although all too often still ignored by doctors; the need is perhaps particularly great after a malformed infant has been born, and insensitive or inadequate management at this stage can seriously affect the parents' attitude to subsequent pregnancies and to genetic counselling. Frequently, a mother may not have seen the baby and may have exaggerated ideas about the abnormalities; most paediatricians now feel that she should see and hold the baby in most circumstances.

With the increasing use of prenatal diagnosis and termination for genetic disorders, it is becoming clear that parents need corresponding help in dealing with the combination of grief and guilt that is inevitable in this situation. The best way to achieve this will vary from family to family, but a sensitive counsellor, not necessarily a genetic counsellor, will probably be able to help most couples to express and to come to terms with their feelings. It seems likely that this more open approach is preferable to attempting to minimize the entire episode. In the past, this activity has often been left to staff of a medical genetics unit because no-one else recognized the need. Fortunately, obstetric departments are increasingly prepared to take on this role themselves, which is appropriate unless there are specifically genetic aspects involved.

INFORMATION SOURCES: GENETICS AND THE INTERNET

The revolution in information technology has been both a blessing and a problem for the field of genetic counselling. Professionals in medical genetics were among the earliest to develop and use computerized databases, not just in terms of genetic registers (see p. 154) but also such information resources as McKusick's *Mendelian Inheritance in Man* (and its on-line successor OMIM); syndrome databases such as the London Dysmorphology Database and POSSUM (see p. 94) and computer-based pedigree drawing and risk estimation programs. Most of these are interactive in nature and are thus of most value to those who are already broadly familiar with the field and have a clear idea as to what information they want.

A further category of useful information for professionals is represented by a rapidly increasing number of databases on the internet, including data on human disease mutations, both general and locus-specific; directories of laboratory genetic services (e.g. Helix; European Directory of Genetics Laboratories); and more general genetic disease information (e.g. GeneReviews). These systems are especially valuable for small or isolated units and those in less developed countries. In theory, they should make books like this redundant! On the other hand, they can create a problem of having too much information; digesting and assessing it can be as much work now as obtaining it was in the past. The Appendix has a list of helpful internet-based and other electronic information resources.

The greatest change in the past few years has been in the amount of information available directly to patients and families. There have always been determined individuals who have consulted textbooks and founded lay societies. Now most of these societies publish valuable information for both families and professionals, while increasingly they have websites, allowing direct access by those affected and at risk, or who are merely interested. More informal groups of patients and others are also developing and can form a valuable link for those who do not wish to become involved personally with specific genetic disease societies.

This rapid development, while undoubtedly beneficial on the whole, can have its drawbacks, apart from the embarrassment of the professional faced with a sheaf of internet information when first meeting a new family. Some of the information encountered may be distressing; for example, a couple searching for information because of a relatively distant history of neural tube defects were immediately confronted with a colour photograph of an anencephalic fetus. Others may be confused or misled by detailed information that would have been better presented as part of a professional consultation. Finally, it must be remembered that there is no data privacy on the internet; professionals and patients alike should avoid giving identifying details of other family members, while no computer with internet access should be used for storing confidential patient-related information unless there is an effective firewall. Whatever one's views, though, those involved in genetic counselling, whether as specialists in medical genetics or in their own disease field, now have to adapt to dealing with a far more informed and articulate clientele than has been the case until recently.

THE BACK-UP TO GENETIC COUNSELLING

Genetic counselling does not take place in a vacuum. The topics of carrier detection and prenatal diagnosis have already been discussed, but there are a number of other practical aspects that arise in connection with genetic counselling and these are dealt with here.

CONTRACEPTION

Ready access to a family planning clinic is essential for any clinician involved in genetic counselling, and it is always wise to enquire tactfully about contraception at an early stage, particularly if the results of investigations are going to take some weeks or months before definitive counselling can be given. It is surprising how often couples aware of the genetic risk and not intending to have children nevertheless take no active measures to prevent pregnancy. The author has more than once had the unhappy experience of seeing such a couple on a follow-up visit, to inform them of a high risk of a serious disorder, only to find that the woman had become pregnant in the meantime. Such an event may not always be as accidental as it seems.

STERILIZATION

Sterilization is often preferable to long-term contraception where a couple has made a definite decision not to have further children. This may apply even to young couples. Before sterilization is undertaken, however, careful consideration must be given to the following points:

- What is the precise genetic risk to offspring? It is not uncommon for sterilization to be requested 'on genetic grounds' when the risks of transmitting a disorder are minimal, e.g. sibs of a patient with an autosomal recessive disorder.

- Is there an alternative, such as carrier detection or prenatal diagnosis, that could reduce or avoid the risk?
- Is it likely that advances in knowledge will change the situation in the next few years?
- Do the couple really agree that sterilization is the best course, and which partner should undergo it?

In general, it is logical to sterilize the affected or at-risk individual in the case of a dominant disease; for autosomal recessive disorders there is no genetic preference. Many couples choose vasectomy on the grounds of simplicity and lower risk. In some instances, the unaffected member of a couple insists on being sterilized; the motivation in such circumstances can be complex. In the case of a fatal disorder, the possibility that the healthy spouse may re-marry and wish to have children must be faced. Divorce and remarriage are also relevant for recessive disorders where the genetic risks in a new marriage will be very low.

Sterilization of the mentally handicapped patient is a difficult and emotive issue. Genetic risks to offspring are often confused with more general questions concerning whether a child could be satisfactorily reared by its parents. Despite arguments over the rights of disabled people to reproduce, sterilization seems a perfectly reasonable course if the retardation is more than mild, the genetic risks are high and the risk of pregnancy is considerable. The right of a child to be born, where possible, into a family able to give care does not seem to have received sufficient emphasis in discussion of this issue. As with most ethical problems, the right course is often clear, provided that each case is considered on its own merits, and the situation is not allowed to degenerate into general polemics.

GAMETE DONATION AND *IN VITRO* FERTILIZATION

This is now technically possible for either sperm or egg, although the latter requires the use of *in vitro* fertilization (see below). Sperm donation (AID) is simpler. The main genetic indications are:

- autosomal dominant disorders where one partner is affected or at risk of becoming so (e.g. Huntington's disease)
- rare autosomal recessive disorders, in particular where prenatal diagnosis is not feasible or termination of pregnancy not acceptable to the couple. Here a mutated gene must be contributed by each parent and an unrelated donor is most unlikely to carry the same mutation.

One should not lose sight of the fact that there may also be implications for the donor. Thus, if a child is born with a recessively inherited disorder, this will imply that the donor is a gene carrier, while if donor screening tests are undertaken for such common recessive disorders as cystic fibrosis, there will be comparable implications. It is not always clear what information is given on such aspects to donors in advance, nor what support is provided if such a result is obtained.

In vitro fertilization

In vitro fertilization (IVF) is now well established as an option for some forms of infertility and offers the prospect of using an ovum from an unrelated donor to avoid serious autosomal dominant disorders in the female line and X-linked recessive conditions such as Duchenne muscular dystrophy. Because (in contrast to AID) potential ovum donors may be sisters or other relatives, great care will be needed to avoid using individuals who might be gene carriers. It is perhaps surprising that this approach has not been more frequently used by couples. This may reflect the increasing feasibility and acceptability of first-trimester prenatal diagnosis, as well as the expense, uncertainty and low success rate still limiting IVF. The topic of pre-implantation prenatal diagnosis is discussed in Chapter 8.

ADOPTION

The question of adoption in relation to genetic counselling arises in two main situations:

- Adoption is being considered as one of the options open to a couple at risk of trans-mitting a genetic disorder.
- A child being placed for adoption has a family history of a genetic disorder and the adoption agency wishes to know how great the risk is before finalizing the placement.

In the past, it was possible to recommend adoption as a possible course of action for couples not wishing to take the risk of having a natural child with a genetic disorder. With increasing use of abortion for social indications and with most single mothers retaining their children, the number of available children has decreased sharply, and couples with a family history of genetic disease will thus find themselves competing with many healthy but infertile couples for a small number of children. In these circum-stances, couples are often discouraged even from considering adoption, but the author feels strongly that this course is wrong and that if a couple want to adopt, they should attempt to do so. They should realize, however, that considerable determination is needed, since a large amount of 'red tape' and bureaucratic inertia may be encountered that will discourage the faint-hearted. The following advice may help:

- Apply early, since a long wait may be inevitable.
- If one agency states that their list is closed try others, in another region if necessary; a serious lack of communication exists between agencies and areas.
- Be prepared to be inspected and questioned, and to fill out a large number of forms.
- If barriers of religion are raised, work through a local authority or other non-denominational agency.
- Be persistent (without being aggressive) if delays occur.
- Consider the adoption of an older child, or one for whom some other reason has made adoption difficult.

Because many couples feel helpless about how to start adopting, further information is included in the Appendix.

One group of people who may have particular difficulty in adopting are those where one partner is at high risk of actually developing a serious genetic disorder, such as Huntington's disease. Here a decision must be made in each case based on a careful evalu-ation of the size of the risk, the chance that the disease will develop while the child is being brought up and the nature of the disorder. For a condition with such serious consequences as Huntington's disease, few adoption agencies will feel able to accept a couple at high risk, except perhaps for placing an older child who would be likely to be grown up in the event of the disorder developing in the adoptive parent.

Adoption and the child at risk

Advice is commonly sought from adoption agencies when a child to be placed for adoption has a family history of a serious disorder. Sadly this advice is rarely sought before the birth of the child, with the result that unnecessary delay may occur, with resulting uncertainty and harm to the infant, natural mother and adoptive parents alike. The estimation of risks is no different from that in other genetic counselling situations, although unavailability (or uncertainty) of the father may cause difficulty. A more difficult problem is where the child results from an incestuous mating (see Chapter 9), where the risks are high for a variety of recessively inherited disorders, not all of which are detectable in infancy. In this situation, it may be wise to defer placement for a few months until the major part of the risk can be excluded.

Where a high risk of a late-onset disorder does exist, many infants are excluded from adoption. This seems unfortunate, because from the child's viewpoint a family would certainly be likely to deal with problems that arise better than an institution would. It is also often overlooked that there are many highly motivated couples who are prepared to adopt or foster in the long term children with even very severe disabilities provided that they are fully in the picture as to what they are taking on; Down's syndrome is a good example. Very few children should be considered 'unsuitable for adoption'.

The development of presymptomatic tests for late-onset genetic disorders has led to requests for children being placed for adoption to be tested, e.g. for Huntington's disease. This raises serious ethical issues (see Chapter 28) and it seems unjustified to undertake such testing unless there are clear childhood medical reasons for doing so.

GENETIC REGISTERS

The keeping of accurate and complete records is an essential (although often neglected) part of all branches of clinical medicine, but the long-term and preventive nature of medical genetics makes this an especially important aspect. Much of the information given in genetic counselling may only be fully used many years later. The sister of a boy with Duchenne muscular dystrophy or the child of a patient with familial polyposis coli may have been too young to be given any information at the time of the initial family study; unless careful records are kept, investigations may have to be repeated. Likewise, it is of great help to know that a person with vague neurological symptoms and a family history of possible Huntington's disease is in fact a member of a kindred in which the diagnosis has been fully established.

A genetic register is something more than an accurate records system. The term 'register' implies that the approach is systematic and at least aiming at completeness, and that the information is actively maintained and updated. Genetic registers may be of several types and vary in complexity, although they will now generally be computer based. Most are specific to a particular disorder or group of disorders.

MANAGEMENT RELATED REGISTERS

This type of register is likely to be of greatest interest to the practising clinician with a special interest in a particular group of inherited disorders, and the register often involves both such a clinician and a clinical geneticist. Here the genetic aspects are only part of the objective, and a register may be of considerable help in overall management and surveillance, as well as in genetic counselling. The familial cancers, notably familial colorectal cancer, provide an excellent example of the value of such a register, especially since the advent of molecular testing now means that many individuals can be effectively excluded from risk at an early age. Such registers are also valuable in audit and applied research, although this is not their primary aim.

CONTACT AND GENETIC COUNSELLING REGISTERS

Here the specific aim is to allow genetic counselling and associated measures such as carrier detection to be offered in inherited disorders where there may be numerous family members at risk who might be unaware of the risks. The most suitable disorders for such a register (Table 10.1) are the late-onset dominant disorders such as Huntington's disease, or X-linked disorders such as Duchenne and Becker muscular dystrophies and fragile-X syndrome. Here an accurate knowledge of affected and at-risk individuals in a region is likely to be of considerable help in ensuring that genetic counselling is provided early rather than when an affected or potentially affected child has already been born. By contrast, autosomal recessive disorders, the common polygenic conditions and chromosomal abnormalities (apart from translocations) are not suitable for this type of register because the risks are either low or confined to immediate family members, who are likely to be aware of them already.

Table 10.1 Disorders worth considering for a genetic register

X-linked recessive
Duchenne muscular dystrophy
Becker muscular dystrophy
Haemophilia (A and B)
Fragile-X mental retardation
Other serious rare X-linked disorders
Autosomal dominant
Polyposis coli (and other inherited cancer syndromes)
Polycystic kidney disease
Huntington's disease
Retinitis pigmentosa (also X-linked form)
Myotonic dystrophy
Marfan syndrome
Chromosomal
Translocation Down's syndrome (and other translocations)

ISSUES TO BE CONSIDERED

How can the register be kept specific and limited?

It is all too easy for the scope of a register to expand until it is out of control. It is better to confine the register to a small number of well-defined conditions and to deal with them thoroughly.

How can the quality of the information be maintained?

An inaccurate or out-of-date register is worse than useless. Accepting data at face value from outside sources is dangerous, and the only person likely to have sufficient sustained enthusiasm to check the information thoroughly is the person actually maintaining the register. It must also be recognized that updating a register entails a great deal of work and that the expense is not negligible.

Confidentiality

Confidentiality is important in all conditions, but in a disorder such as Huntington's disease, it is of the utmost significance. It is essential that no information is given out without the permission of the individuals concerned, that the register is kept securely, and that no identifying details are put on any computerized system that involves transfer of information outside the genetics unit. Permission to place the individual on the register in the first place is also necessary if the register is anything more than a regular records system. In most countries, any computerized register is now subject to data protection legislation, while hospitals and other medical services will have codes of practice that must be carefully followed. The author's experience, gained chiefly from a register of muscular dystrophies and Huntington's disease, is that most individuals are happy to participate provided that they can have a personal relationship with those running the register. If it is under bureaucratic control or any information is divulged without permission, this cooperation would almost certainly be lost.

TREATMENT FOR GENETIC DISEASES

In comparison with other types of disease, such as major infections, nutritional deficiencies or even cancers, most genetic disorders have been relatively unresponsive to treatment or to primary preventive measures. It is this, rather than any absolute increase, that has resulted in their increasing prominence in chronic disorders of childhood and of later life. It would be wrong, however, to give the impression that treatment is not an area of importance to those working with genetic disorders, or that those affected can be offered little of value. The wide range of increasingly effective approaches is summarized in Table 10.2.

Avoidance of serious morbidity or death by early detection of those at risk is now of major importance in many genetic disorders; the familial cancers and myotonic dystrophy are but two examples.

Table 10.2 Approaches to therapy of genetic diseases (the order of the table reflects closeness to the primary defect, not degree of proven effectiveness)

Approach	Example
Replacement of defective gene ('gene therapy')	Inherited immune deficiencies
Replacement of deficient enzyme	Gaucher's disease
Other gene product replacement	Type I diabetes mellitus (insulin), haemophilias (factors VIII, IX)
Dietary modification	Phenylketonuria Galactosaemia
Other medical therapy	Hyperuricaemias (allopurinol) Wilson's disease (penicillamine)
Organ transplantation	Familial amyloidosis (liver transplant) Polycystic kidney disease (renal transplant)
Corrective surgical approaches	Arthrogryposes, limb defects, etc. (numerous orthopaedic measures)
Early detection and surveillance for avoidable complications	Cardiac arrhythmias in myotonic dystrophy

The importance of supportive measures, even when not curative, has already been stressed in this chapter and in Chapter 1. For many structural conditions, corrective surgical and physical procedures may be valuable secondary measures. Increasingly, though, possibilities are developing for specific therapy for disorders where until recently there has been no real prospect of altering the course of the disease. No attempt to give details is made here, though accounts can be found in many of the books cited in Chapter 1.

Clearly the possibility of effective treatment will be of critical importance in genetic counselling, since it will determine the attitude of family members to the disease, as well as whether they are likely to take up options such as prenatal diagnosis. It has to be borne in mind that the physician's concept of 'successful treatment' may not be the same as that of the patient or family member, especially if painful, stressful and prolonged therapeutic measures are involved. Treatment may also change from generation to generation; thus many patients with adult polycystic kidney disease in past generations died from renal failure, while now a combination of dialysis and transplantation offers a much improved outlook. Even within a single sibship, prognosis may alter as a result of early detection and treatment; thus, in congenital adrenal hyperplasia, the first affected sib may die undetected or suffer from serious metabolic problems, while these can be largely anticipated and prevented in subsequent sibs.

Gene therapy deserves a mention, especially in view of the widespread media publicity. It is now possible, when the gene responsible for an inherited disorder has been isolated, to insert a normal copy of it into the DNA of the genetically abnormal cell, and for it to function normally under certain conditions in experimental animals. Clearly there are major practical problems in such an approach, including inserting the gene into the relevant cell types, ensuring that it functions adequately (but not too much), and being as certain as possible that any virus vector used in the process does not itself cause harmful effects (immediate or long-term).

At present, gene therapy remains at the stage of basic research for all genetic disorders (with the possible exception of some rare immune deficiencies). The slow deterioration and variability of many genetic conditions will often make it very difficult to evaluate the success or otherwise of any therapeutic approach. Long-term safety issues remain a major concern. It is much more likely that it will enter clinical practice for serious non-genetic disorders (e.g. cancer) and it is unfortunate that some workers in the field have promoted the view that it is close to becoming a widespread form of treatment for inherited diseases.

A final point that should be noted is that gene therapy as now envisaged will only affect somatic cells and not the germ line, so that there should be no implications for future generations. There is a consensus that any measures to alter the germ line would, at present, be unethical.

FURTHER READING

(See the Appendix for internet addresses and for information on lay societies, adoption and insurance.)

Clinical Genetics Committee of the Royal College of Physicians of London (1998). *Clinical Genetic Services. Activity, Outcome, Effectiveness and Quality*. London, Royal College of Physicians of London.

Dean JC, Fitzpatrick DR, Farndon PA, Kingston H, Cusine D (2000). Genetic registers in clinical practice: a survey of UK clinical geneticists. *J Med Genet* **37**, 636–640.

Dubowitz V (2002). Therapeutic possibilities in muscular dystrophy: the hope versus the hype. *Neuromuscul Disord* **12**, 113–116.

Royal College of Physicians (1998). *Clinical Genetics Services into the 21st Century*. London, Royal College of Physicians.

PART II

Genetic counselling: specific organ systems

Neuromuscular disease

MUSCULAR DYSTROPHIES

Too often patients are still referred for genetic counselling or, even worse, for prenatal procedures, with a label of 'muscular dystrophy' and no indication as to the type of dystrophy concerned. Many lay people (and some doctors!) still have the impression that all muscular dystrophy affects boys, but is carried by girls. The first task in genetic counselling is thus to establish the precise diagnosis beyond all reasonable doubt, something that is now normally possible using a combination of clinical, histological and molecular approaches. Table 11.1 lists the major categories of muscular dystrophy and their inheritance. Reviews listed under 'Further reading' give details of the genetic and molecular aspects, knowledge of which has been entirely transformed by recent developments. It is important to recognize that, in some types, DNA analysis of blood is the primary confirmatory test, while in others this needs to follow immunohistochemical studies of specific muscle proteins.

DUCHENNE MUSCULAR DYSTROPHY

Duchenne muscular dystrophy (DMD) is one of the major problems in genetic counselling for paediatricians and neurologists, as well as for clinical geneticists. Its X-linked recessive mode of inheritance means that numerous female relatives may be at risk of being carriers, even with a single case in the family. It is essential that they are advised

Table 11.1 The major progressive muscular dystrophies

	Type	Molecular basis
X-linked	Duchenne	Dystrophin (usually absent)
	Becker	Dystrophin (usually present but altered)
	Emery–Dreifuss	Emerin (protein function unknown)
Autosomal recessive	Early-onset 'Duchenne-like' girdle	17q;13q. Adhalin/α-sarcoglycan; γ-sarcoglycan
	Limb girdle (late-onset types)	Very heterogeneous (different sarcoglycans; calpain 3)
	Congenital muscular dystrophy	9q; 6q (merosin/laminin α-2 chain)
Autosomal dominant	Facioscapulohumeral	4q deletions (gene unknown)
	Distal	Heterogeneous (titin, dysferlin)
	Emery–Dreifuss	Lamin A/C
	Oculopharyngeal	14q (trinucleotide repeat mutation)
	Adult-onset limb girdle	5q
	Myotonic dystrophy	19q Expanded trinucleotide repeat

accurately and that all available information is used correctly in determining carrier status. At present this is still not always the case, and the resulting misinformation may lead to disastrous results for the family concerned, although this is less of a problem with the increasing feasibility of specific molecular analysis.

This disorder has seen important progress over recent years and has served as a prototype for other genetic disorders. The gene, located on the short arm of the X chromosome, was isolated by the positional cloning approach (see Chapter 5); it is one of the largest known human genes (around two million base pairs). The size of the gene makes recombination within it frequent, so that even DNA markers within the gene can have a significant error rate of up to 5 per cent. However, a high proportion of cases (around two-thirds) result from large partial gene deletions, so that specific prenatal diagnosis and, in most cases, carrier detection are now feasible, provided that DNA from an affected male in the family is available to determine the nature of the mutation.

The protein product of the DMD locus, dystrophin, was entirely unknown before isolation of the gene. It is largely muscle-specific, with an alternative form present in brain. It is usually absent in typical cases of DMD, in contrast to Becker muscular dystrophy (see below), where it is present but altered in structure or amount, and other dystrophies where it is generally normal. Immunological assays on muscle biopsy sections now form an important part of the investigation of suspected DMD; properly stored frozen muscle may be used for this.

Prenatal diagnosis of DMD by first-trimester DNA analysis is now feasible in the great majority of cases. Every effort should be made to establish the precise molecular defect or genotype of an affected family member in advance of prenatal diagnosis being required, along with the risk that the mother is indeed a carrier. A 'multiplex' PCR-based approach allows prenatal detection of most gene deletion cases, but those due to point mutation or gene duplication are a greater problem, requiring more difficult forms of DNA or RNA analysis. Linked markers are still required in some non-deletion cases.

Carrier detection remains a considerable problem in some female relatives and has been less completely resolved by molecular advances than might have been anticipated. It thus remains important to start from basic principles of pedigree analysis and to use all available information in risk estimation, including creatine kinase information, rather than relying on DNA results in isolation. This particularly applies to relatives of an isolated case, and where a specific mutation has not been identified.

The general problems of calculating risks for a lethal X-linked disorder have already been discussed (see Chapters 2 and 7). A woman with two affected sons or with one affected son and another affected close male relative should be considered as an obligatory carrier, with a 50 per cent risk of further sons being affected and of daughters being carriers. Detailed examples of risk estimation in DMD can be found in Chapter 2 of this book (p. 45), and in the books of Young and Emery (see 'Further reading').

Population screening

The exceptionally high levels of serum creatine kinase seen in presymptomatic cases of DMD leave no doubt that the great majority of affected males (not carriers) can be detected soon after birth. Cord blood values are too variable for this, but population screening of males can be undertaken using the newborn samples collected on filter paper for phenylketonuria testing. There is debate as to whether this approach is justified as a service at present, for a number of reasons. There is no effective treatment; thus the justification would be to offer genetic counselling to families at risk of having a second affected child. Whether the distress likely to be caused in these families (and in the families whose tests prove to be false positives) is outweighed by the resulting benefits needs careful consideration.

Evaluation of newborn DMD screening programmes is currently in progress (notably of a programme in Wales) and it will be important to ensure that full information and support are built into any such development being introduced into services. It must also be remembered that around two-thirds of cases (the first in a family) will not be avoidable, however effective the newborn screening programme may be.

BECKER MUSCULAR DYSTROPHY

While we now know that Becker muscular dystrophy (late-onset X-linked dystrophy) is determined by mutations at the same locus as DMD, it is valuable to consider this form separately, because the clinical and genetic problems are somewhat different. Onset and course vary greatly from family to family and asymptomatic males must be checked carefully, even in adult life, before being pronounced unaffected. Isolated male cases can be distinguished from other muscular dystrophies by the use of DNA analysis on blood and dystrophin analysis of muscle.

Most patients with Becker muscular dystrophy (BMD) develop symptoms in adolescence and remain ambulant into adult life, though with increasing disability. This creates a totally different genetic counselling situation to DMD, since many patients will reproduce, and all their daughters will be obligatory carriers. Since no offspring will be affected, the genetic risks may well be forgotten or ignored by the time grandchildren at risk are born. Levels of creatine kinase (CK) in carriers are more frequently normal than in DMD; obligatory carriers may be erroneously reassured on the basis of such testing.

OTHER PROGRESSIVE MUSCULAR DYSTROPHIES

The main forms are listed in Table 11.1.

Emery–Dreifuss muscular dystrophy

This is usually X-linked, determined by a specific gene for the protein lamin, allowing specific mutation testing in some families. Affected males and some carrier females are at risk of serious cardiac conduction defects, even though weakness is often mild. Some clinically similar families follow autosomal dominant inheritance and are due to defects in the gene for the muscle protein lamin A/C.

Facioscapulohumeral dystrophy

This is a variable autosomal dominant disorder which is often mild but is seriously disabling in 15 per cent of cases. Although the gene is 95 per cent penetrant by early adult life, careful examination to exclude minimal signs is essential in counselling asymptomatic family members. Serum CK levels are often normal in mild or presymptomatic cases. The gene has been mapped to distal 4q, with closely linked markers, the closest of which shows a specific change in most affected individuals, even though the actual gene has not yet been isolated. This allows presymptomatic detection or exclusion, as well as prenatal diagnosis, although this is requested by only a minority of families.

Autosomal limb girdle dystrophies

Molecular studies have greatly helped to resolve this confusing and heterogeneous group; most are recessively inherited and due to defects in molecular components of the muscle membrane and contractile complex. The severe and extremely rare (except in North Africa) autosomal recessive dystrophy clinically resembling DMD should be considered, along with X-chromosome abnormalities, in any apparent case of DMD in a girl. More common are the later childhood-onset types of autosomal recessive limb girdle dystrophy, although in most populations this group is considerably less common than Becker dystrophy. It is essential to avoid confusion between female cases and manifesting DMD carriers.

Finally, occasional families with limb girdle dystrophy, often following a benign course with adult onset, show autosomal dominant inheritance.

In investigating this whole group, analysis of muscle by immunohistochemistry is essential in distinguishing the different types. Mutation analysis is only helpful once the particular protein involved has been determined.

Table 11.2 Congenital myopathies

Type	Inheritance	Gene location or defect
Nemaline myopathy	Autosomal recessive (severe congenital)	Nebulin
	Autosomal dominant (milder type)	α-tropomyosin (1q)
Centronuclear (myotubular) myopathy	X-linked recessive lethal neonatal type (see text); rarely autosomal dominant or autosomal recessive	Myotubularin
Central core disease	Autosomal dominant	Ryanodine receptor (19q)
Congenital fibre type disproportion	Uncertain (probably not a distinct entity)	–
Congenital muscular dystrophy	Autosomal recessive (heterogeneous)	Merosin, fukutin
Congenital myotonic dystrophy	Autosomal dominant (maternally transmitted)	See text

CONGENITAL MYOPATHIES

Unless the pattern of inheritance within a particular family is clear-cut, genetic counselling for the heterogeneous group of congenital myopathies (Table 11.2) should not be undertaken without an accurate muscle biopsy and, where possible, molecular diagnosis from an expert centre. Variation in severity within families may be marked, and both autosomal dominant and recessive inheritance have been recorded for the main types. The X-linked form of lethal centronuclear (myotubular) myopathy is more common than previously thought as a cause of neonatal death and is easily confused with congenital myotonic dystrophy; muscle biopsy and molecular analysis can distinguish the two. The term 'congenital muscular dystrophy' should be reserved for those specific forms that are progressive, as well as having congenital onset; they may also show CNS involvement.

METABOLIC MYOPATHIES

Specific metabolic defects are being found for an increasing number of myopathies, as shown in Table 11.3. This emphasizes the need for full biochemical and ultrastructural investigation of any obscure case of muscle disease before genetic counselling is given. The relevant individual chapters of the textbooks given in 'Further reading' provide details on the different forms.

Mitochondrial myopathies, which may present as muscle disorders or as central nervous system degenerations with wider system involvement, may be determined by

Table 11.3 Metabolic myopathies

Type	Inheritance
Mitochondrial myopathies (heterogeneous)	
Infantile cytochrome oxidase deficiency	Autosomal recessive
Late onset with ophthalmoplegia	Autosomal dominant (some families)
Hypermetabolic (Luft type)	Sporadic or mitochondrial
With retinal and other changes (Kearns–Sayre type)	Uncertain; usually sporadic
Carnitine palmityl transferase deficiency	Autosomal recessive
McArdle syndrome (glycogenosis type V)	Autosomal recessive
Other glycogenoses (except type VIII)	Autosomal recessive

nuclear genes and follow mendelian inheritance, or may be maternally transmitted following the general principles of mitochondrial inheritance.

MYOTONIC DYSTROPHY

Myotonic dystrophy is an autosomal dominant disorder, for long a special interest of the author. It ranks second only to Duchenne dystrophy as a major genetic counselling problem in inherited muscle disease and is the most common muscular dystrophy of adult life. Its extreme clinical variability adds special difficulty.

Definitely affected people have a 50 per cent risk for affected offspring. Affected women, even if mildly affected, have a considerable risk (Table 11.4) that an affected child will have the severe congenital form of the disease, which may result in neonatal death or severe respiratory problems after birth and severe physical and mental handicap in survivors. The risk is especially high where a woman has already had such an affected child and very low when no neuromuscular abnormalities are present. The risk of this form in the offspring of affected males is minimal, although childhood onset may occur.

Both genetic counselling and our general understanding of myotonic dystrophy have been entirely transformed as a result of the identification of the gene and specific mutation on chromosome 19. An unstable trinucleotide repeat sequence is involved, with expansion in a specific CTG repeat found in virtually all cases so far studied. The expansion correlates broadly with severity of phenotype, and tends to increase from generation to generation, thus explaining the progressively earlier onset and greater severity (anticipation) characteristic of this disorder. The gene itself codes for a previously unknown protein, which shows protein kinase activity. Unlike DMD, there does not appear to be absence of myotonin protein kinase in patients – the mutation is in an untranslated part of the gene and its effects appear to be related to its size. An effect on the function of other genes at the RNA level is involved, and the cell biology of the disorder is complex.

Individuals carrying a minimal change in the gene usually show little or no muscle disease, but they may have cataract. All patients may have originated from a few, even a single ancestral mutation, which may have been relatively stable for many generations, progressive instability resulting once expansion has passed a critical point. As with

NEUROMUSCULAR DISEASE 167

Table 11.4 Risks (approximate) of a congenitally or severely affected child with myotonic dystrophy in relation to clinical status of the mother

Maternal status	Risk (%)
Established neuromuscular disease	10–30
Neuromuscular disease minimal or absent	<5
Risk after birth of one congenitally affected child	40

Note: all groups have the same chance (50%) of a child being genetically unaffected.

Huntington's disease and other trinucleotide repeat disorders, asymptomatic individuals with borderline expansions form a reservoir of gene carriers who may transmit clinically significant disease to their offspring.

Although these molecular advances should not become an excuse for omitting a careful clinical assessment, asymptomatic relatives at risk can now be confirmed or excluded as having the mutation by specific molecular analysis, while this is also useful in situations of uncertain diagnosis. Electromyography and eye examination for lens opacities should now be regarded as means of assessing clinical, rather than genetic status. Prenatal diagnosis is also feasible by molecular analysis. Testing of samples from extended relatives in the older generation or from children should not be done without careful consideration of the implications, since we remain uncertain of the closeness of correlation of mutation with phenotype and of the risk for instability in family branches where overt disease has not occurred. The reason why congenitally affected cases are exclusively maternally transmitted appears to be that expansions over a certain size cannot be transmitted by sperm. The varying risks of severe disease according to the clinical status of the mother (Table 11.4) can now in part be logically explained by the size of the mother's DNA expansion and its likelihood for further progression in the child.

Presymptomatic testing should be done with full genetic counselling, as for other disorders, and should be avoided in healthy children in whom clinical examination is normal. Because the disorder is largely penetrant by adult life, the risk of an abnormal result in a clinically normal person is only around 10 per cent.

Type 2 myotonic dystrophy

A small number (around 1 per cent in UK) of myotonic dystrophy patients fail to show the expected chromosome 19 mutation and it is now known that a separate gene (on chromosome 3) is involved, also with an unstable mutation (CCTG), causing the disease. This type 2 myotonic dystrophy is the same as the disorder known as **proximal myotonic myopathy (PROMM)** and shows more proximal weakness, no childhood form, but similar systemic features to the classical 'type 1' form. Inheritance is autosomal dominant.

OTHER MYOTONIC SYNDROMES

Other myotonic syndromes (Table 11.5) are rare in comparison with myotonic dystrophy, which must be carefully excluded. Myotonia congenita (Thomsen's disease) is

Table 11.5 The myotonic disorders

Syndrome	Inheritance	Mutation or gene involved
Myotonic dystrophy (type 1)	Autosomal dominant	Expanded CTG repeat
Progressive myotonic myopathy (PROMM, type 2 myotonic dystrophy)	Autosomal dominant	Expanded CCTG repeat
Myotonia congenita		
Thomsen's disease	Autosomal dominant	Skeletal muscle Cl^- channel
Recessive type	Autosomal recessive	Skeletal muscle Cl^- channel
Paramyotonia congenita	Autosomal dominant	Skeletal muscle Na^+ channel
Periodic paralysis		
Normo/hyperkalaemic (adynamia episodica)	Autosomal dominant	Na^+ channel
Hypokalaemic	Autosomal dominant	Ca^{++} channel
Chondrodystrophic myotonia (Schwartz–Jampel syndrome)	Autosomal recessive	Perlecan (HSPG2)

heterogeneous and at least half the cases are recessively inherited, despite the prominence of some large dominantly inherited families. The two types show clinical as well as genetic differences. Because new mutations for this benign condition are likely to be rare, it is wise to give a 1 in 4 risk for further children born to healthy parents of an isolated case. Correspondingly, the risk of such an isolated case in the absence of a molecular diagnosis transmitting the condition is small. Careful neurophysiological tests by an expert are important in distinguishing the different disorders in this group.

The molecular advances in myotonic dystrophy have been equalled by corresponding progress in the non-progressive myotonias, but instead of a previously unknown gene and protein, the defects have proved to be those predicted by physiological and pharmacological studies. Following cloning of the adult muscle sodium and chloride channel genes, the former (on chromosome 17) has been shown to be responsible for both paramyotonia and myotonic periodic paralysis, while different mutations in the chloride channel gene on chromosome 7 occur in the dominant and recessive forms of myotonia congenita.

HYPERPYREXIC MYOPATHY

Hyperpyrexic myopathy (malignant hyperthermia) is a particularly important dominantly inherited disorder to recognize in those at risk. It gives a subclinical myopathy (often with muscle hypertrophy and raised CK levels), and also profound contracture with hyperthermia following anaesthesia. Detection of carriers at risk remains unsatisfactory. The previously used *in vitro* contractural test on muscle biopsy is invasive, has proved unreliable and, in the author's opinion, should be abandoned. Unfortunately

DNA analysis is not yet service-ready outside families with an established mutation. In some families the condition is due to defects in the ryanodine receptor (chromosome 19), but the condition is heterogeneous.

MYASTHENIA GRAVIS

In the usual adult form of myasthenia gravis associated with antibodies to the acetyl-choline receptor, genetic risks are extremely low. In one series of over 400 patients, one pair of affected sibs was the only familial case. A risk of around 1 per cent for myasthenia gravis is appropriate for first-degree relatives, along with an increase in autoimmune thyroid disease. It is of interest that an association has been found between myasthenia gravis and the antigens HLA-DRw3 and HLA-B8. This is a good illustration of the fact that such associations do not necessarily imply high risks to family members. Transient congenital myasthenia gravis is seen in about 20 per cent of the offspring of affected mothers, but, unlike the corresponding situation in myotonic dystrophy, rarely has permanent effects. The only group showing a clear genetic basis is that comprising the rare forms with onset in infancy which consist of several types of receptor deficiency, and are mostly autosomal recessive; antibodies are absent.

SPINAL MUSCULAR ATROPHIES

PROXIMAL SPINAL MUSCULAR ATROPHY

The spinal muscular atrophies are a group of anterior horn cell disorders which require careful distinction on clinical, electromyographic, histological and molecular grounds from primary myopathies. The great majority of all childhood proximal types follow autosomal recessive inheritance, so that sporadic cases should be counselled as such in terms of risk for sibs, even if it is difficult to assign them to a particular type. All the major forms appear to be allelic, with a locus identified on chromosome 5q that now allows prenatal diagnosis. Two adjacent genes appear to be involved, variable combinations of deletion resulting in differing severity and age at onset in over 95 per cent of cases.

In **type I**, or severe infantile spinal muscular atrophy (Werdnig–Hoffman disease), onset is at or shortly after birth, with death invariably before 2 years and usually before 18 months. Severity in other affected sibs is closely correlated, so that couples taking the 1 in 4 risk of recurrence can be told that the risk of a severely disabled but surviving child is minimal and that a sib apparently healthy at 6 months old will almost certainly remain normal, something that can be confirmed by DNA analysis. DNA analysis or banking on the first affected child is vital to allow subsequent prenatal diagnosis.

Type II, or intermediate spinal muscular atrophy, includes cases with childhood onset, but survival beyond 2 years. The majority are severely disabled during childhood, and this may occur in sibs of mild cases. Variability between sibs is greater than for the infantile type, but apparently healthy sibs will have passed through 90 per cent of their risk by the age of 12 years. The same molecular analysis can be used in prediction as for type I.

In **type III**, or benign spinal muscular atrophy (Kugelberg–Welander disease), most cases follow autosomal recessive inheritance, and are determined by the same 5q locus as types I and II. A few isolated cases may be environmental or represent new dominant mutations. Offspring of affected individuals will usually be normal, but where an isolated case is of adult onset, the possibility of dominant inheritance gives a risk to offspring of around 1 in 20.

OTHER TYPES

Distal spinal muscular atrophy is more likely to be confused clinically with Charcot–Marie–Tooth disease (see below) than with the types described above, which are proximal in distribution. Inheritance is usually autosomal dominant, even in childhood-onset cases; the course is often very slow. It is important to explain to families the very different prognosis and inheritance to the proximal spinal muscular atrophies.

Some forms of lethal arthrogryposis are due to spinal muscular atrophies with onset *in utero*; one type is X-linked. A number of cases are difficult to categorize, and since isolated cases may rarely be new dominant mutations, a risk for offspring of around 5 per cent should be given for such atypical spinal muscular atrophies until they are better understood.

MOTOR NEURONE DISEASE

Motor neurone disease is generally sporadic; risks to first-degree relatives in two un-selected series were under 1 per cent, although these studies need extending in the light of molecular advances. Rare familial types have been recorded, following autosomal dominant inheritance, and due to mutations in the superoxide dismutase gene on chromosome 21 in some families; familial clustering also occurs in specific geographical areas (e.g. Guam). Kennedy's disease or X-linked bulbospinal atrophy, more common than previously recognized and usually following a more prolonged course, must also be distinguished. This disorder is due to a mutational defect (a CAG repeat) in the androgen receptor, which can be recognized in the isolated case by mutation analysis and by features of mild androgen deficiency.

MOEBIUS SYNDROME

The diagnosis of Moebius syndrome of multiple cranial nerve palsies is frequently misapplied to children with other myopathies (e.g. myotonic and FSH dystrophies) or anterior horn cell disorders presenting with facial and ocular palsies. If these can be excluded, the recurrence risk is probably low (1–2 per cent).

CHARCOT–MARIE–TOOTH DISEASE

The majority of cases of Charcot–Marie–Tooth disease (also termed peroneal muscular atrophy, hereditary motor-sensory neuropathy) are autosomal dominant. Cases in families previously thought to be recessive probably mostly result from germ-line mosaicism. Nerve conduction studies allow two main groups to be distinguished, although there is overlap phenotypically. The nomenclature and classification still remain fluid.

TYPE I (DELAYED NERVE CONDUCTION)

A specific and unusual molecular defect has been found in many families with the type I disorder, with duplication of a small region of chromosome 17p detectable by DNA probes, although not usually visible microscopically, so that affected individuals have three functioning copies of the segment. In most families with apparently normal parents but multiple affected children, the disease can now be shown to result from mosaicism in a parent. The specific gene involved is that for peripheral myelin protein (PMP22). This defect provides a specific diagnostic and presymptomatic test, applicable even to isolated cases. A few families show no abnormality of or linkage to chromosome 17 and some severe cases are due to changes in a separate myelin gene (*P0*); interestingly, deletions of the *PMP22* gene produce a different clinical disorder, 'hereditary liability to pressure palsies'.

The X-linked form of Charcot–Marie–Tooth disease must be borne in mind when considering an isolated male case or a pedigree suggested of X-linkage. Molecular defects in connexin 32 have been found in this type. Nerve conduction is often variable in this form, and usually normal in heterozygous females, who may be variably affected clinically.

TYPE II (NORMAL NERVE CONDUCTION)

Type II disease, with an underlying pathology of axonal degeneration, is clinically similar to type I, though often milder. This group is very similar to the distal spinal muscular atrophies. Asymptomatic relatives need careful examination to exclude minimal features before they can be given a low risk. In most families with multiple affected sibs but normal parents, inheritance is probably still autosomal dominant but with either mosaicism or undetected parental disease. No helpful molecular tests exist as yet in diagnostic service but this should change soon, as specific genes are isolated.

OTHER HEREDITARY NEUROPATHIES

Now that specific molecular tests are becoming available, it is becoming possible to distinguish other hereditary neuropathies with greater confidence, and to identify isolated cases with a specific genetic basis. The group of autosomal dominant familial amyloidoses (often characterized by central nervous system, cardiac and other systemic involvement as well as neuropathy) have been shown to result mainly from defects in transthyretin or gelsolin, with different mutations resulting in different phenotypes, often showing marked geographical variation. Recent evidence suggests that liver transplantation may reverse or prevent progression of the disorder. It should be noted that most cases of primary amyloidosis are not familial, but no clear figure exists to put the proportion that is heritable into perspective.

Familial dysautonomia (autosomal recessive) has highly specific features and is most frequent in those of Ashkenazi Jewish origin, while neuropathy may form an important pattern of such metabolic disorders as Refsum's disease and the porphyrias (see Chapter 23).

Rare forms of pure hereditary sensory neuropathy (usually autosomal recessive) may result in disabling trophic changes.

FURTHER READING (see also list in Chapter 12)

General

Emery AEH (ed.) (1998). *Neuromuscular Disorders: Clinical and Molecular Genetics*. Chichester, Wiley.
Engel AG, Banker BQ (eds) (2004). *Myology*, 3rd edn. New York, McGraw–Hill – this comprehensive book contains a series of chapters on all the principal inherited muscle diseases.
Karpati G, Hilton-Jones D, Griggs RC (eds) (2001). *Disorders of Voluntary Muscle*, 7th edn. Cambridge, Cambridge University Press – another excellent and comprehensive book.
Young ID (2000). *Introduction to Risk Calculation in Genetic Counselling*, 2nd edn. Oxford, Oxford University Press.

Muscular dystrophies

Bushby K (2001). The limb girdle muscular dystrophies. *Eur J Paediatr Neurol* 5, 213–214.
Coelho T (1996). Familial amyloid polyneuropathy: new developments in genetics and treatment. *Curr Opin Neurol* 9, 355–359.
Emery AEH (2003). *Duchenne Muscular Dystrophy*, 3rd edn. Oxford, Oxford University Press.
Emery AEH, Emery MLH. (1995). *The History of a Genetic Disease: Duchenne Muscular Dystrophy or Meryon's Disease*. Oxford, Oxford University Press.
Harper PS (2001). *Myotonic Dystrophy*, 3rd edn. London, Saunders.

Neuropathies and spinal muscular atrophies

Murakami T, Garcia CA, Reiter LT, Lupski JR (1996). Charcot–Marie–Tooth disease and related inherited neuropathies. *Medicine (Baltimore)* 75, 233–250.
Siddique T, Nijhawan D, Hentati A (1996). Molecular genetic basis of familial ALS. *Neurology* 47, S27–S34.
Zerres K, Wirth B, Rudnik-Schoneborn S (1997). Spinal muscular atrophy – clinical and genetic correlations. *Neuromuscul Disord* 7, 202–207.

Central nervous system disorders

Disorders of the nervous system, both central and peripheral, make up a remarkably high proportion of genetic counselling referrals, around 50 per cent in the author's experience and in reports from many other centres. This partly reflects the large number of conditions that follow mendelian inheritance, but is also likely to be due to the severe burden resulting from many neurological disorders and the consequent concern of relatives to avoid recurrence, if possible. Awareness of the genetic aspects has recently been heightened by isolation of many of the genes responsible, a field in which inherited neurological disorders have led the way, and which is rapidly increasing our understanding of many conditions in terms of their molecular basis. The availability of molecular analysis allowing accurate prediction makes it particularly important that families in which an inherited neurological disorder has occurred have access to accurate genetic counselling.

HUNTINGTON'S DISEASE

Huntington's disease (HD), in the author's opinion (unchanged since the first edition of this book), represents the most difficult genetic counselling problem among the mendelian disorders of adult life. The severe burden imposed on families by the disease and by fear of it, the present inadequacy of preventive and therapeutic measures (although current research on transgenic animals and cell implantation gives reason for optimism), and the very real possibility that hasty or insensitive genetic counselling or inappropriate testing may do more harm than good, all add to the difficulties. The advent of accurate molecular presymptomatic testing has provided a particular challenge in ensuring appropriate genetic counselling and support, and Huntington's disease has become a model for presymptomatic testing in serious late-onset disorders overall.

Huntington's disease, although regularly autosomal dominant in its inheritance, is late and very variable in its onset, and most of the difficulties arise from this. To advise affected individuals or their spouses that children have a 50 per cent risk is arithmetically simple, but most individuals requiring advice are the healthy offspring themselves.

Although molecular testing can now resolve whether a relative at risk carries the mutation or not, most decide against this, and in any event it is vital that decisions regarding testing and other aspects are made in the context of an accurate general risk estimate. Fortunately, the careful use of all available genetic information and knowledge of the distribution of ages at onset can be of considerable help in this, as shown in Table 12.1. Although drawn up for a particular population, this table is of general application. Figure 12.1 shows the more general risk curves for first-degree relatives, corresponding to the data shown in Table 12.1. Tabular data for second-degree relatives are summarized in Table 12.2. This information is especially valuable where a parent at risk has died relatively young but apparently healthy. Risk estimates for limited periods at different ages are also available [see Harper and Newcombe (1992), cited in Table 12.2] and may be useful in situations relating to employment or fostering and adoption. Figure 12.2 gives a practical example of how the use of age-modified risks can alter the situation for a second-degree relative.

A difficult question, not confined to Huntington's disease, is to what extent ages at onset are correlated within families. The variation within a family and our recent understanding of the unstable nature of the mutation are such that unless information is available from many members, it is better to rely on the overall curve. However, sibs of juvenile cases have passed through about half their risk by the age of 25 years and virtually all of it by the age of 40 years.

Juvenile HD disease is rare, but well documented. It is almost always paternally transmitted (the opposite to myotonic dystrophy) and results from large expansions (commonly 60–100 repeats) in the HD gene. It often presents atypically, with general neurodegeneration and rigidity rather than chorea. Familial chorea occurring in childhood is unlikely to be due to HD, and other conditions such as benign hereditary chorea or one of the dystonias (see below) should be considered. Molecular testing must be handled with great caution if juvenile HD is suspected, and other possible causes ruled out first; otherwise presymptomatic detection of a mutation unrelated to the symptoms may inadvertently result.

Table 12.1 Risk for a healthy subject at 50 per cent prior risk of Huntington's disease (HD) carrying the HD gene at different ages

Age (years)	Risk (%)
20.0	49.6
22.5	49.3
25.0	49.0
27.5	48.4
30.0	47.6
32.5	46.6
35.0	45.5
37.5	44.2
40.0	42.5
42.5	40.3
45.0	37.8
47.5	34.8
50.0	31.5
52.5	27.8
55.0	24.8
57.5	22.1
60.0	18.7
62.5	15.2
65.0	12.8
67.5	10.8
70.0	6.2
72.5	4.6

From Harper PS, Newcombe RG (1992), *J Med Genet* **29**, 239–242.

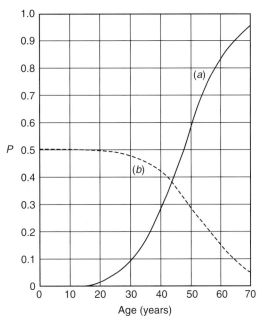

Figure 12.1 Probability that (*a*) an individual possessing the gene for Huntington's disease will have developed the disorder by a certain age; (*b*) the healthy child of an affected parent has the Huntington's disease gene at a particular age. (Based on Harper PS, Walker DA, Tyler A *et al.* (1979), *Lancet* **ii**, 346–349, with additional data provided by Dr Robert Newcombe.)

ISOLATED CASES

Most isolated cases of HD prove, on careful investigation of living family members and records of previous generations, not to be isolated at all. In some cases, early death of parents and lack of records make it impossible to exclude transmission of the disease, or paternity may be in doubt, but often a parent (usually the father) may have had a gene expansion in the borderline range giving no symptoms, but expanding in the next generation to give full HD. Most cases of progressive adult-onset chorea prove to be HD. Diagnostic molecular testing can now resolve the situation for most atypical or isolated cases, although autopsy should also be performed on such individuals to confirm the diagnosis, as well as on apparently unaffected relatives dying of other causes in order to exclude it. It is possible, however, for early clinically evident HD to show no neuropathological changes at all unless special cell counting techniques are used.

Table 12.2 Risk estimates (per cent) for second-degree relatives of a patient with Huntington's disease (HD). The table shows the residual risk of a healthy second-degree relative carrying the HD gene at various combinations of age for the individual and the intervening parent

Age of second-degree relative (years)	Age of parent (years)										
	20–	25–	30–	35–	40–	45–	50–	55–	60–	65–	70–
70–	1.6	1.5	1.5	1.4	1.2	1.0	0.8	0.6	0.4	0.3	0.1
65–	3.8	3.7	3.5	3.3	3.0	2.5	1.9	1.5	1.0	0.7	0.3
60–	5.6	5.4	5.2	4.9	4.3	3.7	2.8	2.2	1.5	1.0	0.4
55–	8.5	8.3	7.9	7.4	6.7	5.6	4.4	3.4	2.3	1.6	0.7
50–	11.2	10.9	10.5	9.8	8.9	7.5	5.8	4.6	3.1	2.1	0.9
45–	14.9	14.6	14.0	13.2	11.9	10.1	7.9	6.2	4.2	2.9	1.3
40–	18.1	17.8	17.0	16.1	14.6	12.5	9.8	7.7	5.3	3.7	1.6
35–	20.6	20.2	19.4	18.4	16.7	14.3	11.3	9.0	6.1	4.3	1.8
30–	22.2	21.8	20.9	19.9	18.1	15.5	12.3	9.8	6.7	4.7	2.0
25–	23.5	23.1	22.2	21.0	19.2	16.5	13.1	10.4	7.2	5.1	2.2
20–	24.2	23.7	22.8	21.7	19.7	17.0	13.6	10.8	7.4	5.2	2.3

From Harper PS, Newcombe RG (1992), *J Med Genet* **29**, 239–242.

Where the individual at risk has an affected grandparent, but the intervening parent is healthy, the risk can be found in the table from the age of the individual and the age of the parent at risk.

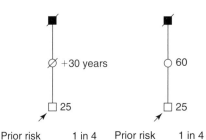

Prior risk   1 in 4   Prior risk   1 in 4   **Figure 12.2** Use of age-modified risks for a
Modified risk ≃ 1 in 4   Modified risk 1 in 14   second-degree relative in Huntington's disease.

ASSOCIATED ASPECTS

Calculating the risks is perhaps the least difficult task in the genetic counselling of families with Huntington's disease. It is the range of more general problems that provides the challenge.

In the past, ignorance of the genetic nature of the disorder was a major problem in relation to genetic counselling of those at risk for Huntington's disease, and while there is no specific legal or professional duty to inform the wider family, the author believes that all adults at high risk have a right to know that they are at risk, preferably before having children. Some parents protect their children from the knowledge well into adult life, with long-term consequences that are often disastrous for them, resulting in deep family discord. An increasingly open attitude to the disease, partly due to active lay groups, seems to be decreasing this problem, but increasing mobility may be having an opposite effect in decreasing awareness of the family background.

When the information should be given will vary from family to family, but the best time for the subject to be raised is probably the early to mid-teens, or before this if the child asks questions or is an early maturer. In this way, further, more detailed discussion can occur when relationships and family are planned, without this coming as a disruptive shock at this time.

It cannot be too strongly stressed that individuals at high risk for HD need support to help them cope with the information that they have been given. This is particularly the case when the disease is newly diagnosed in a family, or when the individuals concerned are being seen as part of an extended family investigation rather than having actively sought advice themselves. Wherever possible, the initial information should come through a responsible family member or sympathetic family doctor, with the genetic clinic providing the opportunity for a fuller and more independent discussion. Where this is not feasible (all too often), the clinician giving advice, whether neurologist or geneticist, must ensure that support is provided. There is no substitute for an experienced genetic counsellor or comparable professional in this respect; any success the author may have had in this field is due largely to the availability of such colleagues.

The confidentiality of records and registers, while important for all disorders, is a special problem in Huntington's disease, as the information may be exceedingly damaging to prospects for careers or insurance. Such information must be severely restricted to clinicians directly involved with the family; access by others should not be allowed without the specific written consent of the individual concerned. This need for consent should include enquiries from other centres about living relatives.

Reproductive options have increased since prenatal exclusion testing and specific prenatal diagnosis have become feasible (see below), although these are only used by a minority of couples. For those who decide not to reproduce, it is important to find alternatives. Adoption is usually ruled out by the severity of the disorder, although adoption or fostering of an older child may be possible, based on a low risk of the disorder developing before such a child has become independent. Gamete donation (see Chapter 8) could potentially be a valuable option, but has not been widely used so far. Pre-implantation diagnosis, as yet only established in one or two centres, may also prove useful.

GENETIC TESTING FOR HD

Although genetic testing using linked markers was possible for almost a decade before the HD gene itself was isolated, the discovery of its specific molecular basis has greatly affected the practical aspects of testing, as well as increasing our understanding of the disease and its possible treatment.

HD results from the expansion of a trinucleotide repeat sequence in a specific gene. Most normal individuals have fewer than 30 repeats, while HD is associated with 39 repeats or more. Age at onset correlates (though only approximately) with repeat length, juvenile cases having the largest repeats (often 60–100) while late-onset cases may be close to the borderline. The instability of the expanded repeat gives a tendency for the mutation to increase and the disease onset to become earlier in successive generations (anticipation), especially when transmitted by males.

The repeat sequence (CAG) appears as polyglutamine in the protein (huntingtin) produced by the HD gene, and it is now clear that this has a direct effect on cellular pathology, which can be reproduced in transgenic mice and which is similar to that of other CAG repeat disorders such as the ataxias. These major advances in understanding could well lead to therapeutic possibilities in the not too distant future.

The practical consequences of this major advance are as follows:

- Essentially all cases of HD show the same mutational basis, so both diagnostic and presymptomatic testing can be done by a single test, regardless of geographical origin or family structure.
- Presence of the mutation correlates very closely with neuropathology of HD. It is wise to ensure that either the mutation or typical neuropathology is present in an affected family member, but testing no longer depends on this.
- The number of repeats is too variable to be of use in predicting onset in an individual (except in the juvenile range).
- Prenatal testing is feasible (though not commonly requested). Pre-implantation testing is becoming available in one or two centres worldwide (see Chapter 8).

Specific mutation testing rapidly replaced indirect testing by linked markers, and there has now been extensive experience of it (almost 5000 presymptomatic tests in the UK up to the beginning of 2004). Some of the main points are summarized below:

- Presymptomatic testing for HD should only be done within a framework of adequate preparation, information and support. Almost all centres use two separate interviews before giving results.
- Important information needing to be given, and thought through, includes implications of an abnormal test result (on individuals and their family members, for insurance, employment etc.); information on the disorder itself (not all those being tested will have had personal experience of HD); sources of support and approaches to coping with an abnormal result.
- Serious adverse reactions have so far been few and seem to reflect the nature of the individual rather than whether the result was abnormal or normal. This is probably because testing has been done cautiously, with ample opportunity for those who wish to change their mind before testing is done, rather than only realizing the consequences afterwards.
- The reasons for requesting testing vary, but commonly involve the wish to resolve uncertainty and to remove risk from children, whether already born or planned for the future.
- It is generally agreed that presymptomatic testing of young children, requested by parents, should not be carried out, the view being that individuals have the right to decide for themselves, as adults. Requests from adolescents are few, and these need sensitive discussion before any decision is made.
- It has become generally accepted that presymptomatic testing for HD is something that should be done by clinical geneticists, in contrast to diagnostic testing of symptomatic individuals, which is becoming part of the practice of neurologists, psychiatrists and other involved clinicians. It is important that the difference between these two categories of genetic testing is fully appreciated (see Chapter 5), as there are major practical considerations involved.

One issue in presymptomatic testing that has arisen since specific mutation analysis became possible is the testing of those at 25 per cent risk, i.e. individuals whose parent is at risk but healthy. If the mutation is detected in the younger generation, then this will imply that the parent also carries it, and will probably be much closer to onset of the disease. How should one respond to such a request if the parent does not wish to be tested themselves, or does not know about their offspring's request? Fortunately, data from both the UK and elsewhere show that such difficult scenarios are rare, probably because the situation is resolved by sensitive genetic counselling. In this area, and many others, HD not only highlights an issue which is relevant to presymptomatic testing in general, but also shows how important it is that presymptomatic testing is not isolated from the general genetic counselling process or regarded as an activity purely for the laboratory.

PARKINSON'S DISEASE

Most cases of Parkinson's disease are idiopathic rather than secondary to arteriosclerosis or encephalitis, and a prevalence of around 1 in 10 000 is seen in most European countries. Most cases are sporadic, or at least non-mendelian, but a few large early-onset dominant families have been recorded and some of these have shown mutations in the alpha synuclein gene on chromosome 4q.

One study has shown that the risk to sibs varies with age at onset in the proband, being around 1 in 12 when age of onset is under 45 years; 1 in 20 when it is 45–55 years; and under 1 in 50 when it is over 65 years. It would seem reasonable to use the above figures in the absence of other affected family members, but they may be an overestimate, since another study has shown no difference between sibs and controls, while two twin studies have shown low concordance in both monozygotic and dizygotic twins, although the rate is higher if new functional imaging studies are used. The very rare juvenile Parkinson's disease, in which molecular defects have also been identified in a gene termed **parkin**, is autosomal recessive in inheritance.

OTHER INVOLUNTARY MOVEMENT DISORDERS

Essential tremor is a common and benign disorder, inherited as a late-onset autosomal dominant, and is important mainly as a condition to be distinguished from other movement disorders, particularly Parkinson's disease. At the other extreme of life, there are several benign dominantly inherited tremors of head and chin beginning in infancy.

Torsion dystonia follows autosomal dominant inheritance in most cases, though with incomplete penetrance in some gene carriers and minimal expression in others; the disorder is more common in Ashkenazi Jews. A single mutation in a specific gene on chromosome 9 has been found to be responsible for almost all typical cases, Jewish and non-Jewish, including most sporadic early-onset cases. DOPA responsive dystonia, due to a separate molecular defect, is an important form to recognize, even though it is very rare.

Hereditary benign chorea is characterized by non-progressive chorea present from infancy, without mental retardation. Inheritance is autosomal dominant, with reduced penetrance in females. It is most important not to confuse this benign condition with Huntington's disease. A separate locus and specific gene have been identified in some families.

Familial paroxysmal choreoathetosis shows intermittent symptoms, as its name implies. It is autosomal dominant.

Chorea-acanthocytosis (neuroacanthocytosis), described mainly from Japan, is autosomal recessive and can be distinguished by the red blood cell changes.

DRPLA (dentato-rubro-pallido-luysian atrophy) shows a variable combination of chorea, myoclonus and ataxia and is due, like HD, to a specific expanded CAG repeat. It also is relatively common in Japan.

A variety of other hereditary movement disorders exist, including a number of rare striatonigral degenerations, while metabolic disorders such as Wilson's disease and Lesch–Nyhan syndrome must be considered.

THE HEREDITARY ATAXIAS

Genetic heterogeneity and confused classification of the hereditary ataxias have now started to resolve with molecular advances. Careful family documentation and clinical assessment allow correct genetic counselling to be given in most cases, even when the diagnosis remains uncertain. The following broad framework is a starting point:

- Hereditary ataxia may form part of a generalized syndrome: over 50 such syndromes have been identified, many from a single family.
- Classic Friedreich's ataxia, with absent reflexes, cardiac involvement and early onset, is autosomal recessive, and the risk for offspring of affected individuals is minimal in the absence of consanguinity. The gene has been isolated and the mutation found to be a trinucleotide repeat expansion, but this is not in the coding region of the gene, in contrast to the dominant ataxias. Prenatal diagnosis is now feasible.
- Other ataxias with congenital or childhood onset, a very heterogenous group, are generally autosomal recessive, including congenital cerebellar ataxia with aplasia of the vermis (Joubert syndrome) and ataxia telangiectasia (the gene for which has been isolated). Metabolic causes must be excluded.
- Late-onset ataxia accompanied by upper motor neurone signs (spinocerebellar ataxia) is a heterogenous group and has been found to result from trinucleotide repeat (CAG) expansions in specific genes; the repeat appearing in the protein as polyglutamine (as in HD) and probably directly responsible for the disease pathology. The group is now classified by its specific numbered genetic types, all autosomal dominant, and this largely replaces the previous names (e.g. type III for Machado–Joseph disease). The phenotype of the different forms overlaps extensively; all show a relationship between clinical phenotype and size of repeat expansion, with anticipation present (see p. 27). In addition to molecular diagnosis, presymptomatic testing is now increasingly feasible and a comparable protocol to that used for HD is advisable.
- X-linked cerebellar ataxia is very rare, but well documented – cases are too infrequent to affect counselling for isolated male cases of ataxia. However, it has recently been recognized that a proportion of fragile-X pre-mutation carriers may develop a progressive, late-onset neurodegeneration with ataxia, something that has wide implications for genetic counselling in fragile-X syndrome (see Chapter 13).

A number of patients will fail to fit into any of the above groups. If the particular pattern of inheritance in the family is characteristic, this should be the basis for counselling; for isolated cases, it is wise to assume autosomal dominant inheritance for adult cases unless there is evidence to the contrary.

HEREDITARY SPASTIC PARAPLEGIA

Hereditary spastic paraplegia is often very benign in its course: autosomal dominant inheritance is usual, but X-linked and, rarely, autosomal recessive inheritance has occurred in several families. Several different loci have been identified for the dominant types, with one specific gene (*spastin*) isolated on chromosome 2. It is impossible to exclude a high risk for offspring of an isolated case and parents should always be studied carefully because manifestations can be very mild, especially in females. Confusion with anoxic cerebral palsy and the dystonias is still frequent.

MOTOR NEURONE DISEASE

This has been considered in Chapter 11 (p. 170), but it should be noted here that some affected families may show a wider range of phenotype overlapping with other CNS degenerations.

OTHER INHERITED DEGENERATIONS WITH DEMENTIA

These are considered in Chapter 13 (p. 193), but the close parallels with HD in terms of presymptomatic testing issues deserve note here.

MULTIPLE SCLEROSIS

Familial occurrence (not necessarily genetic) in multiple sclerosis is well documented, but uncommon. The risk to first-degree relatives is low (around 2–3 per cent from birth and only around 1 per cent by age 30); even monozygotic twin pairs are usually discordant (risk 20–30 per cent). One study has subdivided the risk categories but it is not clear how valid this is. In the rare families in which two first-degree relatives (usually parent and child) are affected, risks are considerably increased (around 5 per cent for subsequent children). It is likely that the major aetiological factors will prove to be immunological and possibly infective, but that a specific genotype may be required for susceptibility. An association with specific HLA antigens exists, but is too weak to be used in genetic counselling. For familial cases presenting with optic neuropathy, care must be taken to exclude Leber's optic atrophy and related mitochondrial disorders.

SYRINGOMYELIA

Recurrence of syringomyelia in a family is unusual.

NEUROFIBROMATOSIS

Several forms of neurofibromatosis can be distinguished, the most common being type I (von Recklinghausen's disease). Inheritance is autosomal dominant, with new mutations representing one-quarter to one-half of all cases. Careful examination of apparently unaffected family members is essential before pronouncing them to be unaffected. The presence of six or more pigmented spots over 1.5 cm in diameter and of the characteristic appearance is an indication that the gene is present. Young children frequently show only inconspicuous signs of the disorder, but careful examination can usually exclude the disorder by the age of 1 year, and exclude it with confidence by the age of 5 years. Lisch nodules (harmless hamartomatous lesions) in the iris are a helpful confirmatory clinical sign. There is no evidence that particular families with neurofibromatosis are free from serious effects. Most surveys have shown that around one-third of affected individuals have one or more serious problems (including optic glioma, various cerebral and spinal tumours, and mild or moderate mental retardation), while two-thirds are mildly affected. The gene for von Recklinghausen's disease has been isolated and shown to produce an important protein (neurofibromin) regulating cell division and differentiation. Mutations can only be identified in a minority of patients so far.

Type 2 (bilateral acoustic or central) neurofibromatosis is a separate, much rarer dominantly inherited abnormality, which also produces multiple Schwannomas and meningiomas, with characteristic lens opacities, but has relatively few skin lesions. The gene has been isolated, allowing genetic testing in families for this serious condition.

VON HIPPEL–LINDAU SYNDROME

Von Hippel–Lindau syndrome is characterized by haemangiomatous cysts and tumours of the retina, brain (especially cerebellum), kidney and other viscera. Inheritance is autosomal dominant. Penetrance is age-dependent, so apparently unaffected members require periodic medical review and cannot be completely reassured until late in adult life. Renal ultrasonography, MRI brain scan and ophthalmological assessment are essential. The need for recurrent assessment of both patients and relatives makes this disorder (like other familial tumour syndromes) especially suitable for a genetic register. The gene is located on chromosome 3, and has been isolated. Mutations can now be detected in around 75 per cent of cases.

TUBEROUS SCLEROSIS

Tuberous sclerosis follows autosomal dominant inheritance, but causes considerable problems in genetic counselling because of its variability. The classic skin lesions (multiple depigmented patches, adenoma sebaceum, shagreen patches and subungual fibromas) may be the only abnormalities present in some patients, while others may develop epilepsy or may be severely retarded from cerebral involvement. Computed tomographic (CT) scan or magnetic resonance imaging (MRI) are particularly helpful in showing intracerebral lesions; many patients have renal cysts, while affected infants may have cardiac tumours. The birth of a severely affected child to a mildly affected parent cannot be excluded, and since individuals who reproduce are less severely affected than average, their offspring are likely to be more severely affected than themselves.

About 60 per cent of cases appear to represent new mutations, in which case the risks of recurrence in future children of normal parents will be small, although the possibility of mosaicism leaves a small residual risk (around 3 per cent). Careful study of such parents, including examination of the skin under ultraviolet light for depigmented patches, and, if doubt exists, brain CT or MRI scans and renal ultrasonography, should be made before concluding that the case is likely to represent a new mutation. These tests are now being progressively replaced by specific molecular testing.

Two specific tumour suppressor genes on chromosomes 9 and 16 have been identified, allowing molecular prediction in many cases. The chromosome 16 form may be more likely to be associated with mental handicap. Some patients also have involvement of the adjacent polycystic kidney disease gene (see p. 292) and these may have serious renal disease.

EPILEPSY

About one person in 20 has an epileptic attack at some time, while the prevalence of recurrent epileptic attacks is around 1 per cent in North America and is probably similar in the UK.

Seizures may be secondary to a variety of environmental or hereditary disorders, in which case the primary cause is the determining factor for genetic risks. Some forms of primary epilepsy have a major genetic contribution and several of the genes have now been mapped and isolated, particularly for some of the rare mendelian types which are proving to be due to ion channel mutations. So far, specific genes have not been recognized in common primary epilepsy.

SIMPLE ABSENCE EPILEPSY

When accompanied by the typical 'spike and wave' electroencephalographic (EEG) pattern this type of epilepsy is probably controlled by a major gene following autosomal dominant inheritance. Close to 50 per cent of first-degree relatives show the EEG defect when studied in adolescence, but penetrance is much reduced in both early childhood and adult life. Not all those with an abnormal EEG have clinical attacks; the empiric risk for sibs is around 6 per cent.

FEBRILE CONVULSIONS

These are extremely common in the general population (2–7 per cent in various studies). The risk to sibs is increased threefold (8–29 per cent), the highest figures coming from Japan.

BENIGN NEONATAL CONVULSIONS

Although most cases are sporadic, a clear autosomal dominant form is relatively frequent, with the gene isolated on chromosome 20. Convulsions cease after infancy in around 90 per cent of patients.

INFANTILE SPASMS

Infantile spasms are rarely familial (recurrence risk for sibs around 2 per cent), provided that underlying conditions such as tuberous sclerosis or metabolic disorders have been ruled out.

MYOCLONIC EPILEPSY

Rare progressive cases may form part of general neurodegenerative disorders, usually autosomal recessive; one gene (cystatin B) for a specific form (Unverricht–Lundborg epilepsy) has been isolated on chromosome 21. The possibility of an underlying mitochondrial disorder (see Chapter 2) should also be considered. A benign form of recurrent childhood myoclonic epilepsy is autosomal recessive and is HLA-linked.

PARTIAL BENIGN EPILEPSY OF CHILDHOOD

Partial benign epilepsy of childhood is a variable disorder which may follow an autosomal dominant pattern. The prognosis is good with appropriate treatment.

PRIMARY IDIOPATHIC GENERALIZED EPILEPSY

Numerous surveys of primary idiopathic epilepsy have been carried out, with diverging results, probably depending on the severity of disease in the patients studied and on the social attitudes at the time. Most of the studies were done 20–40 years ago, and, although they included massive numbers, the earlier ones did not have the benefit of EEG classification.

More recent studies have shown both higher population frequencies and higher risks to relatives, partly as a result of using the cumulative incidence of epilepsy rather than the prevalence (see 'Further reading').

Table 12.3 Genetic risks in idiopathic epilepsy

Individual affected	Cumulative risk of clinical epilepsy up to age 20 years (febrile convulsions excluded) (%)
Monozygotic twin	60 (approx.)
Dizygotic twin	10 (approx.)
Sib	
Onset < 10 years	6
Onset > 25 years	1–2
Overall	2.5
Parent	4
Parent and sib	10 (approx.)
Both parents	15 (approx.)
General population (variable)	1

The risks given in Table 12.3 reflect these higher estimates for both relatives and controls and represent the cumulative risk of epilepsy up to the age of 20 years. The relationship between risk to sibs and age at onset in the proband should be noted. In giving the risks for offspring, the possible teratogenic effects of antiepileptic drugs must be remembered. These are likely to be as important as, or more important than, the actual genetic risks (see Chapter 26). It is possible that current pharmacogenetic research may prove helpful in improving control by anti-epileptic drugs and in minimizing effects.

NARCOLEPSY

Individuals with narcolepsy show a marked excess of the HLA haplotype DR2. Some families show a pattern suggestive of autosomal dominant inheritance, but a study of unselected patients has shown only 1 per cent of first-degree relatives of an isolated case to be affected, much less than the figure of 14 per cent for offspring found in a previous study, providing a good example of the limitations of genetic susceptibility testing. Somnolence may be confused with epileptic absences and can also result from other genetic disorders (e.g. myotonic dystrophy).

CEREBRAL ANEURYSMS AND STROKE

Occasional family clusters of cerebral aneurysm suggestive of autosomal dominant inheritance have been recorded, but in general these aneurysms are rarely familial (they are, however, associated with polycystic kidney disease). The same is true for most cerebral angiomas (provided that von Hippel–Lindau syndrome has been excluded). The possibility of a connective tissue disorder (e.g. Ehlers–Danlos syndrome type IV) should be considered. Autosomal dominant microaneurysms with cerebral haemorrhage have also been associated with mutations in the beta-amyloid precursor protein gene.

Table 12.4 Single gene causes of stroke and related vascular disorders

Cause	Inheritance
Connective tissue disorders	
Pseudoxanthoma elasticum	AR or AD
Ehlers–Danlos syndrome (type IV)	AD
Marfan syndrome	AD
Metabolic disorders	
Sickle cell disease	AR
Homocystinuria	AR
Fabry's disease	XR
Thrombotic factor disorders	Various (see Chapter 24)
Others	
Hereditary haemorrhagic telangiectasia	AD
CADASIL	AD
Moya Moya disease	Uncertain (most sporadic)

AD, autosomal dominant; AR, autosomal recessive; XR, X-linked recessive.
Based on Markus H (2003) (see 'Further reading').

Table 12.4 lists some of the more important mendelian causes of stroke; all are rare and make up only 1 per cent of all stroke cases. Gene mapping studies in the Icelandic population have recently defined a locus involved in susceptibility to common stroke, but this will need confirming independently.

MIGRAINE

This exceedingly common condition is frequently familial, but specific genes have not yet been identified in common migraine. However, a specific ion channel gene on chromosome 19 is now known to underlie the rare familial hemiplegic migraine and intermittent ataxia in some families, with a dominant inheritance pattern.

CEREBRAL PALSY

A diagnosis of cerebral palsy should be mistrusted. All too often it merely camouflages ignorance of a variety of neurological disorders, some of which are genetic. The question to be asked first is whether sufficient evidence of perinatal anoxia, prematurity or other factors exists to explain the observed clinical problems. If the answer is 'yes', then genetic risks are likely to be small, although it must be remembered that an underlying genetic disorder could compromise neonatal respiratory function. If the answer is 'no', then one should ask whether sufficient investigation has been done to identify any specific primary neurological disorder such as familial specific paraplegia (see p. 181).

The problem lies less with newly diagnosed patients, carefully studied in a good centre, than with those families in which a relative in a previous generation has been labelled as having 'cerebral palsy' with little or no investigation. It may be necessary to reassess the original patient if accurate genetic counselling is to be given.

One early but thorough British study showed an overall recurrence risk of only 1 per cent, but as environmental factors are progressively reduced, it is likely that genetic risks for remaining cases have increased. Several subgroups have been noted to have a higher risk, notably congenital ataxia and symmetrical tetraplegia occurring without definite external cause. In both of these conditions, the recurrence risk is about 10–12 per cent for sibs, which includes a number of recessive disorders such as Joubert syndrome (see earlier) and disequilibrium syndrome. The athetoid type, formerly associated strongly with kernicterus, may also have a largely genetic basis when no external factors exist, in which case a similar recurrence risk is appropriate. We do not yet have adequate figures for offspring risk in any of the groups.

NEURAL TUBE DEFECTS

Despite much work and many hypotheses, the aetiology of neural tube defects remains incompletely understood. Their incidence varies greatly even within restricted geographical areas, and it is recognized that a high proportion of affected fetuses are lost as spontaneous abortions. Nutritional factors, notably folic acid, form an important environmental component; genetic factors may prove to involve folate metabolism (e.g. the folate receptor gene, MTHFR). Segmental developmental genes (see Chapter 6) do not seem to play a major role outside specific syndromes and no clearly mendelian subset has yet been defined.

Neural tube defects may occur as part of chromosomal and other severe malformation syndromes, including the recessively inherited Meckel syndrome (see below). There is an increased frequency in association with congenital heart disease, diaphragmatic aplasia and oesophageal atresia.

All studies agree that anencephaly and spina bifida are closely related genetically and in pathogenesis. It is essential that this is indicated to families seen for genetic counselling, because a high risk of recurrence of the invariably fatal anencephaly is acceptable to some, whereas a surviving but handicapped child with spina bifida might not be. In general, the recurrence risk is equally distributed for anencephaly and spina bifida, regardless of which condition the index case had. The possibility that low sacral lesions form a separate group is still debatable.

The recurrence risks for neural tube defects are summarized in Table 12.5. The sex of the index case or individual at risk does not appear to alter the risks greatly. A detectable increase in risk is not seen for a relationship more distant than first cousins. The 5 per cent risk for sibs given in early editions of this book is probably now an overestimate in the light of the marked fall in incidence in recent years. Where accurate recent incidence data are available, a risk of 10 times the incidence is a reasonable one, i.e. 2.5–3 per cent for most of North America and Europe.

The situation for families at risk has been completely changed by the widespread use of prenatal diagnosis, based originally on amniotic fluid alpha-fetoprotein (AFP) and

Table 12.5 Anencephaly and spina bifida: approximate recurrence risks (per cent) in relation to population incidence

Individual affected	Population incidence		
	1/200	1/500	1/1000
One sib	5	3	2
Two sibs	12	10	10
One second-degree relative (uncle/aunt or half-sib)	2	1	1
One third-degree relative	1	0.5–1	0.5
One parent	4	4	4

acetylcholinesterase assessments (see Chapter 8), now largely superseded by high-resolution ultrasound scan. These will detect virtually all subsequent cases of anencephaly and at least 95 per cent of cases of spina bifida, those undetected being covered defects or small open ones. Thus, the risk of an undetected neural tube defect in the offspring of a couple with an affected child is extremely low.

The use of radioimmunoassay for maternal serum AFP as a screening test for all pregnancies in the detection of neural tube defects has been adopted in many areas of high incidence, while high-resolution ultrasonography is now comparably sensitive provided that the operator is experienced (not always the case). As discussed in Chapter 8, it is now possible to detect almost all cases of anencephaly and over 90 per cent of cases of open spina bifida in this way, although the organization and social problems of such a screening approach are considerable (see Chapter 27).

Data are now available for the offspring of patients affected with spina bifida, and show a risk of around 3–4 per cent regardless of which parent is affected. Amniocentesis and careful ultrasound screening should be offered for such pregnancies. No increase in other abnormalities has been noted.

The primary prevention of neural tube defects has been greatly helped by the finding that preconceptional folic acid supplementation appears to reduce the recurrence risk for women with one affected child to around 1 per cent. To what extent this approach can be applied on a population basis as well as to high-risk groups is still uncertain, but it certainly strengthens the view that dietary advice is important in preconceptional counselling.

SPINA BIFIDA OCCULTA

Spina bifida occulta is a term applied both to individuals with spinal dysraphism, showing a significant spinal defect, usually lumbosacral and often associated with a pigmented or hairy patch of skin, and to individuals with radiological absence of one or two vertebral arches, without a visible lesion, usually discovered incidentally following radiography for backache or other unrelated symptoms (sometimes termed uncomplicated spina bifida). The first group shows an increased incidence of overt neural tube defects in their offspring and sibs, with a risk similar to that for overt spina bifida, and it is reasonable to offer them prenatal testing. The second group, amounting to around 5 per cent of the general population, shows no evidence of any increased risk and it is unfortunate that the term 'spina bifida' is used at all here, as women aware that they have this variant may be seriously alarmed at the possibility of clinical spina bifida occurring in their children. Amniocentesis is not justified in this situation.

HYDROCEPHALUS

Hydrocephalus frequently accompanies spina bifida, and a careful check should be made before assuming that hydrocephalus is an isolated and primary phenomenon. The great majority of families do not follow a mendelian pattern; an X-linked type with aqueduct stenosis exists but is extremely rare, and counselling as for an X-linked trait should only be given if the pedigree pattern is clearly X-linked or if the other characteristic features of this type are present. Mutations have been shown in this form in the *LCAM* gene, involving a neural cell adhesion protein. The general recurrence risk for sibs of an isolated case of hydrocephalus is 1–2 per cent, 4–5 per cent for male sibs of an isolated male case, and around 8 per cent where two sibs are affected. Where an isolated male case is due to aqueduct stenosis, the risk to male sibs has been shown to be somewhat higher, possibly 5–10 per cent, although the author suspects that this is an overestimate.

Ultrasound scanning is now able to detect some cases of hydrocephalus in early pregnancy, especially early developing types with spina bifida, and the severe hydranencephaly, for which the recurrence risk is similar to hydrocephalus, unless syndromal. The Walker–Warburg syndrome, with associated retinal changes, is a rare autosomal recessive cause of hydrocephalus, as is the hydrolethalus syndrome. The combination of hydrocephalus with hypoplasia of the cerebellar vermis (Dandy–Walker syndrome) may be part of several more general disorders, but otherwise recurrence risks are similar to those in isolated hydrocephalus.

OTHER STRUCTURAL CENTRAL NERVOUS SYSTEM MALFORMATIONS

ENCEPHALOCELE

Encephalocele should probably be regarded as part of the anencephaly–spina bifida complex and risks given as such. An important association to recognize is the autosomal recessive Meckel syndrome, in which encephalocele and hypoplasia of the olfactory lobes are accompanied by a variety of other malformations, notably cleft lip or palate, polydactyly, renal cystic disease and eye defects (coloboma, cataract, microphthalmos).

MICROCEPHALY

This diagnosis is best restricted to individuals whose head circumference is more than two standard deviations below the mean. The obvious but poorly resolved heterogeneity present in microcephaly, together with its severe consequences and high overall recurrence risk, makes this a particularly difficult area for genetic counselling. The book by Baraitser listed in 'Further reading' (see especially pp. 17–18) provides some valuable cautionary notes, although the identification of specific genes for some of the recessive types is beginning to unravel some of the complexity.

Microcephaly may result from a variety of intrauterine factors, including congenital infections, teratogens and maternal phenylketonuria. It may also be part of many genetic malformation syndromes, including the more severe autosomal trisomies and deletions, and is a striking feature of the autosomal recessive Seckel syndrome. Occasional mild dominantly inherited families have been recorded. Isolated severe microcephaly with a normal facial structure is often inherited as an autosomal recessive; the overall recurrence risk has been 10–20 per cent in different studies. Where no specific cause can be found, a recurrence risk of 10–15 per cent is appropriate, but this is 25 per cent if consanguinity is present. Ultrasound monitoring should be seriously considered in a pregnancy at risk for the severe forms, but recognition is not always possible until late in pregnancy.

MACROCEPHALY

Macrocephaly (to be distinguished from hydrocephalus) may be part of a neurological disorder (e.g. neurofibromatosis, various cerebral degenerations), part of a more general growth disorder (e.g. Sotos syndrome) or an isolated feature, usually not associated with serious consequences, and commonly autosomal dominant. Fragile-X syndrome should be excluded.

HOLOPROSENCEPHALY

In holoprosencephaly there is a variable failure of development of the forebrain with associated facial features. It is usually lethal, especially the extreme forms of cebocephaly and cyclopia. The condition may be isolated or it may be part of trisomy 13. Apart from Meckel syndrome (see above), cases of autosomal recessive inheritance have been reported, as well as occasional dominant inheritance with a very mildly affected parent, so caution, chromosome analysis and thorough pathology are needed. The recurrence risk after an isolated non-syndromal case is relatively low (4–5 per cent). The human counterpart of a specific *Drosophila* developmental gene (SHH) on chromosome 7q shows mutations in some dominantly inherited cases.

LISSENCEPHALY AND RELATED NEURONAL MIGRATION DEFECTS

This group contains various disorders affecting cerebral gyral development, including microdeletions of chromosome 17p (Miller–Dieker syndrome) and an important X-linked recessive type. It is important to base a specific diagnosis on a combination of neuroradiological, molecular and clinical criteria. Sib recurrence risk is around 7 per cent when specific causes have been carefully excluded. Older diagnosis in this heterogenous group should be reassessed, as a more specific and accurate diagnosis may well affect genetic counselling.

AGENESIS OF CORPUS CALLOSUM

Agenesis of the corpus callosum may occur as part of a more general cerebral maldevelopment or it may be isolated. Most isolated cases have been sporadic, although occasional families following an apparently X-linked recessive pattern have been recorded. Aicardi syndrome, recorded only in females and possibly an X-linked dominant lethal in males, is associated with infantile spasms and retinopathy. Several syndromes with limb defects (acrocallosal, Neu–Laxova) are autosomal recessive.

DEGENERATIVE METABOLIC DISORDERS OF THE CENTRAL NERVOUS SYSTEM

Where degenerative metabolic disorders of the central nervous system are part of systemic metabolic conditions, these are considered in Chapter 23. An important group of disorders is largely confined to the nervous system (Table 12.6). Most are mendelian, making the

Table 12.6 Degenerative metabolic disorders of the central nervous system (see also Chapter 23)

Disorder	Enzyme or molecular defect	Inheritance
Leucodystrophies		
Metachromatic leucodystrophy	Arylsulphatase A	AR
Adrenoleucodystrophy	Long-chain fatty acid defect	XR
Pelizaeus–Merzbacher disease	β-myelin protein	XR
Krabbe's disease	β-galactosidase	AR
Neuronal storage disease		
Gangliosidoses (including Tay–Sachs, Sandhoff's diseases)	See Chapter 23	All AR
Batten's disease (infantile neuronal lipofuscinosis)	Main gene now isolated (see text)	AR
Kuf's disease (adult lipofuscinosis)	Unknown	AD
Canavan's disease	Aspartoacylase	AR
Others		
Menkes disease	Copper metabolism	XR
Neuroaxonal dystrophy (previously known as Hallervorden–Spatz disease)	Pantothenate kinase (PANK2)	AR
Leigh's encephalopathy (heterogeneous)	Pyruvate metabolism (some cases)	AR, also mitochondrial

AD, autosomal dominant; AR, autosomal recessive; XR, X-linked recessive.

recognition of a specific biochemical diagnosis, and increasingly the use of molecular techniques, of great importance in relation to genetic counselling. Frozen tissue or stored cultured cells are often crucial where the only affected individuals are dead. Isolation of the principal gene for infantile Batten's disease on chromosome 16p (*CLN3*), with one particular mutation predominant in several populations, has been a development of especial importance in view of the lack of any previously known metabolic defect.

FURTHER READING

General

Aicardi J (1992). *Diseases of the Nervous System in Childhood*. Oxford, Oxford University Press.
Baraitser M (1997). *The Genetics of Neurological Disorders*. Oxford, Oxford University Press.
Ptacek LJ (1997). Channelopathies: ion channel disorders of muscle as a paradigm for paroxysmal disorders of the nervous system. *Neuromuscul Disord* **7**, 250–255.
Wells RD, Warren ST (eds) (1998). *Genetic Instabilities and Hereditary Neurological Diseases*. London, Academic Press.

Neurodegenerations

Bates G, Harper PS, Jones L (eds) (2002). *Huntington's Disease*, 3rd edn. Oxford, Oxford University Press.
Hammans SR (1996). The inherited ataxias and the new genetics. *J Neurol Neurosurg Psychiatry* **61**, 327–332.
Jarman PR, Warner TT (1998). The dystonias. *J Med Genet* **35**, 314–318.
Klockgether T, Dichgans J (1997). The genetic basis of hereditary ataxia. *Prog Brain Res* **114**, 569–576.

Epilepsies

Berkovic SF, Scheffer IE (1997). Epilepsies with single gene inheritance. *Brain Dev* **19**, 13–18.
Callenbach PM, Brouwer OF (1997). Hereditary epilepsy syndromes. *Clin Neurol Neurosurg* **99**, 159–171.
Gardiner RM (2000). Impact of our understanding of the genetic aetiology of epilepsy. *J Neurol* **247**, 327–334.

Other

Gomez MR, Sampson JR, Whittemore VH (eds) (1998). *Tuberous Sclerosis Complex*. Oxford, Oxford University Press.
Huson SM, Hughes RAC (1994). *The Neurofibromatoses*. London, Chapman and Hall.
Markus H (ed.) (2003). *Stroke Genetics*. Oxford, Oxford University Press.
Tolmie J (2002). Clinical genetics of neural tube defects and other congenital malformations of the central nervous system. In: Rimoin DL, Connor JM, Pyeritz RE, Korf B, eds. *Emery and Rimoin's Principles and Practice of Medical Genetics*, Edinburgh, Churchill Livingstone, pp. 2975–3011.

CHAPTER 13

Disorders of mental function

Psychiatric genetics has a long history of experimental studies, but until recently these impinged relatively little upon genetic counselling for mental illness, nor was there significant contact between clinical geneticists and workers in psychiatric genetics. The past few years have seen a striking convergence, largely because it is becoming possible to identify some of the specific genes involved in key processes, but also because investigators have developed rigorous diagnostic criteria that can help in the analysis of family data.

Four main groups of disorders are covered in this chapter: the dementias, mental retardation, behavioural disorders and major psychiatric illnesses. Some of these might, with justification, be placed in the preceding chapter as neurological disorders; their location in this book has been determined more by the groups of professionals most involved than by biological factors. As with other disorders, requests for genetic counselling rise sharply when it is perceived that, as a result of advances, more specific genetic information can be offered than broad risk categories. Such an increase can be anticipated for all the groups of disorders outlined here, and there is an urgent need for psychiatrists and associated staff to become familiar with how to identify and handle well the genetic and family aspects of this difficult and sensitive group of disorders.

THE DEMENTIAS

It is now recognized that most of the major dementias have a significant familial and genetic component (Table 13.1). At present, dementias following strict mendelian inheritance are few (Huntington's disease has already been considered in Chapter 12), but susceptibility loci are beginning to be identified in some of the non-mendelian forms.

ALZHEIMER'S DISEASE

Alzheimer's disease is the most common dementia of old age, and increased survival makes it a major problem for society as well as for individual families. Certain diagnosis

Table 13.1 Major dementias with a significant genetic component

Disorder	Inheritance	Gene or chromosome involved
Huntington's disease	AD	Chromosome 4P. Unstable CAG repeat
Alzheimer's disease		
Rare dominant early-onset (<65 years) form	AD	Beta amyloid precursor protein (APP), chromosome 21; also chromosomes 1 and 14 (presenilin loci)
Later-onset cases	Unclear	Apolipoprotein E susceptibility locus (see text)
Pick's disease (frontotemporal dementia)	Unclear	Tau protein (occasional families)
Amyloid cerebrovascular disorders	AD	Mutations on chromosomes 21 and 9 (some families)
Familial multi-infarct dementia (CADASIL)	AD	Human homologue of *Drosophila* 'Notch' gene
Creutzfeldt–Jakob disease (and related spongiform encephalopathies)	AD (when mendelian)	Prion mutations (chromosome 20) in some familial cases
Mitochondrial encephalopathies	Mitochondrial or sporadic	Various mitochondrial DNA mutations

AD, autosomal dominant.

is only possible at autopsy and rests upon the demonstration of large numbers of senile plaques and neurofibrillary tangles in the brains of sufferers. A specific locus on chromosome 21 was suggested by the occurrence of Alzheimer's disease in most older Down's syndrome patients, and by the location of the gene encoding beta-amyloid precursor protein (the major constituent of the senile plaques) on this chromosome. Specific mutations have now been identified in this gene in a few families showing dominant inheritance of early-onset Alzheimer's disease, but in rather more such families the disease is determined by mutations in the *presenilin 1* gene on chromosome 14, and in a second *presenilin* gene on chromosome 1.

Families where the disease shows clear autosomal dominant inheritance are rare (around 1 per cent of all cases) and onset is usually early (under 65 years). For these rare mendelian families, a small minority even of early-onset cases, presymptomatic testing may be feasible if a specific mutation can be identified in an affected individual. The issues involved in such testing and the type of protocol involved are closely comparable to those for Huntington's disease.

For the great majority of Alzheimer cases not showing mendelian inheritance, which includes almost all those of late onset, genetic risks to relatives are not greatly increased (Table 13.2). These cases are strongly age-dependent, as also shown by a Canadian study of a series including all non-mendelian cases, which found a risk to first-degree relatives of 2 per cent at age 75, rising to 4 per cent by age 80. Put in a different way, the chance of such a relative *not* having Alzheimer's disease (if they live to this age) is around 95 per cent.

Table 13.2 Genetic risks in Alzheimer's disease

	Risk of dementia before age 75 years (%)
Sib affected (onset over 65 years)	2
Sib affected (onset under 65 years)	4–12
Sib and parent affected (onset over 65 years)	4–5
Sib and parent affected (onset under 65 years)	16–22

Based on Bundey S (1992), *Genetics and Neurology*. Edinburgh, Churchill Livingstone.

The accidental finding that common normal variants of the lipoprotein gene *ApoE* showed an association with Alzheimer's disease led to suggestions that this marker might be used in prediction. Further evidence shows that the association is less strong than first thought – a two- to threefold increase for those with one *ApoE* 4 allele and a 10-fold increase for the rare homozygotes for this. A series of consensus meetings in both the USA and the UK has firmly concluded that this should not be used in either prediction or diagnosis. The need for caution is further strengthened by the finding that the association may actually be reversed in some populations so that the E4 allele could actually be protective in these. The whole *ApoE* story shows how complex such interactions are likely to be in multifactorial disorders (see Chapter 3) and how unwise it is to rush into using genetic susceptibility factors in prediction.

OTHER FAMILIAL DEMENTIAS

While all of these are rare, they represent an important group because of the mendelian inheritance (usually dominant) and high risks to relatives. Increasingly, detectable specific molecular defects allow presymptomatic testing, which should follow a procedure comparable to that for Huntington's disease.

FAMILIAL MULTI-INFARCT DEMENTIA ('CADASIL')

This rare, but probably under-recognized dominantly inherited disorder is due to mutations in a specific gene on chromosome 19q, homologous to the *Drosophila* gene known as 'Notch'.

PICK'S DISEASE (FRONTOTEMPORAL DEMENTIA)

This is much less clearly defined and understood in both clinical and pathological terms than is Alzheimer's disease, and genetic risks are poorly defined. The term frontotemporal dementia is now more generally used. As with Alzheimer's disease, only a small subset is likely to follow mendelian dominant inheritance, but in some of these, mutations have been recognized in the *tau* gene on chromosome 17.

PRION DEMENTIAS AND CREUTZFELDT–JAKOB DISEASE

The group of disorders comprising the prion dementias and Creutzfeldt–Jakob disease (CJD) is now recognized to be more common and to have a broader and more variable phenotype than was first thought. The late-onset but rapidly progressive dementia known as Creutzfeldt–Jakob disease is familial in around 15 per cent of cases, showing clear autosomal dominant inheritance in a small proportion of these. Mutations in the prion protein gene on chromosome 20 have been shown to be present in most of these rare families, as well as in some families in which cerebellar involvement predominates with a more protracted course (Gerstmann–Straussler syndrome). An unusual phenotype known as fatal familial insomnia has also proved to be due to a specific prion mutation. Other cases may be of a particular susceptible genotype, but no significant increase in risk to relatives of an isolated case exists unless a prion mutation is present. Analogy with scrapie in sheep (and human kuru) had suggested that human Creutzfeldt–Jakob disease might be mostly dietary in origin, a matter of considerable concern in relation to the recent UK epidemic of bovine spongiform encephalopathy (BSE). There is now clear evidence for this being responsible for the (so far) small number of 'new variant' CJD cases, but it seems unlikely that there is any dietary basis for CJD overall.

Testing for prion mutations is clearly important in the context of an unexplained familial dementia, but may have serious consequences. Widespread testing of all dementias for these mutations, as with those for Alzheimer's disease, would identify high genetic risks for families of some cases not thought to be familial, while testing of samples from relatives should only be done if specifically requested, and only then within a counselling framework comparable to that developed for Huntington's disease. Testing of healthy children is clearly unethical and relatives at risk should not be tested as part of a research study without specific consent.

MENTAL RETARDATION

Mental retardation has traditionally been divided into two principal categories:

- moderate or severe mental retardation (IQ 50 or less) – prevalence about 3 per 1000
- mild mental retardation (IQ 50–70) – prevalence about 30 per 1000.

All IQ levels above 70 are generally considered as part of the normal range. The importance of this division stems from the fact that mild mental retardation behaves genetically as the lower end of a normal distribution, so that the IQ levels in sibs or offspring are closely influenced by those of the parents (see below). By contrast, in severe mental retardation, parental intelligence is usually normal and a sharp discontinuity is seen between family members who are affected and the normal members, with little increase in mild retardation in between. It is also in severe mental retardation that specific causes are most likely to be found, whose accurate recognition is essential for genetic counselling.

SPECIFIC CAUSES OF MENTAL RETARDATION

The number of specific recognized disorders of which mental retardation is an integral or major component is exceedingly large and is growing steadily, a fact which makes it important to reassess individuals who have not received thorough recent investigation. Some of the disorders have been found to have a definite aetiological basis, which may be biochemical, chromosomal or environmental; in most cases the underlying cause remains unknown, but the occurrence of a constant series of physical abnormalities may allow the delineation of a clinical syndrome.

One major group of specific disorders needing to be recognized is that following mendelian inheritance, for it is here that the risks of recurrence in sibs are highest, particularly the autosomal recessive and X-linked recessive disorders. Table 13.3 lists some of the major causes; many are considered in more detail in other chapters.

Among the non-mendelian causes of mental retardation (Table 13.4), chromosomal disorders are particularly important to recognize (see Chapter 4). Almost all unbalanced autosomal disorders are associated with mental retardation; in older patients said previously to have been chromosomally normal, it is worth investigating further with the more sensitive banding techniques. Molecular analysis and in-situ hybridization are beginning to identify small, invisible deletions in some cases. Unless a parent also has a chromosomal rearrangement, the recurrence risk for such a disorder will be low, in particular those with syndromal features. Techniques of studying chromosome telomeres for submicroscopic rearrangements are proving of particular importance, identifying defects in around 5 per cent of cases.

If an environmental cause can be identified, recurrence is unlikely, provided that the harmful agent is not still operating. Care must be taken not to attribute mental retardation falsely to perinatal anoxia or other factors which may be the result of the underlying disorder rather than its cause.

The less constant association of mental retardation with a large number of specific physical disorders is of extreme importance in genetic counselling, since many couples who would accept the risk of physical handicap in an affected child are unwilling to accept the additional risk of mental handicap. Unfortunately, bias of ascertainment or reporting often makes the frequency of mental retardation in genetic disorders difficult to assess. Duchenne and myotonic dystrophies are examples where there is a true association, while in other situations where the association has been suggested (e.g. histidinaemia, X-linked ectodermal dysplasia), it is now considered unlikely.

SEVERE NON-SPECIFIC MENTAL RETARDATION

Despite the most careful study, close to half of severely mentally retarded children have no clear underlying causative factor or associated syndrome, and there is often no relevant pedigree information. Here one is forced to use the older general empiric recurrence risks (see *Genetics and Neurology* by Bundey, listed in 'Further reading', for details), even though many such cases are likely to prove in the future to have their own specific basis. Fortunately, a number of studies have been carried out with broadly similar results; the overall recurrence risk to sibs appears to be a little under 3 per cent (i.e. about 10 times

Table 13.3 Mendelian disorders causing or frequently associated with mental retardation

Autosomal dominant
Apert syndrome
Mandibulofacial dysostosis (not constant)
Myotonic dystrophy (particularly early-onset and congenital cases)
Neurofibromatosis type I (not constant)
Tuberous sclerosis

Autosomal recessive
Ataxia telangiectasia
Bardet–Biedl syndrome
Canavan's disease (spongy degeneration of white matter)
Carpenter's acrocephalopolysyndactyly
Galactosaemia
Homocystinuria
Marinesco–Sjögren syndrome
Microcephaly (some forms)
Mucopolysaccharidoses (types I, III)
Neurolipidoses (including Tay–Sachs, Gaucher's, metachromatic leucodystrophy and numerous others)
Phenylketonuria
Seckel syndrome
Sjögren–Larsson syndrome
Wilson's disease
Xeroderma pigmentosum (some forms)

X-linked
Alpha-thalassaemia X-linked mental retardation syndrome
Adrenoleucodystrophy
Cerebral sclerosis with Addison's disease
Cerebral sclerosis, Pelizaeus–Merzbacher type
Coffin–Lowry syndrome
Duchenne muscular dystrophy (not constant)
Fragile-X syndrome
Hunter syndrome (MPS II)
Incontinentia pigmentia (male lethal, X-linked dominant) some cases
Lesch–Nyhan syndrome
Lowe (oculocerebrorenal) syndrome
Menkes syndrome
Norrie's disease
Orofaciodigital syndrome type I (male-lethal, X-linked dominant) some cases
Rett syndrome (male-lethal, X-linked dominant)
X-linked aqueduct stenosis with associated anomalies, MASA syndrome
X-linked 'non-specific' mental retardation without fragile-X

Table 13.4 Non-mendelian and chromosomal syndromes associated with mental retardation

Major chromosomal abnormalities (see Chapter 4)
Down's syndrome
Other autosomal abnormalities (numerous)
XXY (Klinefelter) syndrome (variable)
XXX syndrome (and other multiple X)
XXXY syndrome
Hypomelanosis of Ito (mosaicism in some cases)

Chromosome microdeletions (*not in all cases*) (see Chapter 4)
Prader–Willi syndrome
Angelman syndrome
Rubinstein–Taybi syndrome (molecular deletions of locus on chromosome 16p)
Williams' (infantile hypercalcaemia) syndrome.

No consistent chromosomal defect detectable at present
(some may prove to result from new dominant mutations)
de Lange syndrome
Noonan syndrome
Sturge–Weber syndrome
Hallerman–Streiff syndrome
Hydrocephalus and hydranencephalus

Environmental factors (see Chapter 26)
Congenital infections (rubella, cytomegalovirus, *Toxoplasma*)
Teratogens (alcohol, phenytoin)
Anoxia
Brain damage associated with prematurity
Intrauterine growth retardation syndromes
Maternal phenylketonuria
Congenital hypothyroidism (heterogeneous)
Trauma (non-accidental)
Lead poisoning

the population risk). The somewhat higher risk to male sibs in some series probably results from a generally greater susceptibility of males as well as from inclusion of X-linked families (see below). Table 13.5 gives approximate risks suitable for counselling. These figures assume that a careful search has been made for the fragile-X syndrome. Exclusion of this disorder is essential, even in an isolated case of either sex, in view of its high frequency. Additional family information may modify the risk estimate. Thus consanguinity in the parents increases the likelihood of autosomal recessive inheritance, giving an empiric risk of 1 in 7 for sibs of such cases.

Where two affected sibs exist, a risk of close to 1 in 4 to future sibs is appropriate, regardless of sex, unless a pattern suggesting X linkage is present in previous generations.

Risks to offspring of affected individuals are not a significant problem in severe mental retardation; no estimate of risk can usually be deduced from the rare examples

Table 13.5 Genetic risks in severe 'non-specific' mental retardation (IQ 50 or less)

Affected	Individual at risk	Risk
Isolated case, male or female	Sib (both sexes)	I in 35
	Male sib	I in 25
	Female sib	I in 50
Two sibs, regardless of sex	Sib of either sex	I in 4
Isolated case, male or female, parents consanguineous	Sib of either sex	I in 7
Affected male with affected maternal uncle	Male sib	I in 2 (X linkage probable)
	Female sib	Low
One affected parent (either sex)	Child of either sex	I in 10
One affected parent, affected child	Child of either sex	I in 5
Two affected parents	Child of either sex	I in 2

of reproduction in such cases. The risk to second-degree relatives, i.e. the offspring of healthy individuals who have a mentally retarded sib or sibs, is a considerable worry to families. This is especially difficult to resolve where a healthy woman has a retarded brother or brothers, a situation in which the possibility of X-linked inheritance must be seriously considered. If a maternally related affected male is also present in a previous generation, this is strong support for X linkage. Where the affected individuals are females, or females and males, an X-linked recessive basis is less likely, and risks for second-degree relatives are small. Third-degree relatives are unlikely to be at significant risk unless the family pattern is clearly X-linked.

FRAGILE-X MENTAL RETARDATION

Fragile-X syndrome is a frequent cause of inherited mental retardation, with a frequency of around 1 in 5000 males (less than earlier estimates). Its recognition is crucial to genetic counselling and to the prevention of recurrence in mental retardation as a whole. The delineation of its clinical and genetic basis and the recognition of the underlying molecular defect represent advances of the greatest importance.

At a clinical level, the retardation varies from mild to severe in males and mild to moderate in females. Accelerated growth, characteristic facies and, in postpubertal males, macro-orchidism, are all valuable clinical signs. The visible chromosome fragile site consists of a constriction near the end of the long arm of the X chromosome (Xq27), with partial detachment of the distal portion.

The defect in this disorder is now known to be the result of expansion in a specific DNA triplet repeat (CGG) in a gene whose function is still unknown. The size of the expansion correlates with the degree of mental retardation and is usually progressive from one generation to the next. Thus males with a minimal expansion are mentally normal, but will transmit the mutation to their daughters, who will all be carriers, though again clinically normal. Their offspring have a high risk of mental retardation (Table 13.6), owing

Table 13.6 Fragile-X mental retardation

	Clinical features	Risk to children	Cytogenetic results	DNA results
Index cases (male of female)	Mental retardation and typical facies	Rarely reproduce	Fragile site present, frequent	Large DNA expansion
Normal transmitting male	Normal (but see text)	All daughters, carriers; sons normal	Fragile site not normally seen	Small expansion pre-mutation
Carrier daughters of normal transmitting male	Normal (but see text)	Around 75% of affected sons and 1/3 affected daughters	Fragile site absent or occasional	Small to moderate expansion (heterozygous)
Carrier sister of affected male	Variable; 1/3 retarded	All affected sons and half affected daughters retarded	Fragile site usually present	Moderate to large expansion (heterozygous)

to expansion of the DNA sequence, although some of their daughters will also be clinically normal carriers, and some sons will also be carriers. For those female carriers who have affected brothers, the sons inheriting the mutation (50 per cent) will almost all be retarded, as will half of those daughters who are heterozygous for the mutation.

This previously puzzling pattern of inheritance, particularly the normal male transmitters and the anticipation in successive generations, is satisfactorily explained by the expansion of the unstable sequence. At a practical level, it is now possible not only to give a more accurate range of risks, but also to offer specific molecular tests for carrier detection and prenatal diagnosis and for detecting the minimal mutation in chromosomally normal individuals. Cytogenetic analysis remains a useful primary diagnostic test in retarded patients, but has been superseded by molecular testing for carrier detection. It should be remembered that there are rare cases of fragile-X mental retardation due to different fragile sites (Frax E and F), and where molecular tests for the usual form (Frax A) will be normal.

The possibility now exists technically of using these advances in the general screening of mentally handicapped individuals, or even of the general population, raising important ethical issues, especially since many heterozygous females are only mildly retarded or in the normal range. Until further experience has been obtained, it seems preferable to concentrate on the complete identification of affected individuals and the offering of counselling and appropriate testing to their relatives.

A recently recognized complexity is that a proportion of male pre-mutation carriers appear to develop a late-onset neurodegeneration with ataxia, while some female pre-mutation carriers develop premature ovarian failure. This is still further reason against widespread screening for fragile X and must be carefully considered even when undertaking testing of relatives.

OTHER FORMS OF X-LINKED MENTAL RETARDATION

Apart from a number of well-defined syndromes (see Table 13.3), there are several forms of non-specific X-linked mental retardation that are distinct from the fragile-X disorder. Fortunately molecular and cytogenetic studies now allow this distinction to be made with confidence. Collectively, they are likely to account for around a third of the cases of X-linked mental retardation. Gene mapping suggests as many as 50 different loci, some of which have begun to be isolated.

RETT SYNDROME

Rett syndrome is a poorly understood disorder, almost exclusively affecting females and almost always sporadic in occurrence. It is characterized by deterioration of mental function after normal early development, with autistic behaviour and subsequently stereotypic hand movements; the course often levels out for some years. Other neurodegenerative disorders must be carefully excluded before the diagnosis is made. The condition is determined by an X-linked dominant gene, lethal in the male, but the recurrence risk is very low. A few males with X-linked mental handicap are now proving to show mutations in this gene as well.

OTHER DISTINCT GROUPS IN 'NON-SPECIFIC' MENTAL RETARDATION

In addition to families showing X-linked inheritance, there are other groups with sufficient distinguishing features to give risk figures different from those in Table 13.5. A particularly high risk is that of symmetrical spasticity with mental retardation; here the recurrence in sibs seems to be around 10 per cent. By contrast, the recurrence risk for other forms of cerebral palsy associated with mental retardation is low, although this should be restricted to cases with clear evidence of anoxia (see p. 186).

Another important low-risk subgroup is that of idiopathic infantile spasms. A similarly low risk has been found for mental retardation associated with slight microcephaly. This contrasts with the autosomal recessive inheritance of the specific type of severe microcephaly with normal facial structure (see Chapter 12).

MILD MENTAL RETARDATION

It has already been stated that in contrast to severe mental retardation, mild mental retardation behaves as part of the normal distribution of intelligence, as a polygenic trait. One or both parents are commonly retarded and the intelligence of future children will be distributed between the mid-parental and general population mean. Correspondingly, the risk of an intelligent couple having a further mildly retarded child is low.

Nevertheless, a careful search should be made for specific causes that may underlie mild mental retardation and which, if found, may radically alter the genetic risks. The heterozygous state for the fragile-X syndrome should be considered in females, especially if there is a history of more severely retarded male relatives.

NORMAL INTELLIGENCE

When faced with an enquiry about the inheritance of normal intelligence, the initial reaction of the physician, daily seeing patients with inherited causes of severe mental and physical handicap, is to tell parents to be content with the fact that their child is normal. Nevertheless, intelligence is undeniably an attribute of the highest importance and is not so completely under the control of the environment as some would wish to believe. The following general comments may be helpful if answering questions about families:

- The mating pattern is highly assortative for intelligence, i.e. intelligent people tend to marry each other, as do the less intelligent.
- On average, the intelligence of a child is likely to be intermediate between that of the parents and the general population mean, with a considerable scatter around this.
- It is possible for the intelligence of a child to be outside the range between the parental IQ levels; the greater the departure from the mid-parental point, the less likely this will be.
- Too much reliance should not be placed on the results of single IQ tests, especially in early childhood. (One of the author's patients with Marfan syndrome, initially investigated in infancy for 'mental retardation', later studied astrophysics after winning scholarships to three separate universities!)

Current research attempts to identify specific genes involved in normal IQ do not seem, in the author's view, to have given proper consideration to the important societal issues involved and should only be pursued with public awareness and support. Perhaps fortunately, it seems likely that any genes involved will contribute only very small amounts individually to the variance, making it improbable that genetic testing will prove meaningful at an individual level.

BEHAVIOURAL DISORDERS

Under the heading of behavioural disorders are grouped various abnormalities that cannot be regarded as diseases, but which may result in considerable functional disability. While long recognized as being frequently familial, studies to localize the genes are in progress, in relation both to the disorders and to normal function.

This, like the genetics of IQ, is a highly sensitive area, something which not all research workers in the field appear to appreciate. The social stigma often involved and the tendency for entrenched attitudes regarding the role of environmental and genetic factors add to the difficulties. At present, genetic counselling is rarely requested, but this could change if genetic tests become feasible, something that will present society, as well as professionals, with difficult issues. Any suggestions that specific genes identified in this group should be used for prediction or diagnosis should be viewed critically and with the greatest caution. This applies also to possible forensic applications (see p. 141). Perhaps fortunately, the genetic basis of common behavioural disorders is proving to be much more complex than previously anticipated and no genetic tests seem likely for the immediate future. A further complexity relevant to genetic counselling is the increasing tendency to 'medicalize' the field by giving diagnostic labels to phenotypes that probably have a largely social basis.

DYSLEXIA (SPECIFIC READING DISABILITY)

A careful family study suggests that, if minor degrees are included, dyslexia may often be transmitted as a variable autosomal dominant trait. No clear molecular basis has yet been identified outside occasional unusual families.

AUTISM

This puzzling and undoubtedly heterogeneous condition requires considerable care in genetic counselling and should be regarded more as a label than a diagnosis. It is essential to exclude specific developmental disorders, including minor chromosome anomalies and fragile-X syndrome. Even though there is no clear mendelian pattern, there is a considerable familial component, as judged from twin and family studies, with a significant (around 5 per cent) recurrence risk for sibs of isolated cases. When onset is abrupt and there are no associated dysmorphic features, a higher sib risk has been suggested, especially for males.

TOURETTE SYNDROME

Tourette syndrome, characterized by a childhood onset of motor and vocal tics, often with behavioural abnormalities, usually runs a fluctuating course and may be determined by a major autosomal dominant gene in some families. The fact that this has not yet been localized, despite extensive study, may reflect inadequate definition of the phenotype and over-diagnosis of the condition.

ALCOHOLISM

Distinguishing environmental and genetic components of the familial tendency to alcoholism is particularly difficult. There is no consensus as to whether a separate genetic subtype exists or whether inherited biochemical variation in alcohol metabolism is relevant.

MAJOR PSYCHIATRIC ILLNESS

Two disorders, schizophrenia and affective disorder (which includes manic-depressive illness or bipolar affective disorder and unipolar disorder with episodes of depression only), account for a considerable proportion of all serious mental illness. They are not only extremely disabling and distressing conditions, often in young people, but also result in a major burden for the community in terms of long-term care. A considerable body of genetic research has been developed over several decades, utilizing carefully planned twin and adoption studies as well as family data. Diagnostic criteria have been standardized to overcome inevitable difficulties of interpretation, while quantitative genetic analysis has been developed to circumvent the lack of any clear mendelian inheritance pattern.

The result of this painstaking research is that for both schizophrenia and manic-depressive illness, a strong familial and genetic basis is clear, but a mendelian basis is not. Biochemical and neurophysiological studies have not provided any clear primary factors either, so it is not surprising that psychiatric geneticists turned to DNA markers as a way of finding specific genetic loci. Unfortunately, early claims of success for both disorders needed to be withdrawn, a salutary lesson for all concerned that molecular methods are no panacea and should be approached (like other new technologies) critically and with scepticism. Large collaborative studies in progress stand a good chance in time of identifying relevant specific genes. Current evidence, at least for schizophrenia, suggests a considerable number of small genetic effects, rather than a few major genes, making it unlikely that the old empiric risks will be superseded by molecular approaches in the foreseeable future.

SCHIZOPHRENIA

When strict diagnostic criteria are used, the risk of anyone developing schizophrenia during their lifetime is close to 1 per cent.

The seriousness of the disease and its high prevalence make schizophrenia a major genetic counselling problem. Numerous surveys have been done on the risks to relatives, and Table 13.7 gives approximate risk figures. It can be seen that the risks are

Table 13.7 Genetic risks (approximate) in schizophrenia and manic-depressive illness

Affected relative	Risk (%)	
	Schizophrenia	Manic-depressive illness
No close family history (general population risk)	1	2–3
Sib	9	13
Parent	13	15
Sib and one parent	15	20
Both parents	45	50
Second-degree relative	3	5
Monozygotic twin	40	70
Dizygotic twin	10	20
First cousin	1–2	2–3

considerable for all first-degree relatives. Several additional points need to be considered in counselling:

- Much of the genetic risk, especially for schizophrenia, is for the early part of life, so that the remaining risk for older relatives is considerably less than the figures given here.
- In addition to the occurrence of classic schizophrenia in relatives, there is an increased frequency of less florid psychiatric states of doubtful classification (so-called schizophrenia-spectrum disorders).
- There is a slight increase of schizophrenia in the sibs of patients with other types of psychosis, but in general, schizophrenia appears to be genetically distinct, particularly when diagnostic difficulties are allowed for.
- Care must be taken to exclude other primary disorders which may present with features suggestive of schizophrenia and which may follow mendelian inheritance, e.g. homocystinuria, Huntington's disease.

Adoption studies in a number of countries have shown an incidence in adoptive children close to that predicted from their natural parents rather than their adoptive parents. This not only suggests that the familial nature of the disorder is predominantly genetic in origin, but is also of direct importance in advising potential adoptive parents. Of particular interest is the observation that where a monozygotic co-twin is unaffected, the risk for offspring is as high as in offspring of the affected twin, whereas this is not the case for offspring of unaffected dizygotic co-twins.

AFFECTIVE PSYCHOSES

Affective psychoses, like schizophrenia, represent a major problem in the community. The expectation of developing a major manic-depressive psychosis in a person's lifetime is around 1 per cent, but if milder depressive states are included, the figure may be as high as 5 per cent. There seems to be a genetic distinction among affective disorders between those that are unipolar, i.e. characterized by recurrent episodes of depression only, and those that are bipolar, i.e. characterized by alternating mania and depression (manic-depressive disorder) or more rarely by hypomania and mania alone. The risk to relatives also appears to be higher where the proband has early onset than when the onset is later (over 40 years).

Table 13.7 summarizes the main risk categories. It should be stressed that different surveys have given a wide range of estimates. Where age at onset in the proband is known, the risk to first-degree relatives should probably be increased to 20 per cent when onset was under 40 years, and reduced to 10 per cent when onset was over 40 years.

Adoption studies, as in schizophrenia, have shown risks for adoptive children corresponding to their natural parents rather than their adoptive parents.

Involvement of X-linked dominant genes in bipolar affective illness has been suggested from the overall female excess and from the inheritance pattern in some large families, but any general linkage with X chromosome markers has now been excluded. No specific major genes have yet been isolated, although certain chromosomal regions seem to be particularly involved.

FURTHER READING

Baker HF, Ridley RM (1996). *Prion Diseases*. New Jersey, Humana Press.

Baraitser M (1997). *The Genetics of Neurological Disorders*. Oxford, Oxford University Press.

Bundey S (1992). *Genetics and Neurology*. Edinburgh, Churchill Livingstone – the sections on mental handicap and its underlying causes are still valuable.

Fisch GS (ed.) (2002). *Genetics and Genomics of Neurobehavioral Disorders*. Totowa, NJ, Humana Press.

Hagerman RJ, Hagerman PJ (eds) (2002). *Fragile X Syndrome: Diagnosis, Treatment and Research*. Baltimore, Johns Hopkins University Press.

McGuffin P, Owen MJ, Farmer AE (1995). Genetic basis of schizophrenia. *Lancet* **346**, 678–682.

McGuffin P, Owen MJ, Gottesman II (2002). *Psychiatric Genetics and Genomics*. Oxford, Oxford University Press.

Nuffield Council on Bioethics (1998). *Mental Disorders and Genetics: the Ethical Context*. London, Nuffield Council on Bioethics.

Nuffield Council on Bioethics (2002). *Genetics and Human Behaviour: the Ethical Context*. London, Nuffield Council on Bioethics.

Piven J (1997). The biological basis of autism. *Curr Opin Neurobiol* **7**, 708–712.

Plomin R, Defries JC, McClearn GE, Rutter M (1997). *Behavioural Genetics*. New York, Freeman.

CHAPTER 14

Disorders of bone and connective tissue

PRIMARY BONE DYSPLASIAS

Genetic counselling in the confusing group of primary bone dysplasias requires special care. Full radiographic and clinical assessments are essential for a firm diagnosis to be reached; even so, many cases remain undiagnosed. In such a situation, one must be guided by the pedigree pattern of the individual family. Most types follow mendelian inheritance, but for an isolated case it is often impossible to distinguish between a new dominant mutation and autosomal recessive inheritance. Few clinicians see many cases of bone dysplasia, so it is unreasonable to expect familiarity with every type. Pooling experience is of great help; the author has had fruitful associations with bone dysplasia groups in different centres involving radiologists, orthopaedic surgeons and paediatricians, as well as geneticists, and there is no doubt that the discussion of problem cases at such meetings has allowed accurate diagnosis and genetic counselling that would not have been possible otherwise.

A special effort should be made to obtain photographic and X-ray evidence on all skeletal dysplasias, particularly stillbirths. It is both surprising and frustrating how often such vital diagnostic information is not obtained or, in the case of radiographs, is destroyed by hospitals. New computerized techniques of storing X-ray images should help to preserve them. Even old family photographs can be of great value in the case of members no longer living. New X-ray investigations should be requested sparingly and selectively, with appropriate gonadal shielding to minimize the mutational load involved. Geneticists have a special responsibility to set an example in this.

Individuals with different (or even the same) forms of dwarfism commonly marry each other, with confusing results in the offspring. Interaction of the genes is to be expected only if the disorders are allelic. The birth of a child of normal stature to such a couple may be unexpected and even pose a difficult problem for them. Many such couples are anxious to adopt children who are also of short stature, and this should be facilitated. Obstetric difficulties in women owing to a small pelvis must not be forgotten.

Ultrasonographic prenatal diagnosis is feasible for a number of the severe neonatal bone dysplasias, especially those with limb shortening, although it can be misleading if used in situations of low prior risk. Specific genes have now been identified for many of the major forms of bone dysplasia, notably those due to collagen mutations, but also mutations in important developmental genes.

Table 14.1 summarizes the inheritance of some of the major types of bone dysplasia and indicates specific gene defects where these have been recognized. More information is available in the 'Further reading' section; a valuable general review is given by Rimoin and Lachman (1993), while various atlases (notably those of Spranger et al., 2003, and Wynne-Davies et al., 1985) show the radiological and clinical features. The book by Gorlin et al. (2001) is especially valuable for disorders with craniofacial involvement. Some specific disorders are mentioned below.

ACHONDROPLASIA

A diagnosis of achondroplasia should never be accepted without checking. True achondroplasia rarely causes problems in neonatal life, although it can be recognized at birth; most fatal cases of 'achondroplasia' are other dysplasias. Inheritance is invariably autosomal dominant, but around 80 per cent of cases are new mutations, with minimal recurrence risk for future sibs (although gonadal mosaicism has been recorded). Homozygous achondroplasia occurs in 1 in 4 of the children of two achondroplastic parents and is lethal soon after birth. Another 1 in 4 of the children of such couples are normal.

The milder disorder, **hypochondroplasia**, is allelic to achondroplasia; 'compounds' have been recorded when one parent has achondroplasia and the other hypochondroplasia. Although most patients with hypochondroplasia have few physical problems and are mentally entirely normal, a small number of cases with mental retardation have been reported.

A specific molecular defect in one of the fibroblast growth receptors (FGFR3) has now been identified in achondroplasia that allows diagnostic confirmation. The same receptor (but a different mutation) is now known to be involved in hypochondroplasia and also in the severe thanatophoric dysplasia.

PSEUDOACHONDROPLASIA

Most cases of pseudoachondroplasia are autosomal dominant. Multiple affected sibs with normal parents may more often be the result of mosaicism than of recessive inheritance. For an isolated case with typical features and no consanguinity, the risk to offspring is close to 50 per cent, while the risk to sibs is low (around 3 per cent). Molecular defects have been found in the collagen-associated protein COMP5.

Table 14.1 Inheritance of major bone dysplasias (see also Table 14.2)

Autosomal dominant
Achondroplasia **FGFR3**
Hypochondroplasia **FGFR3**
Pseudoachondroplasia **COMP5**
Dyschondrosteosis **SHOX**
Osteopoikilosis
Spondyloepiphyseal dysplasia congenita **COL2A1**
Multiple epiphyseal dysplasia **COL9A2; COMP5**
Metaphyseal dysplasia, Schmidt type **COL10A1**
Congenital bowing (Blount's disease)
Craniometaphyseal dysplasia (also AR)
Craniocarpotarsal dysplasia (Freeman–Sheldon syndrome)
Cleidocranial dysplasia **CBFA1**
Diaphyseal aclasis (multiple hereditary exostoses) **EXT 1,2,3**
Progressive diaphyseal dysplasia (also AR)
Nail–patella syndrome **LMX1**
Fibrodysplasia ossificans progressiva (myositis ossificans)
Trichorhinophalangeal dysplasia
Kniest syndrome **COL2A1**
Familial expansile osteolysis

Autosomal recessive
Diastrophic dwarfism **DTST** (sulphate transporter)
Metatropic dwarfism
Sclerosteosis
Pycnodysostosis (cathepsin C)
Van Buchem's disease (most families)
Cartilage hair hypoplasia **RMLP**
Chondro-ectodermal dysplasia (Ellis–van Creveld) **EVC**
Ollier's osteochondromatosis
Jeune thoracic dysplasia
Hypophosphatasia (infantile)
Mucopolysaccharidoses (except type II) (see text)
Weill–Marchesani syndrome

X-linked
Spondyloepiphyseal dysplasia tarda (recessive)
Orofaciodigital dysplasia, type I (dominant, lethal in male)
Vitamin D-resistant rickets (intermediate) **PEX**
Mucopolysaccharidosis II (recessive)
Otopalatodigital syndrome (probably intermediate)
Chondrodysplasia punctata (separate dominant and recessive types)

Variable or uncertain
Russell–Silver syndrome (mostly sporadic). Some cases due to uniparental disomy
De Lange syndrome (risk to sibs around 2%)
Caffey's infantile cortical hyperostosis
Albright's fibrous dysplasia (almost always sporadic)
Paget's disease (probably autosomal dominant with incomplete penetrance)
Melorheostosis (usually sporadic)

Bold type indicates molecular defect, where known.

SPONDYLOEPIPHYSEAL AND SPONDYLOMETAPHYSEAL DYSPLASIAS

The group of spondyloepiphyseal and spondylometaphyseal dysplasias is particularly variable clinically. Most are autosomal dominant, and isolated cases should be considered as dominant, since cases of affected sibs with normal parents, previously thought to be recessive, have transmitted the disorder, probably representing gonadal mosaicism. Defects in type II collagen have been found in some families. The X-linked 'tarda' form should be clearly recognizable, even in an isolated case, by the characteristic radiographic appearance of the spine, with a central 'hump' of bone and relatively normal distal limb bones.

The severe spondyloepiphyseal dysplasia congenita is frequently confused with Morquio syndrome (mucopolysaccharidosis IV) and usually follows autosomal dominant inheritance. Retinal detachment is an important complication.

DYSCHONDROSTEOSIS AND MADELUNG'S DEFORMITY

Most cases of Madelung's deformity of the wrist are part of the mild but generalized dysplasia, dyschondrosteosis, following autosomal dominant inheritance, and due to a specific developmental gene mutation (SHOX). A severe dysplasia may result from homozygosity in the children of two affected parents.

MULTIPLE EPIPHYSEAL DYSPLASIA

Mildly affected individuals may have only moderately reduced stature and the pattern of autosomal dominant inheritance characteristic of most families may be missed as a result. This disorder must be excluded when giving genetic advice to patients with bilateral Perthes' disease. Two specific gene loci have been identified, those for collagen type 9 and the glycoprotein COMP5.

CHONDRODYSPLASIA PUNCTATA (CONRADI'S DISEASE)

Cataract, mental retardation and ichthyosis may all occur. Both autosomal dominant and recessive forms exist (the latter more severe and due to a peroxisomal defect); X-linked inheritance, both dominant and recessive, occurs occasionally. A phenocopy is also produced by maternal warfarin ingestion in early pregnancy and must be excluded before a genetic basis is assumed.

LETHAL NEWBORN DYSPLASIAS

The major causes of lethal newborn dysplasia are listed in Table 14.2. Some are invariably fatal, others not so. Sensitive ultrasound scanning is now of real help in prenatal

Table 14.2 Frequently lethal newborn bone dysplasias

Type	Inheritance
Thanatophoric dwarfism	Usually sporadic; new dominant mutations in *FGFR3*
Achondrogenesis	
Type 1	Autosomal recessive; defects in *DTST*
Type 2	New dominant mutation in type II collagen
Ellis–van Creveld syndrome	Autosomal recessive
Thoracic dysplasia (Jeune)	Autosomal recessive
Majewski and other short rib polydactyly syndromes	Autosomal recessive
Chondrodysplasia punctata	Usually autosomal recessive when severe (but see text)
Metatropic dwarfism	Autosomal recessive
Hypophosphatasia (severe type)	Autosomal recessive
Osteogenesis imperfecta congenita	Usually autosomal dominant (but see p. 217)
Campomelic dysplasia	Mostly new dominant mutations; chromosome analysis needed (some females are XY); mutations of *SOX9* gene in some families
Spondylothoracic dysplasia (Jarcho–Levin)	Autosomal recessive, but heterogeneous; mutations in *DLL3*

diagnosis for this group; serial measurements are of particular value. Radiographs should always be taken of a stillbirth suspected of falling in this group because specific diagnosis may otherwise be impossible. Osteogenesis imperfecta congenita can be easily mistaken for a lethal newborn dysplasia. Although a number of disorders in this group follow autosomal recessive inheritance, the most common, thanatophoric dwarfism, is usually sporadic and shows mutations in the fibroblast growth factor gene *FGFR3* (also involved in achondroplasia). Heterogeneity or mosaicism may well be responsible for the few recurrent cases that have occurred.

OSTEOPETROSIS

A number of conditions are characterized by increased bone density, including pycnodysostosis, sclerosteosis and van Buchem's disease, but true osteopetrosis exists in two forms:

- a mild form, often asymptomatic, following autosomal dominant inheritance
- a severe childhood form with bone marrow involvement, which is autosomal recessive – a specific gene has been identified for this type.

MULTIPLE EXOSTOSES (DIAPHYSEAL ACLASIS)

The inheritance of multiple exostoses follows a classical autosomal dominant pattern, although some individuals have only a few lesions which may not be symptomatic. It may form part of the Langer–Giedion syndrome (microdeletion of chromosome 8q), with mental retardation and features of trichophalangeal dysplasia. Specific genes on chromosomes 8 and 11 have now been isolated. By contrast, enchondromatosis (Ollier's disease) is rarely transmitted to children and is of uncertain inheritance.

LIMB DEFECTS

It is impossible to deal with all the different types here; the books listed under 'Further reading' should be consulted for details. A high proportion of bilateral abnormalities follow mendelian inheritance; many form part of more general syndromes, some of which are summarized in Table 14.3. Unilateral defects, by contrast, are usually non-genetic. Where the recurrence risk is high, sensitive ultrasonography allows prenatal diagnosis of the more severe defects (see Chapter 8). Limb defects are currently receiving much study to identify the specific developmental genes involved, something which is becoming feasible by a combination of molecular techniques and the recognition of homologous mouse models. (See Chapter 6 and its further reading.)

POLYDACTYLY

Isolated postaxial polydactyly is a harmless but common (especially in African populations) autosomal dominant condition, showing incomplete penetrance.

Important conditions with polydactyly include trisomy 13, Ellis–van Creveld and Jeune syndromes and the Bardet–Biedl (Laurence–Moon–Biedl) syndrome.

SYNDACTYLY

Poland syndrome of unilateral syndactyly and pectoral muscle aplasia is an important form to recognize because it appears to be non-genetic in the great majority of cases, possibly vascular in aetiology. Previous suggestions of an epidemiological link with ergot abortifacients have not been confirmed. Bilateral isolated syndactyly of hands and/or feet has several forms, all autosomal dominant. Important syndromes include the orofaciodigital syndrome type I (X-linked dominant, lethal in the male) and the acrocephalosyndactylies (see Chapter 15). The extreme fusion defect of the lower limbs, sirenomelia, is sporadic.

BRACHYDACTYLY

Various distinct types of brachydactyly exist. Inheritance is generally autosomal dominant. Syndrome associations include Albright's hereditary osteodystrophy or

Table 14.3 Syndromes involving limb defects

Syndrome	Inheritance
Polydactyly	
Trisomy 13	Usually sporadic
Ellis–van Creveld syndrome	AR
Jeune thoracic dystrophy	AR
Bardet–Biedl syndrome	AR
Meckel syndrome	AR
Carpenter syndrome	AR
Greig syndrome	AD
Acrocallosal syndrome	AR
Syndactyly	
Poland syndrome	Usually sporadic
Apert syndrome	AD (see Chapter 15)
Other craniosynostosis syndromes	Mostly AD
Orofaciodigital syndrome	XD (male lethal) most common (see Chapter 15)
Brachydactyly	
Albright's hereditary osteodystrophy	AD
Turner syndrome	Usually sporadic
Limb reduction defects	
Thalidomide embryopathy	Non-genetic
Roberts syndrome	AR
Thrombocytopenia–absent radius syndrome	AR
Fanconi pancytopenia	AR
Amniotic bands	Usually sporadic
Holt–Oram syndrome	AD
VATER syndrome	Uncertain
Ectrodactyly	
EEC syndrome	AD

AD, autosomal dominant; AR, autosomal recessive; XD, X-linked dominant.

pseudohypoparathyroidism (variable autosomal dominant, previously thought to be X-linked), and Turner syndrome.

ECTRODACTYLY (SPLIT HAND OR LOBSTER-CLAW DEFECT)

Most isolated bilateral cases of ectrodactyly follow autosomal dominant inheritance. A number of families exist in which multiple affected sibs born to healthy parents have gone on to have affected children themselves. Autosomal recessive inheritance and lack of penetrance seem unsatisfactory explanations and it is likely that germinal mosaicism is operating (see Chapter 2). This means that affected individuals have a high risk of having affected children even if the family pattern does appear to be autosomal recessive. An important syndrome to recognize is the EEC (ectrodactyly ectodermal dysplasia, cleft lip and palate) syndrome, also autosomal dominant.

LIMB REDUCTION DEFECTS

Limb reduction defects may be extremely difficult to distinguish. Some, in particular asymmetrical amputation defects associated with 'amniotic constriction bands', are likely to be non-genetic. Other asymmetrical defects may be associated with oesophageal, anal, cardiac, renal and vertebral abnormalities (the VATER association); again, the recurrence risk is low. Thalidomide was previously a major cause, but no other definite drug-induced defects of this type are known. Claims of association with other drugs are not convincing. The severe symmetrical limb reduction disorder, Roberts syndrome, which shows a characteristic abnormality of chromosomal division, is autosomal recessive. Limb changes in Holt–Oram syndrome (autosomal dominant) are identical to those caused by thalidomide, and may occur without accompanying cardiac defect. The specific gene has now been isolated.

Fanconi pancytopenia and the thrombocytopenia–absent radius (TAR) syndrome (both autosomal recessive) are important generalized syndromes to recognize and to distinguish from each other. The thumb is usually involved in the former, but preserved in the latter.

CONNECTIVE TISSUE DISORDERS

Collagen has always been recognized as fundamental to inherited connective tissue disorders, but it is only recently, with identification of the numerous and often tissue-specific forms of collagen and their genes, that individual diseases can be matched up with particular collagen defects (Table 14.4).

OSTEOGENESIS IMPERFECTA

Many cases of osteogenesis imperfecta are now recognized as defects in type I collagen, whose helix is determined by two separate genetic loci. Although there may be some correlation between phenotype and the type and site of mutation, this is not clear-cut. Unfortunately, this, together with the very wide range of mutations, means that molecular analysis is not regularly available in diagnosis, which remains clinically and radiologically based.

Type I (previously 'tarda')

The great majority of 'classic' non-lethal cases are type I, which varies greatly within and between families and follows autosomal dominant inheritance. Sclerae are usually blue,

Table 14.4 Molecular basis of bone dysplasias and connective tissue disorders

Molecule	Principal site	Disorders
Collagen I (A1 and 2)	Bone	Osteogenesis imperfecta (various types)
		Ehlers–Danlos syndrome (some types)
Collagen II (A1)	Cartilage	Spondyloepiphyseal dysplasias
		Stickler syndrome
		Kniest dysplasia
		Premature osteoarthrosis
		Achondrogenesis type 2
Collagen III	Vascular	Ehlers–Danlos syndrome, arteriopathic
		type (IV)
		Familial aneurysms(?)
Collagen IV	Basement membrane	Alport syndrome (see Chapter 21)
Collagen VII	Skin (see Chapter 16)	Epidermolysis bullosa (one dystrophic form)
Collagen IX		Multiple epiphyseal dysplasia (some families);
		pseudoachondroplasia (some families)
Fibrillin	Vascular; eye	Marfan syndrome
COMP5 glycoprotein	Cartilage	Multiple epiphyseal dysplasia (some families);
		pseudoachondroplasia (some families)

and deafness and osteoporosis may occur in later life, while the number of fractures is extremely variable. Linkage with either of the two type I collagen loci makes application difficult outside large families, unless a specific mutation can be identified. The occasional occurrence of germinal mosaicism means that there is a small risk (around 1 per cent) for sibs of an apparently new mutation case.

Type II

Although the terms 'perinatal lethal' and 'congenita' have been applied to this group, they are not fully accurate. Several subtypes can be distinguished by careful radiological examination:

- *Type IIa* – causes stillbirth or is lethal in the neonatal period, with limb shortening and multiple intrauterine fractures; X-ray shows beaded ribs. Recurrence risk is very low (under 2 per cent) and most cases are due to new dominant mutations in type I collagen, some of which can be recognized by molecular studies
- *Types IIb, IIc* – in these rare types neither long bones nor ribs are thickened. Although mostly due to new dominant mutations, these groups contain recessively inherited forms and the empiric recurrence risks are higher (probably around 10 per cent, but 25 per cent if consanguinity is present); careful discussion with an expert radiologist is needed.

Where no X-ray evidence is available in a perinatally lethal case, the empiric recurrence risk in a thorough survey was found to be around 4 per cent. Recessive forms are definitely a minority in all subgroups; molecular evidence shows that some recurring cases may be the result of germinal mosaicism.

Type III (severe deforming type)

Type III may be difficult to separate from type II in the newborn period, and the distinction may prove artificial. The empiric recurrence risk is around 7 per cent.

Type IV

The term 'type IV' is sometimes applied to severe dominantly inherited forms, but it is doubtful whether this is really separate from type I.

MARFAN SYNDROME

Marfan syndrome is an important disorder now known to be due to deficiency of the connective tissue protein fibrillin, determined by a gene on chromosome 15. This disorder tends to be overdiagnosed in tall individuals of slender habitus but with no cardinal signs, especially rapidly growing adolescents. There is rarely doubt when the presence or absence of the various major features is considered as a whole. Inheritance is autosomal dominant; the occurrence of major aortic complications is unpredictable and many patients live a relatively normal life until aortic surgery is needed or a sudden demise occurs, although others may have severe early orthopaedic and cardiac problems. Around 15 per cent of all patients appear to be new mutations. Penetrance is probably full but apparently healthy family members should be carefully checked (including slit-lamp examination for minor degree of lens dislocation). The isolation of the gene, and recognition of specific mutations in some cases, now gives the possibility of definitive molecular exclusion or confirmation, at least in larger families, as well as prenatal diagnosis if requested. The primary diagnosis remains clinical, however, and if a composite scoring system is used, most cases can be clearly confirmed or excluded. Other disorders to be distinguished include homocystinuria (autosomal recessive), patients with isolated lens dislocation due to spherophakia, who by chance are tall and thin, and neuromuscular disorders giving a 'marfanoid' habitus. A separate dominant syndrome of arachnodactyly with contractures but no internal complications (Beal syndrome) has also been described and appears to be due to a separate form of fibrillin deficiency involving a locus on chromosome 5.

EHLERS–DANLOS SYNDROME

The Ehlers–Danlos group of disorders in which hypermobility of skin and joints, skin fragility and bruising, and rarer vascular, visceral and ocular complications are the main features is extremely heterogeneous. It is important not to confuse the group with the much commoner and essentially harmless benign familial joint hypermobility (also often dominantly inherited). The classification has recently been simplified (Table 14.5). Autosomal dominant inheritance is much the most common. Pregnancy may be dangerous in

Table 14.5 Ehlers–Danlos syndromes

Type	Old classification	Inheritance	Molecular defect
Classical	I and 2	AD	Collagen 5 A1 and 2
Hypermobile	3	AD	–
Vascular	4	AD	Collagen 3 A1
Kyphoscoliotic	6	AR	Lysyl hydroxylase
Arthrochalasia	7	AD	Collagen 1 A1 and 2

the severe forms. The vascular (type 4) form, although rare, is particularly important to recognize on account of the risks of bowel and arterial rupture and aneurysm formation. It results from defects in type III collagen. Other collagen abnormalities are being identified in different forms.

CUTIS LAXA

Cutis laxa may follow autosomal recessive or autosomal dominant inheritance and is even X-linked in a few families, so a high risk for offspring of an isolated case cannot be excluded. Elastin mutations have now been found in some cases.

PSEUDOXANTHOMA ELASTICUM

Most cases of pseudoxanthoma elasticum follow autosomal recessive inheritance, but a few dominantly inherited families have been described, mostly with milder clinical features. Asymptomatic individuals may be detected by the presence of angioid streaks in the retina. Identification of a specific gene should help to clarify the relationship of the different forms.

MUCOPOLYSACCHARIDOSES

All types of mucopolysaccharidoses (Table 14.6) follow autosomal recessive inheritance except for the X-linked type II (Hunter syndrome). The enzymatic basis of the major types is well defined and should be established together with mutation testing where possible, to allow appropriate prenatal diagnosis, which is feasible for all types.

The Hurler and Scheie types are alleles, as are the mild and severe forms of Hunter syndrome. In each case, the two forms run separately in families. Occasional cases intermediate between Hurler and Scheie types probably represent a 'genetic compound' with one allele of each type. The related mucolipidoses are all autosomal recessive in inheritance. Several other rare autosomal recessive lysosomal storage disorders can cause clinical confusion, including mannosidosis, sialidosis and fucosidosis. A detailed account of the individual disorders in this group is given in Scriver *et al.* (see 'Further reading', Chapter 23).

Table 14.6 The mucopolysaccharidoses

Type	Deficient enzyme and inheritance

I(H) Hurler
    Severe course, corneal clouding,
    neurodegeneration
I(S) Scheie
    Mild course, corneal clouding, no
    neurodegeneration, adult survival
	Alpha-iduronidase (autosomal recessive)

II Hunter
    (a) Severe; early onset with
        neurodegeneration
    (b) Mild; late onset, no neurodegeneration;
        skeletal and cardiac problems
	Iduronate sulphatase (X-linked recessive)

III Sanfilippo
    Severe neurodegeneration; less
    severe physical changes; cornea clear;
    several biochemical types not clinically
    distinguishable
	(a) Heparan sulphate sulphatase
	    (autosomal recessive)
	(b) N-Acetyl glucosaminidase
	    (autosomal recessive)

IV Morquio
    Severe spine involvement with dwarfing;
    no neurodegeneration
	Galactosamine sulphate sulphatase (most
	families) (autosomal recessive)

VI Maroteaux–Lamy
    Severe physical course, corneal clouding;
    no neurodegeneration
	Aryl sulphatase (autosomal recessive)

VII Beta-glucuronidase deficiency Physical and mental changes; variable	Beta-glucuronidase (autosomal recessive)

Risks for offspring of healthy sibs are very small except in the X-linked Hunter syndrome, where identification of female carriers is of great importance. Combined enzyme analysis of serum and hair bulbs was used in the past for this but was not fully accurate. Isolation of the gene and recognition of frequent deletions and specific mutations now make DNA analysis the definitive test. In prenatal diagnosis of the various types, amniotic fluid mucopolysaccharide analysis appears to be an accurate and rapid test to complement specific enzyme assay. DNA analysis is likely to be increasingly used in both type I and type II when the specific mutation is known.

ARTHRITIS AND ARTHROPATHIES

The common arthritic disorders are mostly non-mendelian and recurrence risks are relatively low for close relatives, though not well defined. Disorders with an immunological or vasculitic basis often show clear HLA associations, but not of a strength useful in genetic counselling. In some rare forms, abnormalities have been found in type II collagen, which is mainly found in cartilage.

ANKYLOSING SPONDYLITIS

Discovery of the striking association with HLA-B27 has revealed this – or some closely linked gene within the HLA region – to be probably the main genetic determinant in susceptibility, although genetic risks are not high. One family study showed a risk of 5 per cent (7 per cent for males and 2 per cent for females) for clinical disease in first-degree relatives of patients with ankylosing spondylitis. Sixteen per cent showed radiological sacroiliitis. The chance of a B27 child of a B27 patient developing clinical ankylosing spondylitis is 9 per cent, compared with a risk of less than 1 per cent for offspring without this antigen.

The clinical or genetic applications of HLA-B27 testing are actually of very limited value (see Chapter 3 and 'Further reading' to this chapter), since most B27-positive individuals, whether or not there is a family history of ankylosing spondylitis, will not develop clinical features of the disorder, though a B27-negative result will make the diagnosis or future development of the disorder very unlikely. These limitations are a good example of why 'susceptibility testing' for common diseases is generally of little help in genetic counselling.

RHEUMATOID ARTHRITIS

This common disorder (around 1 per cent in most populations) rarely follows a mendelian pattern and the risks of clinical rheumatoid arthritis to relatives are not high; they appear to be around 3–5 per cent for first-degree relatives, although the incidence of radiological abnormalities is considerably higher. As might be expected with multifactorial inheritance (see Chapter 3), the risk appears to be higher for relatives of very severe cases (as high as 10 per cent) and minimal for relatives of mild seronegative cases. The antigen HLA-DRw4 is found in rheumatoid arthritis patients with twice the normal frequency, and is six times more common in familial cases, suggesting that this may be a major genetic determinant in the disorder. The occurrence of positive tests for rheumatoid factor is associated with HLA-DRw3.

A distinct, progressive 'pseudorheumatoid chondrodysplasia' has been recognized which is probably autosomal recessive in inheritance. Generalized contractures and painful swelling can cause confusion with juvenile rheumatoid arthritis. The hand deformities of Freeman–Sheldon syndrome and mucopolysaccharidoses may also be misdiagnosed as arthritis.

SYSTEMIC LUPUS ERYTHEMATOSUS

Association has been found with specific HLA haplotypes and several other genes involved in immune function. There is strong concordance between monozygotic twins (25–75 per cent) but the empiric risk for first-degree relatives (and for dizygotic twins) is around 3 per cent for systemic lupus erythematosus. As with many autoimmune disorders, there appears to be an increased incidence of other autoimmune conditions in relatives, suggesting that a dominantly inherited general predisposition to autoimmunity may be involved.

Table 14.7 Mendelian forms of osteoarthropathy

Type	Inheritance
Interphalangeal osteoarthrosis	Autosomal dominant
Heberden's nodes	Autosomal dominant (see text)
Familial digital osteoarthropathy with avascular necrosis	Autosomal dominant
Hereditary arthro-ophthalmopathy (Stickler syndrome)	Autosomal dominant (type II collagen defect)
Osteoarthrosis, platyspondyly and β_2-globulin deficiency	Autosomal recessive (probable)
Multiple epiphyseal dysplasia	Autosomal dominant
Spondyloepiphyseal dysplasia tarda	X-linked recessive
Other spondyloepiphyseal dysplasias	Mainly autosomal dominant (type II collagen defect)
Premature generalized osteoarthrosis	Autosomal dominant (type II collagen defect)
Hereditary osteoarthritis of the hip	Autosomal dominant
Hereditary chondrocalcinosis	Autosomal dominant or autosomal recessive
Pseudoachondroplasia	Autosomal dominant
Alkaptonuria	Autosomal recessive

Systemic lupus may produce important intrauterine effects, with congenital heart block occurring in some infants born to affected mothers, while the 'lupus anticoagulant factor' (not always associated with overt systemic lupus) may be responsible for recurrent abortion in a small proportion of such cases.

OSTEOARTHRITIS

Osteoarthritis occurs with twice the general population prevalence in first-degree relatives of those suffering from this condition. When associated with Heberden's nodes, the risk is higher, probably threefold. The nodes themselves have been thought to show autosomal dominant inheritance with incomplete penetrance in males, but the fact that they occur more frequently in the relatives of rarer male propositi makes polygenic inheritance likely. No HLA association has been shown.

An unusual concentration of osteoarthritis in a family should arouse suspicion of an underlying bone dysplasia. Dominant inheritance in families with generalized premature osteoarthritis has been reported; some of these cases showed a defect in type II collagen. Table 14.7 summarizes some of the major mendelian causes of osteoarthritis.

CONGENITAL DISLOCATION OF THE HIP

Apart from environmental factors, it is likely that a genetic contribution is provided both by the shape of the acetabulum and by joint laxity. Congenital dislocation of the hip is three times more common in girls, and there is marked social class and ethnic variation.

Table 14.8 Recurrence risks for congenital dislocation of the hip

Individual affected	Individual at risk	Risk (%) Overall	Males	Females
One sib	Sibs	6	1	11
One parent	Children	12	6	17
One parent, one child	Children	36		
Second-degree relative	Nephews, nieces	1		

After Wynne-Davies R (1985), *J Med Genet* **2**, 227–232.

The overall incidence is around 5 per 1000 births. Recurrence risks have been studied by Wynne-Davies, whose data are shown in Table 14.8. Care must be taken to distinguish transient 'clicking hips' in newborns, and other generalized bone, connective tissue and neuromuscular disorders which commonly present with hip dislocation.

PERTHES' DISEASE

True Perthes' disease carries a low recurrence risk, under 1 per cent in sibs and around 3 per cent in children of affected patients. The risks do not appear to be higher in the relatives of patients with bilateral hip disease. Risks for second-degree and third-degree relatives are minimal. Familial concentrations should arouse suspicion that some other disorder, such as multiple epiphyseal dysplasia, may be present.

ARTHROGRYPOSIS (CONGENITAL CONTRACTURES)

There is so much heterogeneity in the group of arthrogryposes that the possible causes cannot be listed (see the review by Hall, 2003, for details). Every effort should be directed to making a primary diagnosis, with a careful pregnancy history (to exclude environmental factors) and family history (relevant neurological or skeletal disorders). Full examination and investigations to determine whether the contractures are part of a general syndrome, or have a neurogenic or myopathic basis, are also essential. If after this no specific cause has been found and the case is isolated, the recurrence risk is likely to be low. Two forms that appear to be specific are distal arthrogryposis (autosomal dominant, often very mild) and amyoplasia, with symmetrical contractures of all four limbs (usually sporadic). Where a parent is affected, even mildly, autosomal dominant inheritance is likely. It should be noted that the prognosis with treatment is generally good when the condition is a secondary deformity.

TALIPES

As with arthrogryposis, there are many primary causes of talipes, in particular neurological defects, which must be excluded. Idiopathic talipes equinovarus occurs in around 1 in 1000 births in the UK, with a male predominance of 3:1. The risk for sibs is around 3 per cent overall, around 10 times the population frequency; the risk for sibs of a male patient is lower (2 per cent) than for sibs of a female patient (5 per cent), as expected on the basis of polygenic inheritance. Full data on risks to offspring of patients are not yet available. Wynne-Davies suggested that the risk may be as high as 25 per cent for further offspring of an affected parent with an affected child. Other forms of talipes (calcaneovalgus and metatarsus varus) appear to run separately in families from equino-varus, and may carry slightly higher sib recurrence risks (4–5 per cent).

IDIOPATHIC SCOLIOSIS

Idiopathic scoliosis may be infantile or adolescent.

Infantile

The incidence of infantile idiopathic scoliosis is around 1.3 per 1000 births in the UK, and much lower in North America. Satisfactory figures for sibs are not available.

Adolescent

The incidence of the adolescent form is around 0.3 per 1000 births in boys and 4 per 1000 births in girls. The overall risk for first-degree relatives is around 5–7 per cent for major defects, but data are insufficient to split by sex and type of relatives.

DUPUYTREN'S CONTRACTURE

When no primary cause is apparent, the inheritance of Dupuytren's contracture is thought to be autosomal dominant, but if this is so, one would expect severe forms due to homozygosity for such a common condition, which have not been recorded.

HEREDITARY DIGITAL CLUBBING

Hereditary digital clubbing is a common and harmless autosomal dominant trait, frequently confused by doctors with acquired clubbing of more serious import. Patients usually correctly recognize its hereditary nature.

VARIOUS SKELETAL SYNDROMES

NAIL–PATELLA SYNDROME

Nail–patella syndrome (autosomal dominant) may present with talipes or hip dislocation in addition to the dysplastic nails and absent patellae. Renal involvement may occur in later life. Linkage with the ABO blood group system was the first autosomal linkage to be discovered on chromosome 9. A specific gene has now been isolated.

CRANIOCARPOTARSAL (FREEMAN–SHELDON OR 'WHISTLING FACE') SYNDROME

The hand deformity superficially resembles severe rheumatoid disease, but the lack of X-ray changes and characteristic pinched face should enable recognition of the syndrome. Inheritance is usually autosomal dominant, but the birth of affected sibs to normal consanguineous parents suggests a recessive form as well.

RUBINSTEIN–TAYBI SYNDROME

Broad thumbs and great toes, short stature, moderate to severe mental retardation and characteristic facies are the principal features of Rubinstein–Taybi syndrome. Recurrence in a family is rare, but patients do not usually reproduce. Molecular studies have recently identified mutations in the CREB binding protein on chromosome 16p, so most cases probably represent new dominant mutations.

LARSEN SYNDROME

A combination of multiple joint dislocation with an unusual facies (and often cleft palate), this syndrome was originally thought to be autosomal recessive, but parent–child transmission has now been reported so the situation is not clear. Heterogeneity is likely.

STICKLER SYNDROME (HEREDITARY ARTHRO-OPHTHALMOPATHY)

Stickler syndrome is a variable autosomal dominant disorder, with characteristic flattened facies, cleft palate, severe myopia with frequent retinal detachment and early osteoarthritis. It has been shown to be due to a defect in type II collagen.

KLIPPEL–FEIL SYNDROME

Many causes of a short neck find their way into this category, but Klippel–Feil syndrome remains heterogeneous even after their removal. Where the case is an isolated one, the risk for sibs is probably low, although minor degrees of cervical vertebral fusion may be more frequent in relatives. The risk for children is significant since some cases are dominantly inherited; no precise figure exists. Congenital heart disease is a common accompaniment in patients. The specific association with severe deafness (Wildervanck syndrome) appears to be confined to girls. Careful clinical assessment and full skeletal survey should allow future delineation of specific entities within this group.

DE LANGE SYNDROME

Low birthweight, dwarfism, mental retardation, characteristic facies with synophrys and a variety of limb defects are the principal features of this rather unsatisfactory syndrome. Although not obviously heterogeneous, de Lange syndrome does not 'hang together' well as a single entity. There is no clear inheritance pattern and no obvious causative factors are known, although a variety of chromosomal defects have been found in a proportion of cases. The risk to sibs is around 2 per cent.

POPLITEAL PTERYGIUM SYNDROME

The multiple pterygia are associated with cleft lip or palate, cryptorchidism and often syndactyly. Inheritance may be either autosomal dominant or recessive (usually the latter in the severe infantile form).

SACRAL AGENESIS

Almost all cases of sacral agenesis are sporadic, but there seems to be a specific relationship to maternal diabetes mellitus. There does not appear to be an association with neural tube defects (see Chapter 12).

FURTHER READING

General

Beighton P (ed.) (1993). *McKusick's Heritable Disorders of Connective Tissue*. Mosby, St Louis.
Gorlin RJ, Cohen M, Hennekam RCM (eds) (2001). *Syndromes of the Head and Neck*. Oxford, Oxford University Press.
Royce PM, Steinmann B (1993). *Connective Tissue and its Heritable Disorders*. Wiley-Liss, New York.
Spranger J (1992). International classification of the osteochondrodysplasias. *Eur J Paediatr* **151**, 407–415.
Young ID (2002). *Genetics for Orthopedic Surgeons*. London, Remedica.

Bone dysplasias

Horton WA (1995). Molecular genetics of the human chondrodysplasias. *Eur J Hum Genet* **3**, 357–373.
Olsen BR (1995). Mutations in collagen genes resulting in metaphyseal and epiphyseal dysplasias. *Bone* **17**, 45S–49S.
Rimoin DL, Lachman RS (1993). Genetic diseases of the osseous skeleton. In: Beighton P, ed. *McKusick's Heritable Disorders of Connective Tissue*. Mosby, St Louis, pp. 557–689.
Spranger J, Brill PJ, Poznanski A (2003). *Bone dysplasias. An Atlas of Genetic Disorders of Skeletal Development*. Oxford, Oxford University Press.
Wynne-Davies K, Hall CM, Apley AG (1985). *Atlas of Skeletal Dysplasias*. Edinburgh, Churchill Livingstone.

Connective tissue disorders

Gray JR, Davies SJ (1996). Marfan syndrome. *J Med Genet* **33**, 403–408.

Pope M (2004). Molecular abnormalities of collagen and connective tissue. In: Isenberg D, Maddison P, Woo P *et al.*, eds. *Oxford Textbook of Rheumatology*, 3rd edn. Oxford, Oxford University Press, ch. 3.2.

Pope FM, Burrows NP (1997). Ehlers–Danlos syndrome has varied molecular mechanisms. *J Med Genet* **34**, 400–410.

Tsipouras P, Devereux RB (1993). Marfan syndrome: genetic basis and clinical manifestations. *Semin Dermatol* **12**, 219–228.

Others

Cran JT, Husby G (1995). HLA-B27 and spondyloarthropathy: value for early diagnosis? *J Med Genet* **32**, 497–501.

Hall JR (2003). Arthrogryposes (multiple congenital contractures). In: Rimoin DL, Connor JM, Pyeritz RE, Korf B, eds. *Emery and Rimoin's Principles and Practice of Medical Genetics*. Edinburgh, Churchill Livingstone.

Rubin LA, Amos CI, Wade JA *et al.* (1994). Investigating the genetic basis for ankylosing spondylitis. *Arthritis Rheum* **37**, 1212–1220.

Oral and craniofacial disorders

For most clinicians, craniofacial abnormality is a confusing area, on the borderline between medicine and dentistry, yet overlapping broadly into other fields. The plastic or maxillofacial surgeon is the person who sees most of the facial disorders, and there is no doubt that genetic counselling is an integral part of management of these patients. Even minor facial anomalies can cause great distress, and accurate information regarding possible risks to offspring will provide considerable relief from worry for such people.

The amount of information available regarding the inheritance of these disorders is considerable. A number of medical geneticists who began their careers as dentists have provided some thorough reviews of the subject (see 'Further reading').

THE TEETH

HYPODONTIA AND ANODONTIA

Hypodontia, or lack of one or a few permanent teeth, is extremely common (5–10 per cent in most surveys) and is often inherited as a variable autosomal dominant trait. It may be the only significant finding in female heterozygotes for X-linked hypohidrotic ectodermal dysplasia (see Chapter 16), where incisors may also be peg-shaped. Complete anodontia is commonly associated with this disorder in males, but can also occur in other ectodermal dysplasia syndromes, in type I orofaciodigital syndrome (X-linked dominant) and with iris dysplasia in Rieger syndrome (autosomal dominant). A single central incisor tooth may be associated with midline abnormalities such as holoprosencephaly.

ENAMEL DEFECTS

Enamel defects are seen in a number of generalized genetic disorders; defects occurring in isolation are termed amelogenesis imperfecta. Classifications have tended to be based on the apparent phenotype, either hypoplasia (a reduction in thickness of the enamel) or hypomineralization (a reduction in the degree of calcification of the enamel), the latter often subdivided into hypocalcification and hypomineralization according to the severity of the defect. In all probability, both hypoplasia and hypomineralization occur together in the majority of cases. Autosomal dominant, autosomal recessive and X-linked modes of inheritance are recognized. In the X-linked forms, characterized by vertical bands of normal and abnormal enamel in heterozygous females, there is evidence of genetic heterogeneity. One locus is the gene coding for amelogenin (the main structural protein of enamel) synthesis in the Xp22 region; another locus lies at the opposite end of the X chromosome in the Xq22–q28 region.

Enamel pits are a characteristic finding in the permanent teeth in tuberous sclerosis.

DENTINE DEFECTS

The most common of the defects of dentine is dentinogenesis imperfecta. This may occur in isolation, inherited in an autosomal dominant pattern, or in the various forms of osteogenesis imperfecta. The teeth are opalescent with an amber or grey colour. The teeth may be subject to attrition and chipping, most probably due to fractures within the dentine. Dentinogenesis imperfecta occurring alone is determined by a gene on the long arm of chromosome 4. When associated with osteogenesis imperfecta, there may be more variation in the severity of involvement, with some teeth being clinically normal, although radiographically and histologically they may show abnormalities.

CLEFT LIP AND PALATE

Before genetic counselling is given, a careful examination must be made to exclude the numerous syndromal associations with clefting. In some of these (e.g. chromosomal trisomies), the other defects are obvious, while in others, e.g. the Van der Woude (lip pits) syndrome (gene isolated on 1q), they may be inconspicuous and even absent in some family members. Maternal teratogens (notably anticonvulsants) must also be considered. The most important syndromes to recognize are those that follow mendelian inheritance (Table 15.1 lists some of the major ones; fuller lists are given in the books listed in the 'Further reading' section). Cleft lip and palate also occur with other malformations in a non-specific manner, and are more common than one might expect. If a careful search for a specific syndrome proves negative, one is forced to use the empiric risks for the abnormalities in isolation.

Numerous studies have shown that cleft palate alone runs in most families (apart from Van der Woude syndrome) separately from cleft lip with or without cleft palate. Table 15.2 summarizes the overall risks. As expected with polygenic inheritance, the presence of other affected family members considerably raises the risks. The population incidence of cleft lip (with or without cleft palate) is 1 in 500 to 1 in 1000, compared with around 1 in 2500 for isolated cleft palate. A small number of undoubtedly X-linked families have been documented with cleft palate and ankyloglossia. While of great interest for isolating the gene involved, they do not affect the general genetic recurrence risk.

Table 15.1 Some major syndromes associated with cleft lip and/or palate

Autosomal dominant
Van der Woude syndrome (lip pits with cleft lip/palate)
EEC syndrome (ectrodactyly, ectodermal dysplasia and clefting)
Hereditary arthro-ophthalmopathy (Stickler syndrome)
Larsen syndrome (originally thought to be recessive)
Retinal detachment, myopia and cleft palate (Marshall syndrome)
Spondyloepiphyseal dysplasia congenita

Autosomal recessive
Chondrodysplasia punctata (Conradi syndrome)
Diastrophic dysplasia
Smith–Lemli–Opitz syndrome
Meckel syndrome
Orofaciodigital syndrome, type II
Fryns syndrome (with diaphragmatic hernia, limb and facial anomalies)
Roberts syndrome

X-linked
Orofaciodigital syndrome, type I (dominant, lethal in male)
Otopalatodigital syndrome
Isolated X-linked cleft palate with ankyloglossia

Chromosomal
Trisomy 13
Trisomy 18
Chromosome 18 deletions
Various other autosomal abnormalities
Velocardiofacial (Shprintzen) syndrome (22q deletion)

Non-mendelian
Pierre Robin sequence
Clefting with congenital heart disease
De Lange syndrome

Table 15.2 Cleft lip and palate – genetic risks in the absence of a defined syndrome or mendelian pattern

Relationship to index case	Cleft lip + palate (%)	Isolated cleft palate (%)
Sibs (overall risk)	4.0	1.8
Sib (no other affected members)	2.2	
Sib (two affected sibs)	10	8
Sib and affected parent	10	
Children	4.3	3
Second-degree relatives	0.6	
Third-degree relatives	0.3	
General population	0.1	0.04

Table 15.3 Genetic risks in cleft lip/palate: effect of severity

Anomaly	Risk to sibs (%)
Bilateral cleft lip and palate	5.7
Unilateral cleft lip and palate	4.2
Unilateral cleft lip alone	2.5

One point to note from Table 15.2 is that the risk for sibs of a patient with cleft lip with or without cleft palate is lower when it can be definitely established that no other relatives are affected (2.2 per cent) than is the overall risk to sibs (4 per cent) found by surveys, which will include some families with other affected relatives of varying closeness. Therefore, this higher risk should be used when family information is unavailable or unreliable. Some data are now available on the influence of severity (Table 15.3) and, as expected, there is a higher risk when the abnormality is bilateral and a lower risk when there is only cleft lip. It is likely that cleft lip and palate are examples of polygenic inheritance; so far, apart from the mendelian and syndromal forms, no major susceptibility genes have been identified.

Median cleft lip should be regarded as genetically separate from the usual types, and may have its own specific syndromal associations (e.g. Ellis–van Creveld syndrome). Lateral and oblique cleft lip and mandibular clefting are likewise due to distinct processes.

PIERRE ROBIN SEQUENCE (CLEFT PALATE WITH MANDIBULAR HYPOPLASIA)

Mandibular hypoplasia, with or without cleft palate and with resulting respiratory obstruction from the tongue, may be part of a variety of skeletal or muscular syndromes, some mendelian (e.g. Stickler syndrome, congenital myotonic dystrophy). In the absence of these, the risk of recurrence is low; the prognosis for patients with careful treatment is good.

OTHER ORAL DISORDERS

RECURRENT APHTHOUS ULCERS OF THE MOUTH

Around 20–25 per cent of the general population suffer from this minor, but tiresome, complaint to some degree, and around 40 per cent of first-degree relatives appear to be affected.

GINGIVAL FIBROMATOSIS

Although most commonly seen as a result of phenytoin treatment, gingival fibromatosis may occur as an isolated autosomal dominant trait, as well as in some more general syndromes.

AGLOSSIA–ADACTYLIA

Recurrence of aglossia–adactylia in sibs has not been noted, but insufficient patients have reproduced to exclude new dominant mutation as the cause.

ATROPHIC RHINITIS

Although most cases of atrophic rhinitis are sporadic, occasional families following a clear autosomal dominant pattern have been documented.

CRANIOFACIAL DISORDERS

CRANIOSYNOSTOSES

Several specific genetic and clinical types of craniosynostosis exist, which are important to distinguish in genetic counselling. Gorlin *et al.*'s *Syndromes of the Head and Neck* (see 'Further reading') provides a detailed list and description. The principal types are listed in Table 15.4. Recognition of the different molecular defects (notably in fibroblast growth factor receptor 2) has been of great importance. All forms except Carpenter syndrome are autosomal dominant, with many cases (almost all in Apert syndrome) due to new mutation.

Table 15.4 Craniosynostosis syndromes

Disorder	Clinical features	Molecular defect
Apert syndrome	Severe craniosynostosis, glove-like fusion of most digits, frequent mental retardation	FGFR2
Saethre–Chotzen syndrome	Milder craniosynostosis; digital fusion, mostly soft tissue and of digits 2–4	TWIST (Drosophila homologue)
Pfeiffer syndrome	Mild acrocephaly with broad thumbs and great toes and partial digital fusion	FGFR2
Greig cephalopolysyndactyly	Broad forehead, characteristic facies and polysyndactyly	GLI3
Acrocephalopolysyndactyly (Carpenter syndrome)	Severe and frequently lethal; autosomal recessive	7p12
Crouzon's disease	Involvement of the orbits and mid-face, as well as the cranium	FGFR2

ISOLATED CRANIOSYNOSTOSIS

Most cases of isolated craniosynostosis are sporadic, regardless of which sutures are involved, and probably represent secondary deformations. Risks for sibs where parents are normal are around 5 per cent for coronal and 1 per cent for sagittal suture fusion, although these will need reassessment in the light of molecular studies. If multiple family members are affected, it is wise to assume that one is dealing with a mendelian type and to consider DNA analysis. Some such families have shown mutations in *FGFR2* or *HOX 8* genes.

MANDIBULOFACIAL DYSOSTOSIS (TREACHER COLLINS SYNDROME)

Severity of the facial abnormality in mandibulofacial dysostosis varies greatly but inheritance is autosomal dominant, with a specific gene isolated on chromosome 5. Deafness is a common feature in addition to external ear defects; mental retardation is said to occur, but is possibly an artefact of ascertainment. Potential parents will tend to be more mildly affected than average and must be warned that an affected child could be considerably more severely affected. High-resolution ultrasonography can detect severe cases. A separate syndrome of mandibulofacial dysostosis with preaxial limb defects (Nager syndrome) usually follows autosomal recessive inheritance.

OTHER CRANIOFACIAL SYNDROMES

Some members of this very extensive group are covered in other chapters and listed in the tables in Chapter 6. A precise diagnosis is often difficult; Gorlin *et al.* (2001) provide a detailed and comprehensive guide. Only a few of the most important are mentioned here.

Hallermann–Streiff syndrome (oculomandibulofacial syndrome; Francois dyscephalic syndrome)

Congenital cataracts, short stature, beaked nose with micrognathia and characteristic facies are all features of the Hallermann–Streiff syndrome. Inheritance is probably autosomal dominant, with most patients being new mutations, but few patients have reproduced. The risk of recurrence in sibs is minimal.

Goldenhar syndrome (oculoauriculovertebral dysplasia)

Goldenhar syndrome must be distinguished from the superficially similar Treacher Collins syndrome. The external ear defects are more marked, mental retardation is common, and epibulbar dermoid cyst of the eye is characteristic. Most cases are sporadic, and the recurrence risk where parents are normal is low.

Hemifacial microsomia

Unilateral hypoplasia of most facial structures is the characteristic feature of hemifacial microsomia; recurrence is exceptional.

Sturge–Weber syndrome

Sturge–Weber syndrome must be distinguished from other angiomatous malformations of the face. The involvement of the ophthalmic trigeminal area and extension to the deep tissue of skull and meninges is characteristic, as is congenital glaucoma. No causative factors are known, but the condition is almost always sporadic.

Orofaciodigital syndromes

Characteristic features of the most common form (type I) are clefting of the jaw and tongue, with digital abnormalities (usually syndactyly) and sometimes mental retardation. Renal cysts may occur and almost all cases are female, suggesting X-linked dominant inheritance lethal in the male (see Chapter 2). A risk of 50 per cent for female offspring of an affected individual should be given. An extremely rare form (type 2 or Mohr syndrome) following autosomal recessive inheritance, and which is clinically distinguishable, has been described; further heterogeneity is likely in the group.

Oculodentodigital syndrome

The narrow alae nasi and small eyes are characteristic of the oculodentodigital syndrome, combined with mild digital curvature and fusion, and dental enamel hypoplasia. Inheritance is autosomal dominant.

Dubowitz syndrome

The autosomal recessive Dubowitz syndrome combines microcephaly and mental retardation with a small face, shallow supraorbital ridges and severe eczema.

Frontonasal dysplasia and median cleft face syndrome

Almost all cases of frontonasal dysplasia and median cleft face syndrome have been sporadic, but affected individuals rarely reproduce.

Aarskog syndrome (faciogenital dysplasia)

Aarskog syndrome is an X-linked recessive disorder combining hypertelorism with digital and spinal abnormalities and characteristic scrotal shape. The Opitz syndrome of hypertelorism and hypospadias is somewhat similar, but follows both autosomal dominant and X-linked inheritance.

FURTHER READING

Cohen MM, Maclean RE (2000). *Craniosynostosis.* Oxford, Oxford University Press.

Gorlin RJ, Cohen MM, Hennekam RJM (2001). *Syndromes of the Head and Neck*, 4th edn. New York, Oxford University Press – this comprehensive and well illustrated volume is the definitive source for both clinical and genetic information, both on well recognized disorders and on incompletely delineated syndromes.

Reardon W, Winter RM (1995). The molecular pathology of syndromic craniosynostosis. *Mol Med Today* **1**, 432–437.

The skin

A high proportion of disorders affecting the skin and its appendages follow mendelian inheritance; because they are readily available for inspection, they are easier than most to document in families. Since skin disorders are rarely fatal and interfere relatively little with reproduction, it is often possible to identify with confidence what mode of inheritance is operating, even if one is ignorant of the precise pathology or aetiology of the condition. It must be remembered, however, that skin lesions may be the external marker for more serious internal or generalized disease, and that their cosmetic effect may be considered much more serious by the patient than by the physician.

For the small but significant number of lethal or seriously disabling skin disorders of infancy, including the epidermolysis bullosa and congenital ichthyosis groups, prenatal diagnosis by fetal skin biopsy is now a proven technique, which has had no serious risks in skilled hands. It is increasingly superseded, though, by specific molecular analysis of a chorion villus sample (see Chapter 8).

Most of the mendelian disorders in this chapter are simply tabulated here, without any attempt to describe them (Table 16.1), although molecular information is included where this is available. Useful sources are given at the end of the chapter. As the major genes involved in skin biology (e.g. keratins, collagens) are progressively isolated, it is becoming possible to identify more of the mendelian skin disorders as due to specific gene defects, although these are proving to be very heterogeneous. Molecular analysis is best carried out in conjunction with expert histological and protein studies and with skilled clinical diagnosis.

SKIN PIGMENTATION AND ITS DISORDERS

Inheritance of skin colour is polygenic, with probably at least five or six gene loci of additive effect. Advice may be sought regarding the offspring of interracial marriages or

Table 16.1 Skin disorders following mendelian inheritance

Disorder	Molecular defect or gene localization
Autosomal dominant	
Acanthosis nigricans	
Acrokeratosis verruciformis	
Angioneurotic oedema	C1 esterase inhibitor
Basal cell naevus syndrome	9q (PATCH homologue)
Blue rubber bleb naevus	
Cutis laxa (also autosomal recessive)	
Cylindromatosis (turban tumours)	
Ectodermal dysplasia, hidrotic types	
Epidermolysis bullosa (most families)	Keratin and collagen defects
Epithelioma, multiple self-healing	9q
Erythrokeratodermia variabilis	
Hailey–Hailey disease (benign familial pemphigus)	ATP 2C2
Ichthyosis hystrix	
Ichthyosis vulgaris	
Keratosis follicularis (Darier's disease)	ATP 2A2
Koilonychia, hereditary	
Mastocytosis, familial	
Monilethrix	Specific hair keratin genes
Nail–patella syndrome	9q (gene isolated)
Neurofibromatosis (von Recklinghausen) type 1	17q (gene isolated)
Neurofibromatosis type 2	22 (gene isolated)
Pachyonychia congenita	Keratin defects
Palmoplantar hyperkeratosis (tylosis)	Various keratin defects
Porokeratosis of Mibelli	
Porphyria (all types except congenital erythropoietic)	Specific enzyme and gene defects
Steatocystoma multiplex	Specific keratin defects
Hereditary haemorrhagic telangiectasia	Specific vascular growth factors
Trichorhino phalangeal syndrome, type 1	TRPS (may also be part of microdeletion syndrome)
Tuberous sclerosis	Specific tumour suppressor genes on 9q and 16p
Autosomal recessive	
Acrodermatitis enteropathica	
Albinism, oculocutaneous (tyrosinase-negative and -positive)	Tyrosinase (genes isolated for both forms)
Ataxia telangiectasia	Specific DNA repair gene isolated
Bloom syndrome	
Chediak–Higashi syndrome	
Chondroectodermal dysplasia (Ellis–van Creveld)	

Table 16.1 (cont.)

Disorder	Molecular defect or gene localization
Autosomal recessive (cont.)	
Cockayne syndrome	Specific DNA repair gene isolated
Cutis laxa (also autosomal dominant and X-linked)	
Epidermolysis bullosa (letalis and some dystrophic forms)	Collagen defect (dystrophic form)
Ichthyosis, congenita and other types	Various keratin defects
Lipoid proteinosis	
Netherton syndrome	
Palmoplantar hyperkeratosis (mal de Meleda and Papillon–Lefevre types)	
Pili torti	
Porphyria, congenital erythropoietic	Specific enzyme defect
Progeria	
Pseudoxanthoma elasticum	
Rothmund–Thompson syndrome	Specific DNA repair defect
Seip lipodystrophy syndrome	Specific DNA repair gene isolated
Trichothiodystrophy	ERCC2 (DNA repair defect)
Werner syndrome	Various DNA repair defects
Xeroderma pigmentosum	
X-linked (recessive unless stated)	
Dyskeratosis congenita	Specific gene isolated (DKC 1)
Ectodermal dysplasia, anhidrotic	Specific gene isolated
Fabry's disease	Alpha-galactosidase (gene isolated)
Focal dermal hypoplasia (?dominant, lethal in male)	
Chronic granulomatous disease	Gene and protein isolated
Ichthyosis, X-linked	Steroid sulphatase (gene isolated)
Incontinentia pigmenti (?dominant, lethal in male)	
Keratosis follicularis spinulosa (dominant)	
Menkes syndrome	Gene isolated (copper transport)
Wiskott–Aldrich syndrome	Specific gene involved in cellular immunity

adoptions, and questions on this subject may merely be the focusing point of a considerable amount of stress, ignorance and latent prejudice. The attitude of other family members such as in-laws or grandparents may be frankly hostile, and it may in fact be not so much skin colour as other racial characteristics, such as hair or facial features, that are the main concern.

In general, children are likely to show skin colour intermediate between that of the parents. Where both parents are of mixed race, this will still apply, but here the likelihood is greater that a child may be either darker or lighter than both parents as a result of inheriting a particular selection of pigment-determining genes.

Light-skinned individuals of mixed race married to a white person may enquire as to whether a child or subsequent descendant might have extremely dark skin colour or African features – in other words, might be a clearly black person who perhaps would not be accepted in the white community into which he or she is born. This is very unlikely, but again it cannot be excluded that the degree of pigmentation, though probably not of other features, might exceed that of the darker parent, especially if the 'white' partner is relatively dark-skinned. Where the partner is blond and light-skinned, this possibility can be discounted.

Where mixed-race origin is known or is a possibility, caution must be advised in predicting later appearance from features present in early infancy. Skin colour may darken significantly and African-type hair may not be apparent for some months after birth. Reed, in the 1955 book *Counselling in Medical Genetics*, dealt in detail with these various features and it is of interest that inheritance of skin colour was the most common reason for seeking genetic counselling at his clinic. Although the climate of opinion has significantly altered since that time, and interracial marriages and adoptions are now more frequent and accepted, one should not underestimate the significance for families of what may, to the physician, appear trivial features.

As the genes involved in skin colour are identified, important and difficult societal questions will arise as to how or whether these should be used as genetic tests for this normal characteristic. It would be wise for society to consider these issues now, rather than wait until misuse of such tests occurs.

ALBINISM

Generalized oculocutaneous albinism is autosomal recessive. Two main types exist: a severe form (tyrosinase negative) with total lack of pigment throughout life, and in which mutations in the tyrosinase gene have now been identified; and a milder tyrosinase-positive form for which the gene has also been cloned (the *p* gene, corresponding to 'pink eye' in the mouse). In the latter type, pigmentation of hair and iris gradually increases and mild cases may easily be missed. The forms are non-allelic, marriages between albinos of different type resulting in all normal offspring; heterozygotes are often detectable by translucency of the iris. A very rare type, associated with a bleeding diathesis (Hermansky–Pudlak syndrome), is also autosomal recessive. Prenatal detection of severe oculocutaneous albinism by fetal skin biopsy may be relevant in tropical countries where the morbidity is high. DNA analysis will be simpler as mutations become recognized. It also seems likely that some of the commoner genetic variants of pigmentation will be relevant to skin cancer susceptibility.

Ocular albinism (see Chapter 17) is X-linked, the gene being mapped to distal Xp.

VITILIGO

Vitiligo is commonly associated with a variety of autoimmune endocrine disturbances, and like them often follows a variable autosomal dominant pattern.

PIEBALDISM

Piebaldism commonly follows autosomal dominant inheritance and has been shown to result from specific mutations in the *c-KIT* oncogene. It may form part of the more generalized Waardenburg syndrome, which is also autosomal dominant in inheritance and determined by the developmental gene *PAX3*. Isolated white forelock may also occur as a dominantly inherited trait.

PSORIASIS

Psoriasis is a common and variable disorder (prevalence around 1–2 per cent) which is frequently familial. Families apparently following all major types of mendelian inheritance have been reported, but it is likely that most of these represent extreme examples of a disorder that is polygenically determined. Susceptibility loci have been identified in the HLA region of chromosome 6, and others have been claimed, but so far none are consistent or strong enough to give any practical genetic test (see Chapter 3).

The risk for first-degree relatives of an isolated case is at least 10 per cent, and probably double this where there are two affected first-degree relatives. Where the disorder appears to follow an autosomal dominant pattern, it is probably wise to give a risk approaching 50 per cent for offspring of an affected member, but it is doubtful whether unaffected members of such pedigrees are completely free from this risk of transmitting it.

The children of two psoriatic patients also have a risk of around 50 per cent of being affected, but there does not seem to be a specially severe form in such children, as might have been expected if homozygosity at a single gene locus were operating.

ATOPIC ECZEMA

Atopic eczema is an extremely common problem, often associated with asthma and other allergic phenomena, and is probably determined by one or more autosomal dominant genes of rather variable expression. The genetics of atopy is discussed in Chapter 19 in relation to asthma and remains confused; a locus on chromosome 11 has been identified, although this is still debatable and may not apply to eczema. No genetic tests are useful in practice at present. The risk of some allergic problem where one parent is affected approaches 50 per cent, and is somewhat higher where both parents are affected, although it does not appear that homozygosity results in a particularly severe clinical picture.

THE ICHTHYOSES

The inherited ichthyoses are listed in Table 16.2. It is usually possible to distinguish different types on clinical and histological grounds as well as genetically, so that, with care, correct counselling can be given even for isolated cases. Thus severe ichthyosis in a neonate, except for the dominant ichthyosiform erythroderma, almost certainly follows

Table 16.2 The inherited ichthyoses

Disorder	Inheritance
Ichthyosis without syndromal association	
Congenital ichthyosis	
Lamellar ichthyosis (collodion baby)	Autosomal recessive
Harlequin fetus (lethal)	Autosomal recessive
Congenital ichthyosiform erythroderma	Autosomal dominant
Ichthyosis hystrix	Autosomal dominant
Ichthyosis vulgaris	Autosomal dominant
X-linked ichthyosis	X-linked recessive
Syndromes associated with ichthyosis	
Refsum syndrome	Autosomal recessive
Ichthyosis with mental retardation and spastic tetraplegia (Sjögren–Larsson syndrome)	Autosomal recessive
Ichthyosis with male hypogonadism	X-linked recessive
Conradi syndrome	Autosomal dominant, recessive or X-linked
Ichthyosiform erythroderma with deafness	Autosomal recessive
Ichthyosiform erythroderma with unilateral limb defects	Autosomal recessive
Ichthyosis congenita with cataract	Autosomal recessive
Ichthyosis with mental retardation and hypogonadism (Rud syndrome)	Autosomal recessive

autosomal recessive inheritance, while mild ichthyosis in a female is likely to be autosomal dominant. A careful general examination to exclude the various generalized syndromes is important. Deficiency of steroid sulphatase has been shown to be responsible for X-linked ichthyosis, in addition to causing post-maturity through placental involvement. The gene has been cloned and a remarkably high proportion of cases (over 90 per cent) found to result from gene deletion, reflecting the localization near the pseudoautosomal region. Several X-linked syndromes with ichthyosis are proving to be due to contiguous gene deletion syndromes in this region, analogous to those around the Duchenne locus.

PALMOPLANTAR HYPERKERATOSIS (TYLOSIS)

Most cases of palmoplantar hyperkeratosis (tylosis) follow autosomal dominant inheritance, and isolated cases thus have a high risk of transmitting the disorder. A variety of specific keratin gene defects have been identified (see Table 16.3). The rare form known as 'mal de Meleda' is autosomal recessive and can occur outside the Adriatic area. The remarkable families with dominantly inherited oesophageal cancer and tylosis have late childhood onset of the skin disorder which appears not to result from a keratin defect. These cases are, however, exceptional, and families with tylosis from early childhood and no history of oesophageal cancer in the family should not be worried unnecessarily by having this possibility raised.

Table 16.3 Hereditary disorders of keratin

Disorder	Keratin type
Epidermolysis bullosa simplex	K5, K14
Epidermolytic hyperkeratosis	K1, K10
Acral type (ichthyosis bullosa of Siemens)	K2e
Palmoplantar keratodermia (hyperkeratosis)	
Epidermolytic type	K9
Non-epidermolytic type	K1, K16
Pachyonychia congenita	K6, K16, K17
Steatocystoma multiplex	K17
Monilethrix (hair defect)	Hb1, Hb6 (hair-specific keratins)

Courtesy of Dr Paul Bowden, Cardiff.

EPIDERMOLYSIS BULLOSA

Epidermolysis bullosa is another exceptionally heterogeneous group of disorders in which genetic differences are supported by the clinical and histological features and where expert clinical and laboratory diagnosis is particularly essential. Thus the neonatal letalis form (now partly treatable by steroids) is autosomal recessive, while the mild simplex types, without scarring, are autosomal dominant; at least one form results from a molecular defect in keratin. The dystrophic forms with scarring may follow either pattern, but most severe cases are autosomal recessive. A defect in type 7 collagen has been found in most families. Junctional forms are due to defects in the basement membrane zone. Prenatal diagnosis of the letalis and dystrophic forms by fetoscopic skin biopsy is possible, but DNA analysis on chorion biopsy is preferable where the molecular defect is known.

ECTODERMAL DYSPLASIAS

HYPOHIDROTIC (ANHIDROTIC) ECTODERMAL DYSPLASIA

Hypohidrotic ectodermal dysplasia is the most common of the ectodermal dysplasias. It is X-linked recessive, with variable expression in female carriers, who may show dental anomalies as well as a reduced sweat pore count and a patchy distribution of the sweating pattern on starch-iodine testing. Isolation of the gene has made carrier detection and pre-natal diagnosis feasible in many families.

OTHER TYPES

Other types of ectodermal dysplasia are autosomal. Both dominant and recessive types have been described, as well as a number of syndromes (e.g. EEC syndrome and chondroectodermal dysplasia).

PIGMENTED NAEVI

When present in a particular site, pigmented naevi commonly follow autosomal dominant inheritance. Multiple pigmented naevi are a feature of Turner syndrome and of the dominantly inherited syndrome of multiple naevi with nerve deafness (LEOPARD syndrome). The autosomal dominant dysplastic naevus syndrome is especially important to recognize in view of the risk of melanomas developing. The skin lesions of neurofibromatosis (see Chapter 11) and tuberous sclerosis must be distinguished, as must lesions overlying a spina bifida.

CAVERNOUS HAEMANGIOMAS

Cavernous haemangiomas of the facial region are usually sporadic, as is the trigeminal area flat vascular naevus of the Sturge–Weber syndrome, and the limb angiomas associated with hypertrophy (Klippel–Trenaunay–Weber syndrome). Somatic mutations have been confirmed in vascular endothelial growth factors in some types. Haemangiomatous and lymphangiomatous lesions of the limbs may be associated with hypertrophy and are usually sporadic, although familial cases are described (see Chapter 25). Rare instances of autosomal dominant inheritance in association with Wilms' tumour have also been recorded. Other specific types of naevus following autosomal dominant inheritance are naevus flammeus of the nape of the neck and the 'blue rubber bleb' multiple naevi.

SEGMENTAL PIGMENTARY DISORDERS

Several unusual disorders of skin pigmentation have been described that follow a patchy or whorled distribution corresponding to Blaschko's lines, and which may be accompanied by mental retardation or other systemic features. Hypomelanosis of Ito, incontinentia pigmenti and focal dermal hypoplasia (Goltz syndrome) are the most clearly defined. Chromosomal mosaicism has been found to underlie many cases previously classed as hypomelanosis of Ito, and should be sought in blood and skin biopsies. Recurrence risk is low unless a parent shows mosaicism. An X-linked dominant (male lethal) gene may be responsible for most cases of incontinentia pigmenti, and the patchy skin distribution may be related to the pattern of X-chromosome inactivation.

BALDNESS

Severe, early male baldness is probably due to autosomal dominant inheritance, with expression of the gene limited to the male unless it is present in homozygous state. The author has never received a genetic counselling request for this innocuous condition, but a specific gene has recently been identified for a form of total alopecia, so it will be interesting to see if this changes the situation. Premature balding is a feature of myotonic dystrophy. Hair loss or scarcity may also result from a variety of ectodermal dysplasias and specific hair disorders (e.g. monilethrix, pili torti). **Alopecia areata** is often associated with autoimmune endocrine disorders.

Isolation of the gene responsible for **red hair colour** (usually autosomal recessive) promises to be more relevant to population genetic studies than to genetic counselling, although perhaps we shall see reports from behavioural geneticists on this topic!

ACANTHOSIS NIGRICANS

Primary acanthosis nigricans starts early in life and follows autosomal dominant inheritance. Acanthosis nigricans may also accompany a variety of other genetic disorders. Onset in later life is commonly an indication of acquired visceral malignancy. The inherited type has no such association.

SKIN TUMOURS

A remarkable number of the rare skin-related tumours follow mendelian inheritance, mostly autosomal dominant, and appear in the lists in Table 16.1 and Table 25.1 (see p. 333). The recessively inherited disorders of DNA repair also frequently present with skin manifestations.

XERODERMA PIGMENTOSUM

Xeroderma pigmentosum (autosomal recessive) is now detectable prenatally as a repair defect of ultraviolet-induced DNA damage. Since several separate types exist, it is important for the cultured cells of the affected sib to be studied before embarking on prenatal diagnosis. Specific DNA repair genes have now been isolated and may simplify prediction.

KAPOSI'S SARCOMA

Most cases of Kaposi's sarcoma are now associated with human immunodeficiency virus (HIV) infection, but for many years a small but well-documented number of families with multiple cases have been recognized. Whether these are truly genetic needs reassessment.

MALIGNANT MELANOMA

Most cases of malignant melanoma appear to be non-genetic, but autosomal dominant inheritance occurs in a few striking families. One type is known as familial dysplastic naevus syndrome. Transplacental passage of malignant cells is also recorded. Several different specific tumour suppressor genes have been found to be involved in the dominantly inherited families.

BASAL CELL NAEVUS (GORLIN) SYNDROME

Basal cell naevus syndrome is a dominantly inherited disorder which may be recognized from skeletal abnormalities, especially jaw cysts, before tumours appear. There may be also an increased risk of cerebral tumours. The gene responsible on chromosome 9 has proved to be a homologue of the *Drosophila* gene *Patch*, involved in cell signalling, and the same gene may prove to underlie the rare and remarkable familial self-healing epithelioma known principally from western Scotland, which is localized to the same region. Isolated basal cell tumours are not known to be genetic.

CONGENITAL FIBROMATOSIS

Congenital fibromatosis is a rare disorder in which multiple spindle-cell fibromatous tumours occur and commonly mature spontaneously. The condition may be fatal if gut tumours occur, but is usually benign. Although autosomal recessive inheritance has been claimed, autosomal dominant inheritance with incomplete penetrance (especially in older individuals) is more probable. Careful search for small lesions in apparently unaffected parents is important.

FURTHER READING

General

Bale SJ (2000). *Genetics for Dermatologists*. London, Remedica – a useful, compact guide with clinical and molecular information.
Moss C, Savin J. (1995). *Dermatology and the New Genetics*. Oxford, Blackwell.
Sybert VP (1997). *Genetic Skin Disorders*. New York, Oxford University Press – this excellent book, profusely illustrated and with molecular details, is an authoritative reference source for all those disorders that are mentioned only briefly (or not at all) in the present chapter.

Specific disorders

Bale SJ, DiGiovanna JJ (1997). Genetic approaches to understanding the keratinopathies. *Adv Dermatol* **12**, 99–113.
Eady RAJ, Dunhall MGS (1994). Epidermolysis bullosa: hereditary skin fragility diseases as paradigms in cell biology. *Arch Dermatol Res* **287**, 2–9.
Paller AS (1996). The genetic basis of hereditary blistering disorders. *Curr Opin Pediatr* **8**, 367–371.
Spritz RA (1994). Molecular genetics of oculocutaneous albinism. *Hum Mol Genet* **3**, 1469–1475.
Spritz RA, Hearing VJ (1995). Genetic disorders of pigmentation. In: Harris H, Hirschhorn K, eds. *Advances in Human Genetics*. St Louis, Mosby, pp. 1–45.

CHAPTER 17

The eye

The study of inherited eye disorders formed a major part of early work on the mendelian basis of genetic disease, largely because their non-lethal nature led to large families with clear inheritance patterns, but also because many generalized genetic disorders have ocular manifestations important in diagnostics. We are now seeing a renaissance as the individual genes are mapped and isolated; there are even future possibilities for localized gene therapy. These rapid developments make it especially important that patients and family members are given accurate and up-to-date genetic information.

Patients with congenital or childhood blindness frequently marry each other, with complex results, although in contrast to congenital deafness it is usually possible to distinguish clinically the precise genetic type of each parent's disorder. The author has found that a clinic at a school for visually impaired children, run jointly with an ophthalmologist, has been of great help to school leavers and their parents. Such schools serve a wide geographical area and allow many patients to be seen who might have been missed through the regular genetic counselling service. Such a system also minimizes the risk of erroneous diagnosis, which a non-specialist is in no position to query alone. The increasing trend for visually impaired children to be educated in regular schools is making provision of this type of service more difficult.

Since this chapter cannot possibly list, let alone discuss, all the hereditary ophthalmic disorders, a selective approach has been adopted, aimed to help paediatricians and

Table 17.1 X-linked eye disorders

Disorder	Changes in heterozygote
Ocular albinism	Patchy fundal depigmentation, translucency of iris
Oculocutaneous albinism with deafness	Partial hearing loss
X-linked congenital cataract	Sutural lens opacities
Choroideraemia*	Retinal pigmentary changes (sometimes symptomatic)
	Abnormal electroretinogram
Colour blindness	Minor defects in colour vision
Deutan*	
Protan*	
Incomplete achromatopsia	
Iris hypoplasia with glaucoma	
X-linked macular dystrophy	
Megalocornea (also rarely dominant)	Corneal diameter increased
Microphthalmos with multiple anomalies (Lenz syndrome)	
Congenital stationary night blindness with myopia	
Norrie's disease (pseudoglioma)*	Some cases due to gene deletion
Hereditary oculomotor nystagmus	Variable; may be fully affected
Oculocerebrorenal (Lowe's) syndrome*	Mild lens opacities
X-linked retinitis pigmentosa*	Patchy retinal pigmentary and electroretinographic changes
Retinoschisis*	

* Indicates gene cloned.

other clinicians who encounter hereditary eye disorders. It is not primarily intended for ophthalmologists, although they may perhaps find some parts helpful. Around 3–4 per 1000 children in developed countries have some form of severe visual handicap and at least half of these are genetic in origin. Mendelian disorders are also prominent in progressive blindness of later onset, while genetic factors are now being identified in such common problems as glaucoma, cataracts and macular degeneration of old age.

A remarkable number of X-linked disorders affecting the eye are known, and these are listed separately (Table 17.1) because they produce special problems in genetic counselling. The carrier state can be recognized in a number of these and they provide direct evidence for mosaicism due to X-chromosome inactivation in the female. Patchy morphological changes can be seen in a number of these carriers, which allow diagnosis of the carrier state in the absence of biochemical tests. Molecular analysis is beginning to provide accurate tests based on genetic linkage and, increasingly, the direct detection of mutations, especially for this X-linked group, but also for autosomal disorders.

CHOROIDORETINAL DEGENERATIONS

A great variety of types exists, characterized by particular features of fundal appearance, by differences in severity and progression, and by different responses to various types of electrodiagnostic investigation. It is most unwise for someone who is not an ophthalmologist to venture into diagnosis, but a valuable contribution can be made by documenting the pedigree pattern and by carefully searching for any associated syndromic features. This information can then be combined with a specific ophthalmic diagnosis to allow accurate counselling. Two broad groups can be distinguished: those mainly affecting peripheral vision (e.g. the retinitis pigmentosa group) and those principally involving central vision (e.g. the macular dystrophies).

RETINITIS PIGMENTOSA

Retinitis pigmentosa is the most common of the retinal degenerations. This group of disorders may follow all three main modes of mendelian inheritance, autosomal recessive forms being the most common (about 50 per cent), with autosomal dominant inheritance accounting for around 25 per cent of families. X-linked cases account for around 15 per cent of the total, but for about 50 per cent of isolated male cases. Marked variation in course occurs in different families, suggesting further heterogeneity.

Carriers of the X-linked form may often (but not always) show visible pigmentary disturbance and an abnormal electroretinogram, a useful distinguishing point from the other forms of inheritance in an isolated male case. The carriers for autosomal recessive forms do not generally show abnormalities, so distinction from a new dominant mutation is often impossible. Clinical features are too variable to help much, while an additional problem is incomplete penetrance of the gene in around 10 per cent of heterozygotes for the dominant form. The empiric risk for an affected child being born to a parent who is an isolated case is around 1 in 8. Should a child indeed be affected, the risk to subsequent offspring would be 1 in 2. Molecular developments in retinitis pigmentosa are now becoming of practical help in those families where a defect is known, with mutations in rhodopsin and peripherin (key molecules involved in retinal function) occurring in a significant proportion of autosomal dominant families; at least three X-linked loci exist, making prediction impossible outside the occasional very large family. Retinitis pigmentosa currently provides a good example of the all-too-frequent situation in genetic testing, of research advances not yet becoming regularly available as a service. Given that there appear to be at least 75 different loci involved, this is hardly surprising.

Choroideraemia is a specific X-linked disorder that may be confused with retinitis pigmentosa, especially in its early stages. Its recognition is particularly important since the gene has been isolated, allowing accurate presymptomatic and carrier detection. Retinoschisis is yet another X-linked disorder, with retinal degeneration associated with a characteristic splitting of the retina. The gene has now been isolated and a variety of specific mutations found.

A number of syndromes with retinitis pigmentosa exist, including the Bardet–Biedl syndrome (with polydactyly, hypogonadism and mental retardation), Hallgren syndrome (with deafness, ataxia and mental disturbance) and Usher syndrome (two types, one with profound nerve deafness), all of which are autosomal recessive.

MACULAR DYSTROPHIES

The macular dystrophies are a heterogeneous group, selectively involving central vision in contrast to the early peripheral involvement in retinitis pigmentosa. This is readily distinguished by an experienced ophthalmologist, but separating the different forms may be very difficult, causing problems in genetic counselling, especially for the isolated case. Many late-onset macular dystrophies, as well as the early-onset Best's macular degeneration (gene isolated on chromosome 11q), follow an autosomal dominant pattern, while the juvenile Stargardt form is autosomal recessive and due to mutations in a specific ion transport gene on chromosome 1. Another rare but treatable recessive type is gyrate atrophy associated with a metabolic defect in ornithine aminotransferase. Cone dystrophies are a further heterogeneous group, associated with deterioration in colour vision. An important recent development has been the finding that some families with dominant macular degeneration in old age are heterozygous for mutations in the Stargardt gene. Since we have no clear idea yet as to the penetrance of this heterozygous mutation or whether this is a generally valid association, clinical use should await this information.

LEBER'S CONGENITAL AMAUROSIS (not to be confused with
Leber's optic atrophy)

Leber's congenital amaurosis is a primary retinal disorder that is one of the most common causes of childhood blindness, and is autosomal recessive in inheritance. The condition can be detected in early infancy by electroretinogram. Occasional families with associated cerebral and renal degeneration are known, but do not overlap with the isolated form. Mutations in a retinal homeobox gene (*CRX*) have recently been identified, while a separate retinal epithelium protein gene (*RPE65*) is also involved.

CONGENITAL STATIONARY NIGHT BLINDNESS

This is usually autosomal dominant or X-linked dominant. An X-linked recessive form with myopia also exists.

NYSTAGMUS

A clear primary diagnosis for nystagmus is essential, because the cases may be neurological or vestibular rather than ocular. Even when the nystagmus is primary, there are a number of causes. Probably the most important ones to recognize are the various types of albinism, congenital stationary night blindness (see above) and the X-linked hereditary oculomotor nystagmus, which shows very variable manifestation in females (see Figure 2.22, p. 41). These last two may prove to be a single disorder.

COLOUR VISION

The common forms of colour blindness, whether protan or deutan in type, are uniformly X-linked recessive in inheritance and occur in about 8 per cent of males.

Because of this high frequency, matings of affected males and carrier females are not uncommon, with a 50 per cent risk of children of either sex being affected. Around 0.4 per cent of women have colour blindness. The genes for red and green colour vision have now been cloned, allowing molecular analysis of colour vision defects.

The rare total colour blindness (monochromatism) is autosomal recessive in inheritance, while the even rarer 'blue cone' type is X-linked. All three disorders should be distinguished from the progressive cone dystrophies.

LEBER'S OPTIC ATROPHY (not to be confused with Leber's congenital amaurosis)

Leber's optic atrophy follows classical mitochondrial inheritance (see Chapter 2), but other genetic and environmental factors modify the primary pattern. The main empiric risks are as follows:

- males are affected more often than females (85 per cent), in Europe, but not in Japan
- males never transmit the disease to descendants of either sex, not even to grand-children or subsequent generations
- where a female is affected or has an affected son, the risk to subsequent sons is 1 in 2, but all her daughters appear to be either carriers (80 per cent) or affected (20 per cent), unlike X linkage.

Mitochondrial DNA analysis can now identify specific germ-line mutations and is especially valuable in cases without a clear genetic pattern. However, as discussed in Chapter 2, the identification of mitochondrial inheritance is of the greatest help in confirming the diagnosis and giving the general pattern of risk, but is singularly unhelpful for the female carrier, since it gives no indication as to whether she will herself become affected, or the risk to particular offspring. An exception is for offspring of a woman who is heteroplasmic for the mutation, i.e. has both normal and mutant DNA; if these offspring show no or very low mutant DNA themselves, their risk of developing the disorder is low. Hopefully some preventive therapy that enhances or spares mitochondrial function may be developed that will help those at risk. Avoiding risk factors such as smoking is important.

OTHER FORMS OF HEREDITARY OPTIC ATROPHY

Several forms exist following both autosomal dominant and recessive patterns. Those of adult life are mostly dominant and a gene locus has been mapped to chromosome 3q. They usually show a slowly progressive course, unlike the subacute onset of Leber's optic atrophy. The Wolfram or DIDMOAD syndrome (diabetes insipidus, diabetes mellitus, optic atrophy and deafness), generally considered to follow autosomal recessive inheritance, has now been shown to result from mitochondrial mutations in some families, so caution is needed in giving risks.

CORNEAL DYSTROPHIES

Numerous types of corneal dystrophy exist. The slit-lamp appearance is often very characteristic (to the expert), and unless a clear pedigree pattern is seen, it is wise to be guided by ophthalmological opinion. Most types are mendelian. Corneal clouding and opacification may be a helpful diagnostic feature in various generalized diseases, notably the mucopolysaccharidoses, but also in lipoprotein disorders and cystinosis.

Some dominant forms of corneal dystrophy have recently been shown to result from molecular defects in different forms of keratin, such as K3, K12, kerato-epithelin and type 8 collagen (see also Chapter 16).

RETINAL DETACHMENT

Retinal detachment is commonly associated with severe myopia, and a significant risk to relatives is only likely when they also have severe myopia. Occasional dominantly inherited families are documented, with one locus mapped. Several other genetic syndromes may be accompanied by retinal detachment, including type II collagen defects such as severe spondyloepiphyseal dysplasia and Stickler syndrome, as well as the related, but distinct, condition known as Wagner's retinopathy, all of which are dominantly inherited.

RETINOBLASTOMA

Retinoblastoma provides an extremely important and difficult area for genetic counselling. All bilateral cases appear to be hereditary, compared with only about 15 per cent of unilateral cases. Further, only 90 per cent of those with the gene develop tumours, and there are instances where the disorder seems to have been suppressed in an entire branch of a kindred. Occasionally, spontaneous disappearance of a tumour may leave a retinal scar as the only feature, so parents of an isolated case should always be examined carefully. Survivors have an increased risk (around 10 per cent) of other neoplasms, notably osteosarcoma, in later life.

Most cases of retinoblastoma are not associated with other malformations, but abnormalities of chromosome 13q may be accompanied by retinoblastoma, a finding that led to localization of the gene on this chromosome.

The gene has been cloned and molecular analysis can be used to provide accurate prediction for those at risk by deletion or restriction fragment length polymorphism (RFLP)

Table 17.2 Genetic risks to offspring in retinoblastoma

Unilateral	Risk (%)	Bilateral	Risk (%)
Affected with affected parent or sib	45	Affected; other family members affected	45
Unaffected; parent and sib or two sibs affected	5	Affected; no other affected family members	45
Affected; no other affected relatives	1		
Unaffected; one affected child	1	Unaffected; one affected child	2
Unaffected; one affected sib	1	Unaffected; parent affected	5

Based on Fuhrmann W, Vogel F (1992), *Genetic Counselling: a Guide for the Practising Physician*. Berlin, Springer. Also on Draper GJ *et al.* (1992), *Br J Cancer* **66**, 211–219.

analysis. Tumour DNA analysis is important in unilateral cases. Retinoblastoma provided the first full vindication of the 'two hit' mutation theory of cancer (see Chapter 25), and tumour DNA analysis shows that the same locus is indeed involved in both germinal and somatic mutations. The lack of penetrance can now be readily explained by absence of the necessary somatic mutation; while the genetic predisposition is dominantly inherited, the developing retinal tissue must be homozygous for the defect if a tumour is to occur. Equally, a germ-line mutation must have been inherited for more than a single tumour to occur in an individual.

The empiric risk estimates given in Table 17.2 need to be reassessed in the light of molecular developments, but remain useful where affected relatives are dead or when DNA analysis is not possible. It should be noted that the risks for some categories have been reduced by comparison with previous editions of this book, in the light of further evidence.

NORRIE'S DISEASE (PSEUDOGLIOMA)

In the past, Norrie's disease was frequently confused with retinoblastoma. The frequent occurrence of mental retardation makes genetic counselling of this X-linked recessive disease of considerable importance. The gene has been identified and some cases are due to deletion. Molecular analysis is thus relevant to carrier identification and prenatal diagnosis.

CATARACT

CONGENITAL CATARACT

Numerous types of congenital cataract exist, with all forms of inheritance recorded. The incidence is around 1 in 250 births. Environmental causes (e.g. rubella) and metabolic and other primary disorders (e.g. galactosaemia and hypoparathyroidism) must be excluded, and syndromal associations (e.g. Conradi's disease) sought.

Because most genetic forms without a metabolic cause follow dominant inheritance, the risk for offspring of an affected person is not far short of 50 per cent. The risks for sibs of an isolated case is probably 10 per cent or less, but more accurate figures are needed.

A number of specific genes, some involving lens crystallin proteins, have been isolated, but are not yet in regular diagnostic use.

CATARACTS IN LATER LIFE

Primary disorders, both mendelian (e.g. myotonic dystrophy) and non-mendelian (e.g. diabetes), must be excluded. Most families showing a clear-cut aggregation appear to follow autosomal dominant inheritance.

LENS DISLOCATION

Lens dislocation is a feature of the Marfan and Marchesani syndromes and of homocystinuria, but may occur as an isolated abnormality due to an abnormally small and spherical lens (spherophakia), usually following autosomal dominant inheritance. The author has seen tall, thin members of one such family persistently misdiagnosed as Marfan syndrome, with much unnecessary worry caused. In some families at least, the same fibrillin locus on chromosome 15 is involved as in Marfan syndrome.

GLAUCOMA

Glaucoma can be a part of a surprisingly large number of genetic syndromes and should be checked for in any ocular assessment of the patient with syndromes involving the eye, since it may be a treatable aspect in an individual without specific ocular complaints. Major advances are occurring in isolation of genes involved with primary glaucoma (see the review by Sarfarazi, 1997), although it is not yet clear how these findings will affect genetic risks for those without a clear mendelian inheritance pattern.

Primary closed-angle glaucoma

Primary closed-angle glaucoma seems to be determined largely by anatomical orbital factors, particularly shallowness of the anterior chamber; 12 per cent of sibs were found to be clinically affected in one study.

Primary open-angle glaucoma

Primary open-angle glaucoma is common in the general population and is found in 1 in 200 elderly people. Studies of sibs have shown between 5 and 16 per cent to be affected; 10 per cent is probably an appropriate risk for clinically significant glaucoma. The risks for children have been lower, but extremely variable. Because the children studied were always much younger than the sibs, it seems likely that the lifetime risk will approach the 10 per cent seen for sibs. The proportion of families that have a mendelian basis is uncertain, but some large families following autosomal dominant inheritance exist, some adult-onset, others juvenile, and have been mapped to specific chromosomes. A specific gene (*TIGR*), with a common single mutation, has been shown to underlie the form on 1q in juvenile and possibly some adult-onset families.

CONGENITAL GLAUCOMA

Congenital glaucoma may be associated with other generalized ocular problems (e.g. Sturge–Weber syndrome). When it is primary, a proportion of families appear to follow autosomal recessive inheritance, but isolated cases are much too common for this mode to explain all cases. The risk to sibs after a single affected child is around 10 per cent; after two affected sibs, a 25 per cent risk should be advised. Risks to children of affected individuals are uncertain. Assuming a mixture of recessive and polygenic forms, a risk of 5 per cent seems appropriate until data are available. A specific cytochrome P450 gene on chromosome 2p has now been shown to be responsible for some recessively inherited families, but other genetic loci also exist.

REFRACTIVE ERRORS

Twin studies show a very close concordance between monozygotic twin pairs, suggesting a high degree of genetic determinance. Individual pedigrees showing all types of mendelian inheritance have been produced for each of the major types of refractive error, but are of little help in deriving general risks for relatives. Studies of unselected families show high correlations for refractive values between both sibs and parents and offspring, suggesting that a polygenic basis is present with genes of additive effect and little dominance or recessivity. The same situation applies to disorders of corneal shape such as astigmatism, keratoconus and cornea plana.

Some regular syndromes of refractive error exist, e.g. myopia and night blindness, which are usually X-linked recessive. Refractive errors may also accompany other primary mendelian disorders, e.g. myopia in Marfan syndrome and some skeletal dysplasias. In isolated cases of severe myopia, a risk of 4–5 per cent for similar severe eye problems in the children has been suggested.

HETEROCHROMIA OF THE IRIS

Heterochromia is frequently an isolated and harmless trait, often autosomal dominant in inheritance. The most important cause of heterochromia to recognize is Waardenburg syndrome (see Chapter 18), in which piebaldness and deafness are major features. Variation in expression of this autosomal dominant disorder is considerable.

EYE COLOUR

In the early medical genetics literature, eye colour was given as one of the most common reasons for requesting genetic counselling, but this rarely seems to be the case now. It is possible that such enquiries were really aimed at establishing paternity. In fact, while brown eye colour in general behaves as dominant to light blue eye colour, the genetic control is considerably more complex than this, and exceptions are sufficiently frequent for this trait not to be used as evidence for or against paternity.

STRABISMUS

Strabismus is a frequent feature of many generalized neuromuscular disorders, which may follow mendelian inheritance (see Chapter 11). Isolated strabismus, whether classified as convergent or divergent, fits a polygenic pattern. Variation between studies results, in part, from the extent to which minor deviations are classed as abnormal. From the viewpoint of counselling, it seems that where parents are normal and one child is affected, the risk for subsequent children is around 15 per cent. Where one parent is also affected, the risk is around 40 per cent.

HEREDITARY PTOSIS

Hereditary ptosis is usually autosomal dominant and may persist unchanged through life. Care must be taken to distinguish more general neuromuscular causes, such as myotonic dystrophy, myasthenic syndromes and the mitochondrial myopathies.

DEVELOPMENTAL EYE DEFECTS

This field provides an excellent example of the value of comparative genetic studies, genes being strongly conserved between species, with an increasing number of mutations recognized in human disorders.

MICROPHTHALMOS AND ANOPHTHALMOS

Microphthalmos and anophthalmos constitute an extremely heterogeneous group. Unilateral cases are frequently non-genetic, but cannot be securely distinguished from genetic forms. Rubella and toxoplasmosis are causes to be excluded for bilateral disease. Mental retardation is frequently associated, and microphthalmos is a feature of severe chromosomal defects as well as mendelian syndromes. The X-linked Lenz syndrome of microphthalmos with cataract, mental retardation and digital and genitourinary abnormalities must be considered. Microphthalmos with coloboma is usually autosomal dominant (in the absence of known external causes). Complete bilateral anophthalmos is generally autosomal recessive. Cryptophthalmos, with absent palpebral fissures, may be part of the above disorders, or may occur with relatively normal eye development, usually following autosomal recessive inheritance. Some cases are part of the more general Fraser syndrome (autosomal recessive), where renal agenesis and laryngeal atresia may be major features, and where a specific developmental gene defect is now known.

CYCLOPS

Almost all cases of this lethal malformation, an extreme form of holoprosencephaly (see Chapter 12), have been sporadic. Chromosomal abnormalities have been found in some cases.

COLOBOMA AND ANIRIDIA

Both bilateral coloboma of the iris and the more severe aniridia usually follow autosomal dominant inheritance; colobomas may form part of more extensive ocular disorders. Because colobomas may vary considerably in extent, a thorough ophthalmic examination of both parents and patient is needed. The rare syndrome of ocular coloboma with anal atresia (cat-eye syndrome) follows an autosomal dominant pattern but is associated with an extra chromosome 22 fragment.

Aniridia may be associated with Wilms' tumour, mental retardation and genital defects, but such cases are generally sporadic, most dominant families being determined by a gene on chromosome 2. A small deletion on the short arm of chromosome 11 is seen in some cases. Detailed molecular analysis of the region has shown that a series of overlapping deletions is responsible for the various syndrome conditions, analogous to those seen in other microdeletion syndromes.

Mutations in the gene *PAX6* and some other developmental genes may occur in aniridia and other anterior chamber abnormalities.

FURTHER READING

Deeb SS, Motulsky AG (1996). Molecular genetics of human color vision. *Behav Genet* **26**, 195–207.

Hackett SE (1997). Leber's hereditary optic neuropathy: a genetic disorder of the eye. *Insight* **22**, 94–96.

Rennie WA (ed.) (1986). *Goldberg's Genetic and Metabolic Eye Disease*. Boston, Little, Brown.

Sarfarazi M (1997). Recent advances in molecular genetics of glaucomas. *Hum Mol Genet* **6**, 1667–1677.

Smith BJ, O'Brien JM (1996). The genetics of retinoblastoma and current diagnostic testing. *J Pediatr Ophthalmol Strabismus* **33**, 120–123.

Sullivan LS, Daiger SP (1996). Inherited retinal degeneration: exceptional genetic and clinical heterogeneity. *Mol Med Today* **2**, 380–386.

Taylor D (1990). *Pediatric Ophthalmology*. Oxford, Blackwell.

Traboulsi EI (1998). *Genetic Diseases of the Eye*. Oxford, Oxford University Press.

Wright AF, Jay B (eds) (1994). *Molecular Genetics of Inherited Eye Disorders*. Chur, Harwood.

Deafness

At least 50 per cent of cases of congenital and childhood deafness may be genetically determined. In the case of non-syndromic deafness, a precise clinical diagnosis may be impossible due to phenotypic overlap with deafness of environmental origin. Careful attention to family history and detailed audiological evaluation, not just of the proband but also of other family members, may help to resolve the question of aetiology in apparently isolated cases. Close consultation with audiological colleagues and others is needed if errors are to be avoided.

Recognition of the specific genes involved in deafness has had a major impact on our understanding of this field and is also now playing a significant role in diagnosis and genetic counselling. For non-syndromic congenital sensorineural deafness, the loci and mutations involved vary considerably between different populations and it is important to know the distribution of molecular defects in the particular population, if possible.

Two groups, in particular, require genetic counselling: parents of a severely affected child wishing to have further children, and young adults with deafness, who frequently marry partners similarly affected.

Even without access to specialized audiological testing, it is often possible to assess the genetic situation accurately if the following points are borne in mind:

- What does the pattern of inheritance in the particular family suggest?
- Is the hearing loss severe congenital deafness, or some milder form?
- If hearing loss is milder, is it static or progressive?
- Is there an identifiable syndrome involving other systems?

Genetic counselling for the profoundly deaf is a service that requires a radically different approach from that in most other fields. The process of communication will usually require an intermediary, unless one has special experience with sign language or other forms of communication. Attitudes to deafness within the community of the profoundly deaf may well be quite different from those of doctors or of normally hearing patients. Genetic counselling may be perceived by some as a threat, unless it is sensitively and appropriately integrated into the overall educational provision for young adults and adolescents.

SEVERE CONGENITAL SENSORINEURAL DEAFNESS

The incidence has been estimated to be around 1 in 1000 births. Care must be taken to exclude external factors such as mild congenital rubella or cytomegalovirus infection.

In the absence of clear evidence of environmental aetiology, there is no doubt that a high proportion of cases result from autosomal recessive inheritance. It is difficult to decide exactly what this proportion is, because the different types are at present clinically indistinguishable. This is changing now that specific genes and mutations have been identified in a significant proportion of cases, but one often remains dependent on older, though well founded, data. Most studies have suggested that 40–50 per cent of the cases are autosomal recessive, with around 10 per cent due to autosomal dominant inheritance and most of the rest due to unknown or undetected environmental (or at least non-mendelian) factors. This would suggest that the risk of deafness in sibs of an isolated case is about 1 in 10. Where consanguinity exists, autosomal recessive inheritance is even more likely, and a 1 in 4 risk should be given. Likewise, should a couple have a second affected child, autosomal recessive inheritance is almost certain. Table 18.1 summarizes the various risks.

The risk for offspring of healthy sibs and other family members is often asked about. This is extremely low (well under 1 per cent) in the absence of consanguinity or of deafness in the family of the other partner.

The risk for offspring of an affected individual who is an isolated case and married to a normal person is low, but not negligible (around 5 per cent). This risk probably results from an inclusion of unrecognized new dominant mutations with the much larger number following recessive inheritance, unless there is consanguinity or other factors suggesting that a recessive gene may have been transmitted by the healthy parent. Although severe, dominantly inherited congenital deafness is rare in comparison to recessive forms and more variable in severity, it nevertheless accounts for the majority of two-generation families. In families with two affected sibs and healthy parents with normal audiograms, where recessive inheritance is almost certain, the risk for offspring of the affected individuals is low (around 1 per cent).

X-linked recessive inheritance is well documented as a mode of inheritance in severe congenital deafness but is not frequent enough to affect the risks for isolated male cases

Table 18.1 Genetic risks in profound childhood deafness of unknown cause

Affected relative	Risk
One child only; environmental factors carefully excluded	1 in 10
One child only; consanguinity present	1 in 4
Two affected children	1 in 4
One parent + one child	1 in 2
One parent only	1 in 20
Parent + sib(s) of parent only	1 in 100
Sib(s) of parent; parent unaffected	<1 in 100

or single sibships containing only affected males. Distinctive findings may be present on cochlear CT scan.

Marriage between two individuals with severe congenital deafness is common, and the offspring of such marriages provide clear evidence for the existence of several non-allelic recessive genes. If all cases were due to the same gene, or to different alleles at the same locus, one would expect all children to be affected. In fact, deaf children only occur in around 15 per cent of marriages between affected individuals and the risk of a pregnancy resulting in a deaf child is only around 10 per cent; in around 80 per cent, all children are unaffected, being heterozygous at each of the two loci involved. Such an outcome may come as a surprise, not without problems, to deaf couples. In only 5 per cent of marriages are all children affected; in the other 10 per cent, some children, but not all, prove to be affected, probably representing the situation where one of the partners has a dominant form of deafness. Figure 18.1 shows the various possibilities, while Table 18.2 summarizes the risks for individual couples. Genetic testing, now becoming available in a service setting, should prove especially useful for this group.

It is important to recognize that the risk for subsequent children of a couple may well be markedly altered by whether their first child proves to be affected or not (Table 18.2), and this should be stressed when genetic counselling is given initially. Most couples are able to understand that the initial risk estimate is a provisional one, being made up of a high-risk and a low-risk element which cannot be distinguished until the couple have actually had a child. A deaf couple whose first child is also deaf have at least a 50 per cent chance of this recurring in the next pregnancy.

Numerous different genes may cause severe non-syndromic deafness. A precise molecular diagnosis is particularly helpful for genetic counselling when both parents

Parents   Offspring

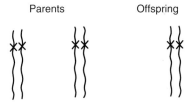

Both parents with same recessive form: offspring all affected

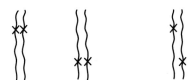

Parents with different recessive forms: offspring all unaffected

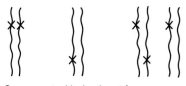

One parent with dominant form, one with recessive: half offspring affected

Figure 18.1 Possibilities for marriages between congenitally deaf individuals.

Table 18.2 Risks for children when both parents have profound childhood deafness (risk for next child)

Number of children already born	0	One unaffected	One affected	Two affected
Parents related	>1/2	1 in 10	All	All
Parents unrelated but from same minority ethnic group	>1/2	1 in 10	All	All
Parents unrelated, not from same minority ethnic group	1 in 10	1 in 20	>1/2	All

are deaf, but not all tests are available outside a research setting. The principal gene responsible for non-syndromic congenital sensorineural deafness is *connexin 26*; mutations in this are responsible for around one-quarter of cases, although the proportion and type of mutations vary considerably between populations. A range of other genes, including other *connexin* genes, may also be involved in some cases; genes causing syndromal types may also be responsible. Mitochondrial mutations are more often involved in less severe or later-onset deafness, but should be considered if there is a maternally inherited family pattern.

MILD-TO-MODERATE DEAFNESS

Partial nerve deafness includes numerous genetic forms of deafness whose effect is confined to the ear but where hearing loss is not sufficient to present as congenital deafmutism. Some forms are present from birth and are static; others are later in onset and progressive, while detailed audiological testing may show loss of particular frequencies. The classification of this group is currently in a state of flux and it is uncertain to what extent clinical, audiological and genetic characteristics can be matched, so expert advice should be sought.

Molecular analysis is now beginning to identify some of the specific genes, notably those on the X chromosome, and is likely to become helpful in resolving the heterogeneity.

Several factors are especially relevant to genetic counselling in this group:

- A considerably higher proportion of cases results from autosomal dominant inheritance than occurs with severe congenital deafness.
- Variability within a family can be considerable – careful testing is required before an individual is pronounced normal.
- Isolated cases are extremely difficult to distinguish from non-genetic forms of hearing loss.
- X-linked deafness of various types is especially important to recognize in view of the risks to the extended family.
- It seems likely that mitochondrial mutations may be involved in predisposition in some families, and also in drug-induced deafness.

OTOSCLEROSIS

Otosclerosis is the most common disorder in this group and can be recognized by its progressive course and mixed conductive and neural pattern. It follows autosomal dominant inheritance with rather incomplete penetrance (around 40 per cent).

DEAFNESS AS PART OF SYNDROMES

The number of syndromes associated with deafness is exceedingly large. Previous editions of this book listed some of the more common syndromes, but readers are now advised to consult Toriello et al. or Tewfik and der Kaloustian (see Further reading) for details, which both contain valuable summary tables as well as full individual descriptions. Hearing problems are most important to recognize in any syndrome since they may be remediable, as well as causing avoidable educational problems that may be mistaken for mental retardation.

Three syndromes (all autosomal recessive) that are of particular importance are mentioned here since they are considerably more common than the others and have serious consequences if overlooked.

Pendred syndrome

This disorder has probably been considerably under-diagnosed. Variable but generally severe nerve deafness occurs with goitre; early thyroxine treatment is important but many patients are euthyroid. The recently isolated gene is involved in ion transport.

Jervell and Lange–Nielsen syndrome

Severe nerve deafness is accompanied by abnormal cardiac conduction. Sudden death may occur (see p. 272 for molecular details).

Usher syndrome

Nerve deafness and retinitis pigmentosa are the defining features, but several forms, all autosomal recessive, are now recognized. In type I the deafness is severe, with vestibular involvement, while this is absent and the deafness moderate in type II. Molecular defects in myosin VII have been found in type 1b.

THE EXTERNAL EAR

Several syndromes, both dominantly and recessively inherited, have been described in which deafness (usually conductive) has been associated with abnormal shape of the external ear as the only visible feature.

External ear malformation is also striking in such craniofacial disorders as Goldenhar syndrome and mandibulofacial dysostosis. Environmental causes include rubella and thalidomide embryopathies, and – usually only in fatal cases – the 'Potter facies' resulting from oligohydramnios secondary to renal agenesis or other causes. Lesser degrees of abnormality form part of the characteristic facies of many genetic syndromes.

Isolated external ear abnormalities, particularly when unilateral, carry a low recurrence risk, but a careful examination should be carried out for minor audiological or branchial arch defects on both sides. The books of Toriello *et al.* and Tewfik and der Kaloustian contain abundant information on this aspect. The latter contains an extensive summary table of congenital anomalies and syndromes involving the ear. The frequent associations with renal abnormalities are especially worth considering.

MÉNIÈRE'S DISEASE

A few familial aggregations of Ménière's disease have been recorded, but one can safely say that the risks to family members of a single case of this common disorder are low.

FURTHER READING

Fischel-Ghodsian N (1998). Mitochondrial mutations and hearing loss: paradigm for mitochondrial mutations. *Am J Hum Genet* **62**, 15–19.

Keats BJB, Popper AN, Fay PR (eds) (2002). *Springer Handbook of Auditory Research: Genetics and Auditory Disorders*. Springer-Verlag, Berlin.

Petit C (1996). Genes responsible for human hearing loss: symphony of a thousand. *Nat Genet* **14**, 385–391.

Reardon W (1998). Connexin 26 gene mutation and autosomal recessive deafness. *Lancet* **351**, 383–384.

Steel K, Brown SD (1996). Genetics of deafness. *Curr Opin Neurobiol* **6**, 520–525.

Tewfik TL, der Kaloustian VM (1997). *Congenital Anomalies of the Ear, Nose and Throat*. New York, Oxford University Press.

Toriello HV, Reardon W, Gorlin RJ (2004). *Hereditary Hearing Loss and its Syndromes*. New York, Oxford University Press.

Internet source

Hereditary Hearing Loss Homepage – *http://dnalab-www.uia.ac.be/dnalab/hhh*

CHAPTER 19

Cardiovascular and respiratory disorders

CARDIOVASCULAR DISORDERS

Cardiovascular disorders provide a large number of genetic counselling problems and, fortunately, have been well studied from the viewpoint of recurrence risks and underlying aetiology. Congenital heart disease is the largest group for which advice is asked, usually regarding the risks for further affected children, but increasingly concerning the offspring of a successfully treated patient. Our knowledge of the genetic basis of congenital heart disease is rapidly increasing through the study of the genes involved in heart development, while the previously confused area of childhood cardiomyopathy has also developed a molecular clarification.

Cardiovascular disease of later life is proving a much more complex area to resolve, and while large-scale genetic–epidemiological studies are beginning to dissect the different genetic and environmental risk components, these are not yet at the stage of affecting risk estimation and genetic counselling. Nor is it clear that this will change rapidly (see also Chapter 3), since a series of complex interactions seems likely that makes attempts at individual risk prediction very uncertain and probably unhelpful, outside those families with a clear mendelian pattern, such as familial hypercholesterolaemia.

CONGENITAL HEART DISEASE

Clinically significant congenital heart disease occurs in around 1 in 200 births (nearer to 1 in 100 if minor cases picked up by investigation are included). Although around 90 per cent of cases are not obviously familial, it seems increasingly likely that important genetic factors are involved in most cases and specific genes and chromosome regions are starting to be identified, notably chromosome 22q. Thus, the first task in genetic counselling of families is to ensure that a high-risk form has been excluded, particularly if abnormalities additional to the cardiac lesion are present. Table 19.1 lists some of the more important mendelian disorders characterized by cardiac involvement that must be distinguished; there are a number of syndromes which do not always follow mendelian inheritance (Table 19.2). Congenital heart disease is also prominent in chromosomal disorders, particularly the autosomal trisomies and Turner syndrome; around 15 per cent of

Table 19.1 Heart disease in mendelian disorders

Disorder	Main extracardiac features	Usual heart defects	Inheritance
Holt–Oram syndrome	Upper limb defects, especially digits and radius	Atrial septal defect	Autosomal dominant
Ellis–van Creveld syndrome	Dwarfism, midline cleft lip, polydactyly	Ventricular septal defect	Autosomal recessive
Noonan syndrome	'Turner-like' phenotype	Pulmonary stenosis	Variable autosomal dominant
Williams syndrome	Facial features, mental handicap	Supravalvular aortic stenosis	Microdeletions around elastin gene; most cases sporadic
Marfan syndrome	Skeletal abnormalities, lens dislocation	Mitral valve prolapse, dilated aortic root	Autosomal dominant
Tuberous sclerosis	See Chapter 12	Intracardiac tumours	Autosomal dominant
LEOPARD syndrome	Nerve deafness, lentigenes	Conduction defects, pulmonary stenosis	Autosomal dominant
Kartagener syndrome	Situs inversus (see p. 277)	Dextrocardia	Autosomal recessive
Jervell–Lange–Nielsen syndrome	Nerve deafness	Congenital conduction defects	Autosomal recessive
Friedreich's ataxia	See Chapter 12	Cardiomyopathy	Autosomal recessive

congenital heart disease is due to chromosomal defects. An important discovery has been that chromosome 22q microdeletions may be responsible for some cardiac syndromes not previously showing a visible cytogenetic defect, possibly around 3 per cent of all congenital heart defects.

Among the identified environmental causes, rubella is still the most important, but congenital heart defects are produced by almost all the less specific teratogens and environmental factors (see Chapter 26), which should be carefully enquired after, even though it may not be possible to prove cause and effect in an individual case. Lithium is specifically associated with Ebstein's anomaly. The offspring of diabetic women also appear to form a high-risk group (see Chapter 20). Monozygous twinning is itself a risk factor for congenital heart disease, such twins having a threefold increase in risk (around 1.5 per cent). Some increase in incidence of congenital heart disease with maternal age has also been shown (excluding Down's syndrome) and a risk of around 1 per cent (twice that for the general population) is appropriate for women aged 40 years or more.

Genetic advice is most frequently sought for future sibs of an affected child, or sometimes for more distant relatives; risks other than for first-degree relatives are low in the absence of multiple cases or an identified mendelian basis. Information is now becoming available for the offspring of affected individuals and there is increasing evidence that risks are higher for offspring of affected females than of males. Overall risks are summarized in Table 19.3, but whenever possible, a specific anatomical diagnosis should be used as the basis for risk estimates. Data for a number of the more common defects, excluding

Table 19.2 Non-mendelian syndromes with congenital heart disease

Disorder	Non-cardiac features	Cardiac lesion	Recurrence risk
Asplenia and polysplenia syndromes	Complex lateralized defects	Dextrocardia and other complex defects	3–5%
VATER association	Oesophageal, anal, vertebral and radial limb defects	Variable	1%
Klippel–Feil syndrome	Fusion and reduction of cervical vertebrae	Cardiac involvement (commonly septal defects) in at least 1/4	
DiGeorge syndrome	Absent thymus and parathyroids	Commonly conotruncal defects Due to 22q microdeletions	Recurrence risk low for sibs if parents normal (see p. 271)
Velocardiofacial (Shprintzen) syndrome	Cleft palate, facial anomalies		
Goldenhar syndrome	Eye, ear and facial abnormalities	Various defects in half	Low
CHARGE association	Ocular coloboma, choanal atresia, ear and genital defects	Commonly conotruncal anomalies	Low
Kabuki syndrome	Characteristic facies	Coarctation	Low

Table 19.3 Overall risks in congenital heart disease (for use when details of specific disorder are uncertain or unavailable)

	Risk (%)
Population incidence	0.5
Sib of isolated case	2–3
Half-sibs or other second-degree relatives	1–2
Offspring of isolated case:	
Father	2–3
Mother	5–6
Two affected sibs (or sib and parent)	10
More than two affected first-degree relatives	50 (approximately)

Table 19.4 Approximate genetic risks for sibs of isolated cases of congenital heart disease

Defect	Risk (%)
Ventricular septal defect	3
Atrial septal defect	2.5
Patent ductus arteriosus	3
Fallot's tetralogy	2.5
Arteriovenous canal defect	2.5
Pulmonary stenosis	2
Aortic stenosis	2
Coarctation of the aorta	2
Transposition of great vessels	1.5
Hypoplastic left heart	3
Pulmonary atresia*	1
Common truncus	1
Tricuspid atresia*	1
Ebstein's anomaly*	1

*Provisional: based on limited data.
Based on multiple studies collated by Nora JJ, Berg K, Nora AH (1991), *Cardiovascular Diseases. Genetics, Epidemiology and Prevention*. Oxford, Oxford University Press.

syndromes, are given in Table 19.4. The data are given for sib risk only, since the figures for offspring in different studies have given widely divergent results and are based on small numbers when broken down into individual types. Where recurrence does occur, the defect is the same as previously in only about half the cases. This is relevant to counselling because it may mean that a sib of a proband with a correctable defect may have a fatal or untreatable lesion, or vice versa.

The increasing resolution of cardiac ultrasound imaging can now identify many structural defects in the later part of pregnancy, but prenatal diagnosis before 18 weeks' gestation is reliably feasible only for the most severe (usually untreatable) defects. Most published data derive from testing in referral centres where many of the pregnancies monitored are already known to be at high risk, so the proven value of ultrasonography in cardiac prenatal screening generally remains limited outside the high-risk situation.

RISKS TO MORE DISTANT RELATIVES

Data are inadequate but the excess risk for second-degree relatives of an isolated case of congenital heart disease is certainly under 1 per cent and it is doubtful if third-degree relatives have a significantly raised risk. Families are not infrequently encountered where there are several affected members, none of whom is a first-degree relative. The possibility of a variable mendelian form should be seriously considered here.

MULTIPLE CASES

Family clusters of congenital heart disease are not uncommon. Their occurrence should prompt a careful search for a mendelian or chromosomal syndrome or teratogenic factor. After two affected children, the risk of congenital heart disease in future sibs is approximately trebled, regardless of whether the affected individuals have the same heart defect or not. This gives risks ranging from 5 per cent for the rare defects to 10 per cent for a common abnormality such as ventricular septal defect (VSD). A similar risk would be likely for future children where an affected parent has an affected child, although data to confirm this are not yet available. Numbers are insufficient to give individual estimates for specific defects. The occurrence of more distant affected relatives does not greatly raise the risks given in Table 19.4. In the occasional families with more than two affected first-degree relatives, risks are likely to approach 50 per cent, even though the factors underlying such occurrences are not understood.

ATRIAL SEPTAL DEFECT

Occasional families following autosomal dominant inheritance exist (one form has been mapped to chromosome 1), as well as dominant syndromal associations such as the Holt–Oram syndrome and atrial septal defect (ASD) with atrioventricular conduction defects. These families are too rare to affect the general recurrence risks, but should be borne in mind when familial clusters of three or more patients are encountered, which should probably be counselled as mendelian. Minimal hand defects should be checked for in such families, to rule out Holt–Oram syndrome, for which the gene has now been isolated and which has proved to be the human counterpart of a previously known mouse developmental gene (TBX5).

VENTRICULAR SEPTAL DEFECT

The figures given in Table 19.4 apply to severe VSDs, mostly those patients requiring surgery. It is doubtful whether the risks are as high for relatives of patients with asymptomatic or transient defects.

PATENT DUCTUS ARTERIOSUS

Congenital rubella must be excluded. The recurrence risk of patent ductus arteriosus varies considerably between series, but 3 per cent seems a reasonable figure for sibs. The similar overall risk to offspring seems to mask a higher maternal risk of around 4 per cent. A rare dominantly inherited form with dysmorphic abnormalities exists (Char syndrome).

CONOTRUNCAL DEFECTS

This is the group where a careful clinical family and molecular search is most likely to show an underlying chromosome 22 deletion (see below). Few such cases are truly non-syndromal, but the features can be subtle.

DEXTROCARDIA WITH ASPLENIA

Absence of the spleen, or the presence of multiple spleens, is an important point to note at autopsy in congenital heart disease, because a combination of defects involving left-sided visceral structures is seen with asplenia, and a corresponding series involving right-sided ones with polysplenia. The recurrence risk overall is probably comparable to other types of congenital heart disease, but there is an X-linked isomerism form for which a gene (*ZIC3*) has been isolated. An important group of developmental defects involving laterality and isomerism is starting to be defined, with the heart prominently involved. Total situs inversus also provides an association with dextrocardia, as in Kartagener syndrome (see p. 277).

ENDOCARDIAL FIBROELASTOSIS

Endocardial fibroelastosis may be secondary to acquired myocarditis or may accompany other congenital heart defects; idiopathic fibroelastosis should only be accepted as the diagnosis with autopsy evidence. A thorough study from Toronto found a recurrence risk of 3.8 per cent in sibs, rather higher than expected from the incidence of the disorder. It is possible that a small subgroup follows autosomal recessive inheritance, but if it exists, it cannot be distinguished from the majority at present.

SYNDROMES WITH CONGENITAL HEART DISEASE

These are numerous and not all show a clear inheritance pattern. The following deserve special note.

Noonan syndrome

The characteristic facies with ptosis and low-set ears, as well as a different cardiac defect (commonly pulmonary stenosis but also hypertrophic cardiomyopathy) from that of Turner syndrome, should allow clinical recognition of this relatively common disorder in either sex. Autosomal dominant inheritance occurs but the risk to sibs of an isolated case with entirely normal parents is low. Mutations in the gene *PTPN II* have been found in about 50 per cent of patients.

22q deletion syndrome

Loss of chromosome material from the proximal part of 22q, involving a number of genes, is now known to be an important syndromal cause of congenital heart disease, particularly conotruncal defects (around 30 per cent of all cases). It combines conditions formerly considered as distinct, such as DiGeorge syndrome (with thymic and parathyroid hypoplasia) and velocardiofacial (Shprintzen) syndrome. Facial features are characteristic but often subtle, and some family members have no heart defect. The precise combination of features probably reflects which genes are involved. Molecular diagnostic FISH testing may show a defect when chromosomes appear normal. The recurrence risk is small if parental tests are normal, but it is close to 50 per cent where a parent has the defect.

Williams syndrome

This combination of supravalvular aortic stenosis with a characteristic facies, mental handicap and variable hypercalcaemia is now known to be a microdeletion syndrome of chromosome 7p, with loss of several genes, including that for elastin, which provides a valuable molecular test. Recurrence is rare if parents are clinically normal and show no elastin defect. Isolated dominantly inherited supravalvular aortic stenosis involves the same region.

CARDIOMYOPATHIES

Cardiomyopathies may form part of primary mendelian disorders such as type 2 glycogenosis, Duchenne and myotonic dystrophy, mitochondrial myopathies and Friedreich's ataxia, as well as specific syndromes. Much adult cardiomyopathy is secondary to external factors such as alcohol.

HYPERTROPHIC CARDIOMYOPATHY

Hypertrophic cardiomyopathy in older children and young adults is not rare (around 1 in 500 prevalence) and appears to be inherited as a variable autosomal dominant. Penetrance is almost complete if the family is studied by echocardiography, but only around 25 per cent clinically, i.e. there is a risk of 1 in 8 for clinical disease in first-degree relatives. Specific mutations at the myosin beta-heavy chain locus have been identified in some families, while others result from defects in tropomyosin and troponin. This may help in the genetic counselling of dominantly inherited families, but the ethical issues of such testing in isolated cases and their asymptomatic relatives are of major importance and need careful consideration. Whether and when to test children is an equally problematic issue, since as yet we have little information on the degree or timing of clinical risk to those carrying such mutations, which appears to vary with the specific gene and mutation involved. Suggestions for the general screening of athletes seem even more unwise. Caution is strongly urged until the situation becomes clearer.

DILATED CARDIOMYOPATHY

This is rarer than hypertrophic cardiomyopathy (around 1 in 2000 births). Most childhood cases have no clear genetic basis or are part of more general metabolic disorders, but specific X-linked and dominant forms are recognized (at least six gene loci mapped), although gene identification has progressed less far than in hypertrophic cardiomyopathy. The X-linked Barth syndrome also shows skeletal myopathy and general metabolic changes. Dystrophin-related cardiomyopathies (also X-linked) are another rare group.

CONGENITAL CARDIAC CONDUCTION DEFECTS

These are important causes of unexpected sudden death. A major recent advance in the long Q–T syndrome has been the identification of specific sodium or potassium ion channel defects for the different forms. All the specific types follow autosomal dominant inheritance, but the form with deafness (Jervell and Lange–Nielsen syndrome) is now known to be due to homozygosity, each parent carrying a mutation (though not necessarily symptomatic). Occasional dominantly inherited families with Wolff–Parkinson–White (WPW) syndrome have been recorded, but most cases are sporadic. As with hypertrophic cardiomyopathy, great caution should be exercised when considering testing healthy relatives, especially children. Familial heart block may very rarely occur congenitally, but an important dominantly inherited form exists with onset in adult life and no early clinical or other detectable abnormalities.

CORONARY HEART DISEASE

The epidemic increase of coronary heart disease in recent decades, now declining in much of North America and Europe, is likely to have environmental causes, but susceptibility has a strong genetic basis, particularly when onset is early. Insurance com-panies have long recognized this, basing their conclusions on extensive actuarial data, but little practical use has yet been made of our knowledge in terms of information to relatives and the application of preventive measures. The risk of death from ischaemic heart disease in relatives of patients with ischaemic heart disease has been known for many years (Table 19.5) and has not been altered by recent studies. As expected, the increase is greater where the index patient is female (see Chapter 3), although the absolute risk figure is greater for male relatives than for females. One-third of monozygotic twin pairs show concordance for coronary heart disease.

Two particular genetic influences have been identified:

- the major gene of familial hypercholesterolaemia and other genetic loci affecting lipid levels
- other genetic factors independent of lipid status.

Table 19.5 Risks of death from ischaemic heart disease between the ages of 35 and 55 years in first-degree relatives of index patients with ischaemic heart disease

	Male index case	Female index case
Male first-degree relative	I in 12 (×5)	I in 10 (×6.5)
Female first-degree relative	I in 36 (×2.5)	I in 12 (×7)

From Slack J, Evans KA (1966), *J Med Genet* **3**, 239–257.

Table 19.6 Risks of heart disease in familial hypercholesterolaemia

Age (years)	Percentage with ischaemic heart disease	
	Males	Females
30	5	0
30–39	24	0
40–49	51	12
50–59	85	57
60–69	100	74

FAMILIAL HYPERCHOLESTEROLAEMIA

This should be suspected whenever a familial aggregation of early coronary heart disease occurs. Many patients will show xanthomas or other cholesterol deposits, but vascular disease may be the only clinical feature. It is most important to recognize that the great majority of lipid abnormalities found in patients with vascular disease are secondary to dietary factors or other disorders and that familial hypercholesterolaemia should only be diagnosed when these have been excluded. Even when only primary cases with typical lipoprotein abnormalities are considered, it seems likely that the majority are multifactorial in origin, rather than following simple mendelian inheritance. Classic familial hypercholesterolaemia, accounting for around 10–20 per cent of early coronary heart disease, is an autosomal dominant disorder, with a heterozygote prevalence estimated to be around 1 in 400 to 1 in 1000, although in some populations (e.g. South Africans of Dutch origin) the prevalence may be as high as 1 in 100. Affected homozygotes with severe childhood disease are well recognized but extremely rare.

The risk of offspring of a heterozygous patient inheriting the gene is 50 per cent, but the risk of heart disease, which is the relevant factor, is considerably lower than this, particularly in females (Table 19.6). The risk to offspring of an isolated case showing this lipid abnormality is also considerably lower than where an established dominant pattern exists in the family, since a proportion of the non-genetic lipid defects are indistinguishable from it, unless a specific mutation has been demonstrated.

The disorder can be reliably detected in early childhood by lipoprotein electrophoresis, and possibly in cord blood by analysis of low-density lipoprotein (LDL) cholesterol. It is still uncertain to what extent early childhood therapy modifies the course of the disorder, or whether newborn testing would be justified. While childhood testing of those at high genetic risk is important, there is certainly no case for population-level cholesterol screening in childhood.

The basic defect is an LDL receptor deficiency, or in some families an alteration of the receptor. The gene itself, located on chromosome 19, has been fully characterized, and a variety of mutational defects found in patients. RFLPs can be used to predict risks in families without an identified mutation.

At a practical level, familial hypercholesterolaemia provides a lamentable example of a neglected opportunity for primary prevention of a common and treatable genetic disorder, despite clear evidence of benefit shown by systemic cascade testing of family members from studies in the Netherlands and the UK. The diagnosis is often missed; families are rarely studied systematically, and even more rarely given proper information and management, while no system of genetic registers exists in most areas. This is probably because the disorder is too frequent to be handled at a regional level by clinical geneticists, while other clinicians and those in primary care are not set up for such a process. The disorder should be a useful indicator as to the success (or otherwise) of moving genetics into regular clinical practice. In 2004, specific programmes of family testing (not population screening) are at last beginning to address the problem in the UK.

OTHER GENETIC INFLUENCES IN CORONARY HEART DISEASE

Apart from familial hypercholesterolaemia, genetic variations exist in a variety of other lipoproteins and their corresponding DNA polymorphisms – e.g. apoAI and AII, apoB, ApoE, Lp(a) – which show correlations with atherosclerosis at a population level, and which may well be important risk determinants. Unlike familial hypercholesterolaemia, their relevance within individual families is not yet well understood and there is no proven case for testing asymptomatic relatives. This may change as we learn more about the mendelian patterns involved and the precise levels of risk. The general issue of cholesterol and related lipid screening is even more questionable.

Familial aggregations of early coronary heart disease are quite often encountered in clinical practice (although rarely referred to genetics clinics), where there is no detectable lipid abnormality or any other primary cause that can be found. Despite extensive genome-wide searches and investigation of possible candidate gene loci (e.g. homocystine and ACE pathways), no clear major risk factors have been conclusively identified and certainly

Table 19.7 Some rare genetic causes of premature vascular disease

Disorder	Inheritance
Pseudoxanthoma elasticum	Autosomal recessive (sometimes autosomal dominant)
Homocystinuria	Autosomal recessive
Progeria	Autosomal recessive
Cockayne syndrome	Autosomal recessive
Werner syndrome	Autosomal recessive
Menkes syndrome	X-linked recessive

none relevant at present to genetic counselling and testing. Some rare causes of premature vascular disease are listed in Table 19.7. They account for only a small proportion of the total problem, but as their molecular basis is now largely known, this may give important clues as to factors involved in more common vascular degenerations.

Venous thrombosis is considered in Chapter 24.

ANEURYSMS AND RELATED VASCULAR LESIONS

Aortic aneurysms and dissection are a feature of Marfan syndrome (see Chapter 14). Large vessel rupture and other serious vascular incidents are also a feature of several of the other primary connective tissue disorders (see Chapter 14), notably those involving type III collagen, such as type IV (vascular) Ehlers–Danlos syndrome and pseudoxanthoma elasticum. Primary cystic medial necrosis may also follow dominant inheritance.

Abdominal aneurysms have been found to involve deficiencies of type III collagen, although it seem unlikely that this deficiency follows a mendelian pattern and such tests should not at present be used as a basis for risk estimation.

Cerebral aneurysms and **stroke** are considered in Chapter 12.

Hereditary haemorrhagic telangiectasia (autosomal dominant) may give serious circulatory problems from pulmonary arteriovenous shunts, as well as the more obvious cutaneous telangiectases and nosebleeds. Two specific genes involved in endothelial growth regulation have been identified.

Cavernous haemangiomas are considered in Chapter 16.

Familial glomus tumours provide an unusual example of autosomal dominant inheritance modified by genetic imprinting (see p. 26), which results in the disorder being expressed only when paternally transmitted.

HYPERTENSION

With rare exceptions, this behaves as a classical polygenic disorder, with around a threefold risk increase for individuals with two or more affected relatives. Despite early reports of angiotensin-converting enzyme (ACE) variants being a risk factor, this has not been confirmed, nor has any other specific locus found to be involved.

Rare, early-onset, dominantly inherited forms of hypertension are seen in the disorders of aldosterone metabolism, Liddle and Gordon syndromes.

Primary pulmonary hypertension is a very rare condition, dominantly inherited in some families, and mapped to chromosome 2q.

LYMPHATIC DISORDERS

Mild lymphoedema of hands and feet may be seen in both Turner and Noonan syndromes. Prenatal onset of oedema may be responsible for a number of dysmorphic features. The most common and most severe form of lymphoedema, Milroy's disease, follows autosomal dominant inheritance and can usually be recognized at birth. It is now known to result from defects in vascular endothelial growth factor (VEGFR3). A milder and later-onset form (Meige's disease) is more variable in inheritance. It is uncertain at present whether the pattern is autosomal recessive or autosomal dominant with variable penetrance.

Two specific autosomal dominant syndromes are lymphoedema with yellow nails and lymphoedema with distichiasis (double eyelashes).

RHEUMATIC FEVER

The recognition of a streptococcal basis for rheumatic fever and its dramatic decline in Western populations should not obscure the fact that susceptibility is strongly influenced by inheritance. Early studies (see pp. 49–52 of Nora et al., 1991) showed a risk of around 10 per cent in sibs and offspring of an affected person developing the condition at some later stage of life, and double this risk when a parent and a sib were affected. The risks are now likely to represent susceptibility rather than actual disease, but may still be appropriate for the many parts of the world where the disorder remains common.

RESPIRATORY DISORDERS

Two important pulmonary disorders, cystic fibrosis and alpha-1-antitrypsin deficiency (the latter discussed in Chapter 20), follow autosomal recessive inheritance and in both there have been major advances relevant to genetic counselling. There is no convincing evidence that the heterozygotes in either disorder are more prone to lung or other diseases.

CYSTIC FIBROSIS

Cystic fibrosis is the most common serious autosomal recessive disorder in northern Europe, where the frequency of the disease is around 1 in 2500 and the carrier frequency is around 1 in 25.

The remarkable recent advances in our understanding of cystic fibrosis (CF) have sprung almost entirely from genetic studies, the gene being the first to be isolated by the positional cloning approach without the help of chromosome rearrangements. Characterization of the protein (the CF transmembrane regulator) promises to lead to therapeutic progress too, but genetic tests are currently based on the gene itself. A single mutation, a deletion of three base pairs (delta F508), is responsible for 60–80 per cent of CF mutations in northern European populations, although it shows a steady decline towards southern Europe and is rare in most non-European populations. Numerous rarer mutations make up the remainder, although some are commoner in particular population groups.

Genetic counselling in CF can now be extremely accurate with use of appropriate mutational tests, making it essential to analyse the mutations present in the particular family, especially any affected individual. Where a couple have had an affected child, with a 1 in 4 risk for future children, early prenatal diagnosis based on DNA analysis can detect or exclude the disorder in most cases; closely linked markers may still be needed if specific mutations cannot be identified.

Carrier detection within families is also now feasible in most cases where the affected individual is available for molecular analysis. Parents and children of a CF patient will be obligatory carriers, but the risk for offspring of sibs (in the absence of consanguinity) is low (1 in 150), and even lower in more distant relatives. In fact, for sibs and for parents of a CF child who subsequently marry other partners, it will be the carrier status of the unrelated partner that will be the major determinant of whether there is risk to a child. Testing for this has been unsatisfactory until very recently and is still not without problems, as indicated below.

Mutational testing for delta F508 of a person with no family history of CF (in northern Europe) will detect around 70 per cent of carriers, leaving a residual risk of being a carrier of a little over 1 per cent for a person with a normal result. In most populations, the testing for three or four further mutations is likely to bring detection close to 90 per cent, leaving a residual risk of under 1 in 200, or 1 in 800 for a child being affected if the partner is a known carrier. These low levels of risk are usually adequate for genetic counselling of CF families and those married into them. Most molecular genetics laboratories will have a battery of tests for the most frequent mutations in the particular populations, which can be supplemented by testing for rare mutations if required. For population screening, the issues are more complex, as discussed in Chapter 27. In southern Europe, the mutational spectrum is different, as it is in non-Caucasian populations as well, while in Jewish populations some specific mutations are prominent.

The different CF mutations show varying degrees of correlation with severity of lung and gastrointestinal problems. Some with minimal systemic effects are being discovered, including isolated absence of the vas deferens (many CF males are infertile because of this; see Chapter 22).

MICROCYSTIC DISEASE OF THE LUNG

Microcystic disease of the lung is a rare disorder which also follows autosomal recessive inheritance.

KARTAGENER SYNDROME

Kartagener syndrome is characterized by bronchiectasis, recurrent sinusitis, dextrocardia and other heart defects, and often asplenia, and has traditionally been considered autosomal recessive. Recent work has shown this disorder to be part of a more extensive group of defects of ciliary function, often accompanied by male infertility. The finding, a recurrence risk in sibs of 13 per cent but no transmission to children, would fit well with autosomal recessive inheritance and penetrance of 50 per cent.

ASTHMA AND ATOPY

The familial tendency for asthma has been recognized for many years, especially in relation to a general atopic sensitivity, including eczema (see p. 241). The commonness of the condition makes it difficult to disentangle a clear genetic basis, since relatives from both parental lines are commonly affected but it is unlikely to follow mendelian inheritance. The risk of intrinsic asthma, with no atopic tendency, is around 5 per cent for first-degree relatives, but for atopic cases the figures are higher, especially if the risk for any form of atopy is considered. Some studies have shown higher risks if the mother is the affected parent, but this is not yet sufficiently established to be incorporated into genetic counselling risks.

The identification of specific genes involved in asthma and atopy remains a controversial area, with conflicting results on earlier findings of a locus on chromosome 11q. There are no genetic tests helpful for counselling at present.

EMPHYSEMA AND CHRONIC OBSTRUCTIVE PULMONARY DISEASE

Even when smoking and other environmental variables have been allowed for, and rare genetic causes ruled out, there is a familial aggregation for this, but no specific genes have yet been identified despite extensive genome searches.

Genetic causes include alpha-1-antitrypsin deficiency (but not its heterozygous state), CF and ciliary dyskinesia syndromes, discussed separately, as well as connective tissue disorders such as pseudoxanthoma elasticum and cutis laxa.

SARCOIDOSIS

Sarcoidosis is occasionally familial, but affected members are usually related through the maternal line. Satisfactory risk figures do not appear to exist.

LUNG CANCER

Lung cancer has long been recognized to have a genetic predisposition, interacting with environmental factors, which include uranium mining, radon and asbestos exposure, as well as smoking. These environmental factors themselves interact. Small-cell lung carcinoma is associated with somatic chromosome changes involving chromosome 3, but whether this is also involved in genetic susceptibility is still unknown. No clear mendelian form has been recognized, possibly because it is submerged by smoking as an environmental factor, but susceptibility loci are being actively sought and should help in understanding the pathogenesis.

CONGENITAL LARYNGEAL AND TRACHEAL DEFECTS

A variety of these have been described, including laryngomalacia, congenital subglottic stenosis, laryngeal atresia and laryngeal clefts. They may be isolated or syndromal. Congenital vocal cord paralysis may also be part of a wider neurological disorder. Very little information is available on genetic risks or specific inheritance patterns, but a useful general review and summary table of syndromes is provided in Tewfik and der Kaloustian (see 'Further reading').

FURTHER READING

Burn J, Goodship J (2002). Congenital heart disease. In: Rimoin DL, Connor JM, Pyeritz RE, Korf BR, eds. *Emery and Rimoin's Practice and Principles of Medical Genetics*. Edinburgh, Churchill Livingstone, pp. 1237–1326.

Caulfield M, Bouloux PM, Munroe P (1997). Progress in determining the genes for hypertension, insulin resistance and dyslipidemia. *Ann NY Acad Sci* **20**, 110–117.

Marian AJ (2000). *Genetics for Cardiologists*. London, Remedica – a compact and useful source of up-to-date information.

Nora JJ, Berg K, Nora AH (1991). *Cardiovascular Diseases. Genetics, Epidemiology and Prevention*. Oxford, Oxford University Press.

Tewfik TL, der Kaloustian VM (1997). *Congenital Anomalies of the Ear, Nose and Throat*. New York, Oxford University Press.

The gastrointestinal tract

Relatively few gastrointestinal disorders follow clear mendelian inheritance, and so genetic counselling is more dependent on empiric risks than is the case for some other systems. Most data of this type have been collected from western European or American populations, so figures must be applied with caution in other areas, particularly where the incidence of the disorder is known to differ significantly.

Gastrointestinal disorders have also proved more treatable than most groups, so that individuals with previously fatal disorders now reproduce. Data for risks to offspring of affected individuals are so far available for only a few conditions, such as pyloric stenosis, and in preliminary form for Hirschsprung's disease and oesophageal atresia.

OESOPHAGEAL ATRESIA

Most cases of oesophageal atresia are combined with tracheo-oesophageal fistula. As many as 55 per cent of cases have been found to be associated with other malformations, notably rectal and duodenal atresia, diaphragmatic hernia, hypoplasia of the radius and renal agenesis. Around 10 per cent of cases are associated with chromosome abnormalities. Despite this, the recurrence risk to sibs in a large series of 345 patients was very low (one affected sib), so that the presence of associated defects (unless part of a specific syndrome) should not be grounds for giving a higher risk. Risk figures for offspring of treated patients are becoming available, and appear to be low, probably not more than 1 per cent.

OESOPHAGEAL CANCER

The risk to relatives is not obviously increased, at least in western Europe. The situation may be different in areas of high incidence such as central Asia and parts of Africa, where striking family clusters have been reported. Environmental factors are probably responsible for the major differences in incidence. The remarkable, but exceedingly rare, families with oesophageal cancer and tylosis (hyperkeratosis of palms and soles; see also Chapter 16) following autosomal dominant inheritance should be borne in mind if a family cluster is found in an area of low incidence. The gene locus is on chromosome 17 (apparently not one of the keratin genes) and it will be of great interest to see if this is also involved in the somatic mutations of common oesophageal cancers.

DIAPHRAGMATIC HERNIA

Although a few instances of affected sibs, most with complete aplasia of the diaphragm, have been reported, the overall risk is extremely low, probably no greater than 1 per cent, even though half the cases in one study had associated defects, most commonly of the nervous system. Diaphragmatic hypoplasia is seen in some primary myopathies (e.g. congenital myotonic dystrophy), and in some specific malformations (e.g. Pallister–Killian syndrome, tetrasomy 12p).

Hiatus hernia, whether in infancy or adult life, does not seem to show any notable increase in incidence in relatives.

INFANTILE PYLORIC STENOSIS

Pyloric stenosis follows the pattern expected for polygenic inheritance, with risks diminishing rapidly outside first-degree relatives, and with relatives of index patients of the more rarely affected sex (female) having a higher risk (Table 20.1).

The overall population incidence for the UK is around 3 per 1000 births (5 per 1000 male births and 1 per 1000 female births). Data on risks for families with more than one affected individual are not available, but such families are not rare and may provide the clue to specific genes involved.

Table 20.1 Risks to relatives of patients with infantile pyloric stenosis

Relative	Male index patients Risk (%)	Increase	Female index patients Risk (%)	Increase
Brothers	3.8	×8	9.2	×18
Sisters	2.7	×27	3.8	×38
Sons	5.5	×11	18.9	×38
Daughters	2.4	×24	7.0	×70
Nephews	2.3	×4.6	4.7	×9.4
Nieces	0.4	×3.6	–	–
Male first cousins	0.9	×1.9	0.7	×1.3
Female first cousins	0.2	×2.3	0.3	×2.6

OMPHALOCELE AND GASTROSCHISIS

Beckwith syndrome of exomphalos, macroglossia, general somatic overgrowth and hypoglycaemia is an important and treatable cause to exclude. Abnormal features may diminish during childhood and are often inconspicuous by adult life. Autosomal dominant inheritance is likely, but paternal transmission is rare, due to genetic imprinting. Microdeletions on chromosome 11p involving the insulin growth factor IGF-2 are responsible for some cases, while others result from loss of the maternal copy due to uniparental disomy (see p. 75).

Isolated omphalocele has a low (under 1 per cent) recurrence risk in sibs, although a few clusters have been reported. It is a cause of raised amniotic fluid alpha-fetoprotein levels requiring distinction from neural tube defects (see Chapter 8); ultrasonography provides help in this situation. This is most commonly an incidental finding in a pregnancy tested for other reasons.

It is most important that such cases detected by alpha-fetoprotein measurement or ultrasound screening are carefully assessed antenatally and postnatally to detect any associated syndrome or chromosome disorder.

BOWEL ATRESIAS AND MALROTATIONS

Most cases are sporadic, possibly resulting from intrauterine vascular occlusions. Familial aggregations are extremely rare – meconium ileus from cystic fibrosis must be distinguished from true atresia. Duodenal atresia occurs with increased frequency in Down's syndrome. Bowel duplications and enterogenous cysts are usually sporadic. 'Echogenic bowel' is an ultrasound finding (not in itself an abnormality) that may, in a proportion of cases, indicate cystic fibrosis or other pathology, although the outcome is normal in the majority.

PEPTIC ULCER

Genetic studies are difficult in a disorder which is common (around 4 per cent of adult males and 2 per cent of adult females in the UK) and where symptoms are often ill-defined. A detailed account of the genetic factors and associations is provided by Rotter *et al.* (2002, see 'Further reading'). Most surveys have shown around a threefold increase in both sibs and offspring. Childhood cases more commonly have an affected relative. The empiric risk for first-degree relations is around 10 per cent, possibly higher if adjusted to a lifetime risk.

Now that infective agents (*Helicobacter pylori*) and high serum pepsinogen levels are established as relevant factors in peptic ulcer, this may help to identify specific genes involved.

Numerous associations exist between peptic ulcer and other primary disorders, some of them mendelian, such as multiple endocrine neoplasia type I. These should be borne in mind, especially when striking familial aggregations are encountered.

GASTRIC CANCER

As with oesophageal cancer, there are considerable geographical variations in incidence, in which genetic factors may play a part (e.g. in the Welsh and Japanese). Unlike colo-rectal cancer, clear mendelian forms are exceptional, although there may be an increased risk in such conditions as HNPCC (see Chapter 25). A few familial cases result from rare mutations in alpha-cadheirin. A modest twofold to fourfold increase has been shown in first-degree relatives of patients.

ATROPHIC GASTRITIS AND PERNICIOUS ANAEMIA

One-quarter of first-degree relatives of patients with atrophic gastritis have histological evidence of the disorder; a similar proportion show parietal cell antibodies. It seems likely that an autosomal dominant gene controlling production of autoantibodies is involved. There is extensive overlap with other autoimmune disorders and autoanti-bodies within families.

COELIAC DISEASE

The risks to relatives depend on the thoroughness with which they are investigated and the criteria for diagnosis, but around 10 per cent would seem the soundest estimate for first-degree relatives based on several series using jejunal biopsy. Risks to second-degree or more distant relatives appear small, not exceeding 1 per cent for overt disease.

Coeliac disease is strongly associated with proteins of the major histocompatibility complex and it is likely that the disease-associated haplotype contains genes coding for specific HLA products which may be necessary for the disease to develop. However, HLA testing is of little help in risk prediction for relatives. A wider genome search for other loci involved is in progress.

GASTROINTESTINAL ENZYME DEFECTS

Gastrointestinal enzyme defects all follow autosomal recessive inheritance and include:

- disaccharidase deficiencies (maltase, sucrase, lactase) – partial lactase deficiency after infancy is normal in most Asian and African populations
- pancreatic enzyme deficiencies (trypsinogen, enterokinase, lipase)
- acrodermatitis enteropathica (possibly due to a defect in zinc metabolism)
- congenital chloride diarrhoea (due to mutations in an ion transport gene related and adjacent to that for cystic fibrosis on chromosome 7).

HEREDITARY PANCREATITIS

Inheritance is autosomal dominant with penetrance around 80 per cent. Hereditary pancreatitis is a rare but important cause of recurrent abdominal pain in childhood and young adults and may predispose to later pancreatic cancer. It is now known to result from mutations in the cationic trypsinogen gene. Genetic testing should be used with considerable caution in view of the great variability of the condition. Type V hyperlipoproteinaemia (autosomal recessive) may also cause recurrent pancreatitis.

CYSTIC FIBROSIS

Cystic fibrosis is discussed in Chapter 19. The diagnostic use of DNA analysis as well as the sweat test in cases of meconium ileus now allows most of such cases where CF is the cause to be recognized.

GALLSTONES

These are only simply inherited when secondary to disorders causing excess haemolysis or disturbed lipid metabolism.

INTUSSUSCEPTION

A risk of 1 in 40 for sibs of childhood cases has been shown, compared with 1 in 750 for the general population. Cystic fibrosis and polyposes may be underlying causes.

INFLAMMATORY BOWEL DISEASE

Overlap within families has been shown between ulcerative colitis and Crohn's disease. Recurrence risks are low in both disorders, with a risk of around 3 per cent for first-degree relatives (possibly around 5 per cent if adjusted to lifetime risks). The risks in Jewish origin families may be somewhat higher.

Recently a susceptibility locus for Crohn's disease (but surprisingly not for ulcerative colitis) has been identified, with mutations in the gene *NOD2* increasing the risk, especially in the infrequent homozygotes. Use of this in practice needs to await more information.

A rare lethal form of enterocolitis in infancy has been described which apparently follows autosomal recessive inheritance. It may well prove to have a metabolic basis.

FAMILIAL ADENOMATOUS POLYPOSIS AND COLON CANCER

These are discussed in Chapter 25.

HIRSCHSPRUNG'S DISEASE

The risks depend on the sex of the index patient and relative, and on the length of the aganglionic segment, as is to be expected in multifactorial inheritance. The male to female ratio in patients is around 3:1, and long segment involvement makes up 13 per cent of all cases. The overall population incidence is about 1 in 5000 births (0.02 per cent).

Table 20.2 combines the results of three major family studies. Risks for offspring of affected patients with short segment disease are now becoming available and are low, probably not over 2 per cent. Risks for second-degree and third-degree relatives are imprecise but are low. An important development has been the finding of defects in the *RET* oncogene in about half of cases, allowing risks to be defined better in these families. Other genes are also involved but the *RET* oncogene appears to be the major determinant, making Hirschsprung's disease one of the rather small number of disorders intermediate between mendelian and truly polygenic inheritance. It is of great interest that the same gene is involved in multiple endocrine neoplasia type 2, and that both disorders relate to neural crest tissue. The risk estimates in the table will need redefining in the light of more systematic molecular studies, but so far do not seem to require significant revision. Molecular analysis is not currently helpful in terms of counselling individual families.

Table 20.2 Genetic risks to sibs in Hirschsprung's disease

	Brothers (%)	Sisters (%)	Offspring (both sexes)
All lengths of aganglionic segment			
Male index patient	5.3	2.3	
Female index patient	11.3	13.6	
Short aganglionic segment			
Male index patient	4.7	0.6	2.0
Female index patient	8.1	2.9	
Long aganglionic segment			
Male index patient	16.1	11.1	High
Female index patient	18.2	9.1	(About 50%)

Based on Passarge E (1972), *Birth Defects* **8**, 63–67; also see Amiel and Lyonnet (2001) (Further reading).

IMPERFORATE ANUS

Imperforate anus is seen in various syndromes, notably with ocular coloboma in association with an extra chromosome 22 fragment (see Chapter 4) and with vertebral and radial limb defects (see Chapter 14). There is no evidence of a high recurrence risk to sibs either in the VATER syndrome or in isolated imperforate anus.

GENETIC LIVER DISEASE

Liver involvement occurs in numerous metabolic disorders, including lipidoses, mucopolysaccharidoses, glycogenoses and galactosaemia. A few require separate mention.

WILSON'S DISEASE (AUTOSOMAL RECESSIVE)

This disorder may present to neurologists or to haematologists as well as with liver disease and is treatable if recognized early. Prenatal diagnosis and carrier detection are both possible now that the gene (on chromosome 13) has been isolated.

HAEMOCHROMATOSIS

This condition, characterized by excessive iron storage in a variety of organs, including liver, pancreas and heart, has traditionally been considered as following autosomal recessive inheritance, but the genetic component should really be considered more as a susceptibility locus than as a true mendelian disorder. It is largely sex-limited to males. Transmission of the full disease by an affected person is rare, but sibs have a higher risk (clinical onset delayed and reduced in females). Although earlier studies suggest this might be as high as 1 in 4, this is likely to be a considerable overestimate in the light of recent research (see below). A close HLA linkage indicating an important and common gene controlling iron storage in this region led to isolation of the gene itself (*HFE*) and represents a major advance. As with cystic fibrosis, one particular mutation (C282Y) seems to be particularly common in northern European populations, with 80–90 per cent of patients homozygous for it.

Application of the findings, however, is going to be complex, and pressure for widespread testing and screening has been both premature and inappropriate. Particularly relevant is the disparity between the high frequency of homozygosity for the main mutation (around 1 in 150 to 1 in 200) and the frequency of the disease, as measured by clinical and pathological studies (around 1 in 5000 to 1 in 6000), 30 times less. Even allowing for underdiagnosis, this can only mean that most homozygotes are, and remain, clinically unaffected, rendering it both unnecessary and unwise for them to be converted into patients and treated by venesection. Thorough studies in both Britain and USA have now confirmed that as few as 1 per cent of homozygotes for the predisposing mutation may develop clinically significant iron overload, although the figure may well be higher for close relatives on account of other shared genes. Heterozygotes (10 per cent of the population in northern Europe) are at no significant risk and it is most important that they are not falsely worried. Until considerably more is known about the relationship between genotype and disorder, in both sexes, genetic testing should be focused on high-risk individuals, i.e. sibs and possibly offspring in particular circumstances. A further complexity is that a considerable proportion of patients with porphyria cutanea tarda are also homozygous for the main haemochromatosis mutation.

ALPHA-1-ANTITRYPSIN DEFICIENCY

This relatively frequent (1 in 2000–4000) autosomal recessive disorder, with the gene isolated on chromosome 14q, is an important cause of neonatal hepatitis and cirrhosis. Some adults develop emphysema, accounting for around 1 per cent of all cases, while others remain healthy. A Swedish newborn screening survey has shown 17 per cent with liver problems as infants, two-thirds of these recovering, the others progressive. This variable prognosis and lack of specific therapy (apart from avoidance of both active and passive smoking) make the disorder unsuitable for population newborn screening. Families tend to be concordant for mild or severe disease. The disorder is rare in black and Oriental populations. Heterozygotes are healthy, with no good evidence of increased risk of either lung or liver disease. Unfortunately they are frequently misinformed and unnecessarily worried as the result of genetic testing, and this may increase with the promotion of DNA-based genotyping as a 'diagnostic' test. Prenatal diagnosis is feasible by molecular analysis but has been rarely used.

HYPERBILIRUBINAEMIAS

The hyperbilirubinaemias are a heterogeneous group, including the following conditions:

- Gilbert's syndrome – probably autosomal dominant; this harmless condition is so common (~5 per cent of the population) that it should be considered a normal variant rather than a disease

- Dubin–Johnson syndrome – variable autosomal dominant; rarely causes significant symptoms
- defective bilirubin conjugation – Crigler–Najjar type 1, type 2 Arias; both probably autosomal recessive
- benign recurrent cholestasis – autosomal recessive
- fatal progressive cholestasis (Byler's disease) – autosomal recessive.

BILIARY ATRESIA

Biliary atresia may occur in chromosomal trisomies or be the result of intrauterine viral hepatitis. Most cases are of unknown cause, and recurrence seems rare in sibs regardless of cause, although no satisfactory figures exist.

ALAGILLE SYNDROME (ARTERIOHEPATIC DYSPLASIA)

Alagille syndrome shows a combination of bile duct hypoplasia with facial anomalies and cardiac defects (commonly peripheral pulmonary stenosis). Microdeletions of chromosome 20 are found in some cases and have led to isolation of a specific gene homologous to the *Drosophila* 'Jagged' gene. Recurrence risk is low if the defect is present in the child but not in a parent. Parents showing partial expression may transmit the disorder.

POLYCYSTIC DISEASE OF THE LIVER AND CONGENITAL HEPATIC FIBROSIS

A variety of forms can be recognized pathologically, depending on the predominance of fibrosis or cystic change and the degree of renal involvement (see Chapter 21). All appear to follow autosomal recessive inheritance. Adult polycystic kidney disease (autosomal dominant) rarely has more than a few hepatic cysts in early life. A separate entity of adult polycystic liver disease without renal involvement may exist, but is rare compared with polycystic kidney disease, so that offspring of patients may have a risk of renal as well as hepatic involvement.

ADULT CHRONIC LIVER DISEASE

In patients with an autoimmune cause, a strong association with other autoimmune disorders and the presence of various autoantibodies suggest the action of a dominant gene affecting immune responses. A few striking familial aggregations of cirrhosis and hepatoma have been found to result from the hepatitis virus and to have been maternally transmitted. Susceptibility to persistence of the hepatitis virus may itself follow autosomal recessive inheritance.

FURTHER READING

General

King KA, Rotter JI, Motulsky AG (2002). *Genetic Basis of Common Diseases*. Oxford, Oxford University Press – the chapter on peptic ulcer is particularly worth consulting.

Scriver CK, Beaudet AL, Sly WS, Valle D (2001). *The Metabolic and Molecular Bases of Inherited Disease*. New York, McGraw-Hill – look at the chapters on specific disorders of carbohydrate metabolism.

Specific

Amiel J, Lyonnet S (2001). Hirschsprung disease, associated syndromes, and genetics: a review. *J Med Genet* **38**, 729–739.

Beutler E, Felitti VJ, Kiziol JA *et al.* (2002). Penetrance of 845 G →A (C282Y) HFE hereditary hemochromatosis mutation in the USA. *Lancet* **359**, 211–218.

Cox DW (1997). Review: molecular approaches to inherited liver disease. Focus on Wilson disease. *J Gastroenterol Hepatol* **12**, S251–S255.

de Paepe A, Dock H, Lechat MF (1993). The epidemiology of tracheo-oesophageal fistula and oesophageal atresia in Europe. *Arch Dis Child* **147**, 1203–1211.

Ellis I, Lerch MM, Whitcomb DC (2001). Genetic testing for hereditary pancreatitis – guidelines for indications, counselling, consent and privacy issues. *Pancreatology* **1**, 405–418.

Eng C (1996). The RET proto-oncogene in multiple endocrine neoplasia type 2 and Hirschsprung's disease. *N Engl J Med* **335**, 943–951.

McCune CA, Ravine D, Worwood M *et al.* (2003). Screening for hereditary haemochromatosis in families and beyond. *Lancet* **362**, 1897–1898.

Mitchell E, Risch N (1993). The genetics of infantile hypertrophic pyloric stenosis: a reanalysis. *Am J Dis Child* **147**, 1203–1211.

Rotter JI, Yang H, Taylor KD (2002). Inflammatory bowel disease. In: Rimoin DL, Connor JM, Pyeritz RE, Korf BR, eds. *Emery and Rimoin's Principles and Practice of Medical Genetics*. Edinburgh, Churchill Livingstone, pp. 1760–1791.

CHAPTER 21

Renal disease

POLYCYSTIC KIDNEY DISEASE

Renal cystic disease may occur in a number of generalized syndromes (Table 21.1). It may also be secondary to obstructive anomalies *in utero* and to end-stage renal disease in later life. Thus, the question to be asked is not just whether the case is one of renal cystic disease, but also what is the cause. Once the various other causes have been excluded

Table 21.1 Genetic disorders associated with renal cystic disease

Autosomal dominant
Tuberous sclerosis
Von Hippel–Lindau disease
Beckwith–Wiedemann syndrome

Autosomal recessive
Meckel syndrome
Cerebrohepatorenal (Zellweger) syndrome
Bardet–Biedl syndrome
Short-rib polydactyly syndromes
Fryns syndrome

X-linked
Orofaciodigital syndrome type I

Chromosomal
Trisomy 13, 18
Turner syndrome
Triploidy

(not always an easy task), primary polycystic disease most commonly falls into two distinct groups:

- adult polycystic kidney disease – autosomal dominant
- infantile polycystic disease – variable but often following autosomal recessive inheritance.

ADULT POLYCYSTIC KIDNEY DISEASE

Autosomal dominant polycystic kidney disease is one of the most common genetic disorders in adulthood (incidence around 1 in 1000), but it is extremely variable. Occasionally, newborn infants present with massive renal enlargement, while mild cases may be found incidentally at autopsy in old age. Genetic counselling of young, apparently healthy, adult family members presents problems. All such individuals should have a careful examination, urinalysis and renal ultrasound scan before being told that they are unlikely to be a gene carrier.

Apparently isolated cases should not be accepted as new mutations unless both parents are alive and have been shown to be normal.

Studies of adult polycystic kidney disease suggest that high-resolution ultrasonography will detect almost all gene carriers of the principal form (PKD1) over 19 years old, the risks of carrying the gene being under 5 per cent for those normal by these tests. There is a strong case for a genetic register for all families in a region, to ensure full ascertainment of families, with information for relatives and access to testing of relatives at risk. A systematic study from Australia has shown that early detection of the disorder in young adults can recognize and often avoid treatable complications, such as those due to hypertension or infection. Intracranial aneurysms are an important cause of mortality. Liver cysts are frequent but not usually of clinical significance.

Both the major genes for adult polycystic kidney disease have now been isolated. The gene for the commonest and more severe type (PKD1) is located on chromosome 16 immediately next to the gene for tuberous sclerosis (TSC2) and some of the renal cystic disease observed in that disorder is due to both genes being involved. Molecular tests are still not feasible for most cases of pure PKD1, so linked markers and renal ultrasound remain the mainstay of family testing. The PKD2 gene, on chromosome 14, is associated with milder disease and later onset, and has probably been under-diagnosed in the past.

The demand for prenatal diagnosis is currently small. It is debatable whether young children should be tested in the absence of clinical indications, whether by ultrasound scan (which can be regarded as a 'genetic' test in terms of its implications) or DNA markers. Certainly this should not be done without careful consideration of the issues, advice that is still too often ignored.

AUTOSOMAL RECESSIVE (INFANTILE) POLYCYSTIC KIDNEY DISEASE

Infantile polycystic disease is a disorder of both the kidneys and liver. The renal cysts are a manifestation of collecting duct ectasia and are accompanied by hepatic fibrosis and biliary dysgenesis.

The predominant presentation is in infancy. More recently, however, onset at later ages and survival into adulthood have been recognized. Generally, sibs show close concordance of onset and severity.

The histological appearance is distinct from that of adult polycystic disease presenting in infancy. Thus it is vital for an accurate autopsy to be done on probands who die, to avoid confusion with early childhood cases of this form and to exclude non-mendelian causes, particularly cystic renal dysplasia. In isolated cases with onset after the neonatal period, ultrasound examination of the liver, spleen and pancreas may be helpful. Increased hepatic echogeneity or dilated biliary ducts are characteristic findings. Although parents are usually clinically normal, both parents should be studied to exclude an asymptomatic case of the dominantly inherited form. Prenatal diagnosis by ultrasonography is now feasible in the more severe types, but false-negative and false-positive results have occurred.

Genetic heterogeneity was originally thought likely, but most cases now appear to be due to a single gene locus on chromosome 6p, with closely linked DNA markers that can be used in prenatal diagnosis. In addition, some severe cases result from deletion of the *PKD1* gene (adult cases result from alteration, not loss of gene function).

CYSTIC DYSPLASIA (MULTICYSTIC KIDNEY DISEASE)

Usually sporadic in occurrence and commonly secondary in aetiology to obstruction or other problems, cystic dysplasia may produce cystic changes and renal enlargement that may be clinically confused with inherited polycystic disease. While high-resolution ultrasonography is making diagnosis easier, careful histological review by an experienced pathologist is wise if there is any doubt.

MEDULLARY CYSTIC DISEASE (JUVENILE NEPHRONOPHTHISIS, MICROCYSTIC DISEASE)

Medullary cystic disease is a heterogeneous group defined by characteristic clinical and pathological features. The kidneys are small and sonographically echogenic. Despite the emphasis on cysts, they appear to contribute relatively little to the functional renal abnormality. Bernstein suggests that these disorders are therefore better regarded as hereditary tubulointerstitial nephritis with three principal subcategories:

- medullary cystic disease with either sporadic or dominant inheritance and a predominantly adult onset
- familial juvenile nephronophthisis with autosomal recessive inheritance and an onset predominantly in children; the gene, on chromosome 2q, has been cloned
- renal–retinal dysplasia with recessive inheritance and retinal degeneration. A comparable renal lesion is seen in Jeune asphyxiating thoracic dysplasia and Bardet–Biedl syndrome.

These types should be distinguished from the benign medullary sponge kidney, where no clear familial tendency has been shown.

Small cortical cysts occur in the rapidly fatal, autosomal recessive **Zellweger (cerebro-hepatorenal) syndrome**. Bernstein provides a useful summary of the many other syndromes associated with renal cortical cysts, although much of the information will require reassessment in the light of molecular advances.

OTHER HEREDITARY NEPHROPATHIES

CONGENITAL NEPHROSIS

Congenital nephrosis comprises a heterogeneous group. In the rare Finnish type (autosomal recessive), prenatal diagnosis is feasible from a greatly raised concentration of amniotic fluid alpha-fetoprotein (AFP; presumably derived from fetal urine). Specific mutation analysis is also now feasible.

IDIOPATHIC (MINIMAL CHANGE) CHILDHOOD NEPHROTIC SYNDROME

A careful family study has shown a 6 per cent risk to sibs.

IgA NEPHRITIS

There is a familial component to IgA nephritis, an immune-mediated disorder that accounts for up to a quarter of primary glomerulonephritis cases in adults. There are some familial clusters of the disease and there is a reported increase in the frequency of HLA-Bw35 or HLA-DR4, or both.

AMYLOIDOSIS

Renal involvement may occur in association with some of the primary amyloid neuropathies (due to defects in transthyretin; see Chapter 11) and with familial Mediterranean fever (autosomal recessive).

ALPORT SYNDROME (HEREDITARY NEPHROPATHY WITH NERVE DEAFNESS)

The mode of inheritance has been much disputed, but if other hereditary nephropathies are excluded, true Alport syndrome is undoubtedly X-linked, with variable expression in females and deafness a variable feature even in affected males. Microscopic haematuria is probably the most accurate clinical detector of heterozygous females. Renal electron microscopic detection of extensive thickening and splitting of the glomerular basement membrane helps to distinguish true Alport syndrome from various other hereditary nephropathies, most of which are dominantly inherited when onset is in adult life. The gene for type IV collagen is now known to be responsible, with specific mutations detected, and accurate carrier detection and prenatal diagnosis are possible.

BENIGN FAMILIAL HAEMATURIA

The haematuria, usually recurrent and painless, sometimes gross or microscopic, is not associated with deafness, ocular defect, hypertension or renal impairment. Moderate basement membrane thinning is sometimes found. Transmission is usually consistent with autosomal dominant inheritance when analysis is done on all available family members. Molecular defects in one of the collagen genes on chromosome 2q have recently been detected.

FABRY'S DISEASE

Fabry's disease is X-linked with partial manifestation in some females. Cardiac involvement, characteristic skin lesions and painful neuropathy are other predominant features, in addition to nephropathy. Isolation of both the gene and the enzyme involved (alpha-galactosidase) allows carrier detection and prenatal diagnosis in most cases.

CYSTINOSIS (CYSTINE STORAGE DISEASE)

Progressive renal failure is one of the main features of cystinosis, which is an autosomal recessive disorder. Positional cloning has isolated a specific gene responsible for a lysosomal membrane protein. The condition must not be confused with the renal transport defect cystinuria (see below).

URINARY TRACT MALFORMATIONS

The review of Gruskin *et al.* (see 'Further reading') gives details of this complex field. Many chromosome abnormalities and other general malformations are associated with structural urinary tract abnormalities, associations which are important to detect in order to avoid preventable obstruction or infection. Ultrasonography is playing an increasing role in the prenatal diagnosis of urinary tract malformations, but needs expert interpretation. In the case of some obstructive uropathies, it has been used in conjunction with intrauterine insertion of shunts, although the results so far have been inconclusive.

RENAL AGENESIS

The estimates of the recurrence risk in sibs range from 3 to 8 per cent for bilateral renal agenesis, which may have associated congenital abnormalities. There may be some additional risk for unilateral agenesis (often undetected without ultrasound). The defect may be part of more general syndromes, including the autosomal recessive Fraser (cryptophthalmos) syndrome, for which a specific developmental gene has recently been isolated.

HYDRONEPHROSIS

Most bilateral cases of hydronephrosis are secondary to obstruction or other disorders. Unilateral hydronephrosis apparently following autosomal dominant inheritance has been recorded, but most cases are not obviously familial.

HORSESHOE KIDNEY

Horseshoe kidney is rarely familial as an isolated defect. It is frequent in Turner syndrome.

BLADDER EXSTROPHY

Recurrence of bladder exstrophy in sibs is very rare (<1 per cent). Prenatal diagnosis may result from a raised serum AFP level detected by a screening test, as well as from ultrasound scan.

SMITH–LEMLI–OPITZ SYNDROME

This autosomal recessive multisystem disorder is due to a primary defect in cholesterol biosynthesis. Hypospadias, other genital defects and a variety of structural urinary tract abnormalities are prominent features, together with mental retardation, characteristic facies and cardiac involvement.

PRUNE-BELLY SYNDROME (ABDOMINAL MUSCLE DEFICIENCY, MEGAURETER, MEGACYSTIS, UNDESCENDED TESTIS)

Almost all cases of prune-belly syndrome are male. Recurrence in sibs is rare (less than 1 per cent) and several discordant monozygotic twin pairs are known. An increasing body of opinion is of the view that the syndrome is a consequence of early urethral obstruction and that the recurrence risk is dependent on the specific cause of the urethral obstruction.

URETHRAL VALVES

Satisfactory risk figures are not available, but the risk is certainly small in sibs.

HYPOSPADIAS

Incidence of hypospadias is at least 1 in 1000 males. The recurrence risk in male sibs is around 10 per cent, and in children of affected males the risk is similar. The risk for off-spring of female sibs of patients is uncertain. Care must be taken to distinguish various intersexual states and mendelian syndromes (such as the autosomal recessive Smith–Lemli–Opitz syndrome and the X-linked Aarskog syndrome). Association with maternal hormone therapy has been suggested and mutations in the androgen receptor have recently been found to be responsible for some cases.

CRYPTORCHIDISM

The recurrence risk in sibs is around 10 per cent. Underlying primary causes must be borne in mind.

VESICOURETERIC REFLUX

A family study of vesicoureteric reflux has shown a risk of around 10 per cent to sibs (about 10 times the population frequency), which is relevant to the early detection and prevention of renal scarring. A similar proportion of parents were affected. In some families, a single dominant gene may be acting; certainly the genetic contribution to reflux is strong.

ENURESIS

This common problem is frequently familial and follows an autosomal dominant pattern in some families, with a locus on chromosome 13q now suggested.

RENAL STONES

Most cases of renal stones, whether calcium, urate or associated with infection, are not mendelian in inheritance. There appears to be an increased risk for close relatives but no precise figures are available. Numerous rare metabolic causes exist for renal stones; some of those due to renal transport defects are listed in Table 21.2. Isolated hyperparathyroidism is rarely familial. In most families showing dominant inheritance, renal stones are due to familial hypocalcaemic hypercalciuria or are part of multiple endocrine neoplasia type 1 (see Chapter 22). Urate stones are frequent in the X-linked Lesch–Nyhan and related hyperuricaemic syndromes.

Cystinuria (see Chapter 23) is autosomal recessive in inheritance, so sibs of affected children deserve careful screening for this relatively common (about 1 in 7000) and readily treatable disorder.

Table 21.2 Inherited renal transport defects

Disorder	Inheritance
Cystinuria (See Chapter 23)	
Xanthinuria	
Renal glycosuria	
Hartnup disease	Autosomal recessive
Dibasic aminoaciduria	
Fanconi syndrome	
(usually secondary to cystinosis)	
Lowe syndrome	X-linked recessive
Familial hypophosphataemia	X-linked
Nephrogenic diabetes insipidus	(variable female expression)
Renal tubular acidosis	Several types; most commonly autosomal dominant (when familial) Occasionally X-linked
Familial hypocalcaemic hypercalciuria	Autosomal dominant

RENAL TRANSPORT DISORDERS

Table 21.2 lists some of the inherited renal transport disorders. As expected with inborn errors of metabolism, most are autosomal recessive, but the three X-linked conditions are all variable in the heterozygous female. Most carriers of Lowe (oculocerebrorenal) syndrome are detectable by lens opacities, while heterozygotes for familial hypophosphataemia may be short in stature and have low serum phosphate levels. Renal tubular acidosis is heterogeneous; many cases are sporadic, but numerous families with autosomal dominant inheritance exist, as well as rarer autosomal recessive and X-linked forms, so careful classification of the precise tubular defect is important.

RENAL TUMOURS

Wilms' tumour and the related syndrome complex are discussed on page 340. An important mendelian cause of adult renal cell carcinoma is von Hippel–Lindau disease (see Chapter 25), which is determined by a specific tumour suppressor gene on chromosome 3. Tuberous sclerosis is another cause, although angiomyolipoma is the more usual renal lesion. In the absence of associated disorders, occasional families with renal cell carcinoma following dominant inheritance have been reported, but most cases are sporadic.

FURTHER READING

Flinter F, Maher ER, Saggar-Malik A (2003). *Genetics of Renal Disease*. Oxford. Oxford University Press.

Griffin MD, Torres VE, Kumar R (1997). Cystic kidney diseases. *Curr Opin Nephrol Hypertens* **6**, 276–283.

Gruskin D, Kanil E, Rimoin DL (2002). Congenital disorders of the urinary tract. In: Rimoin DL, Connor JM, Pyeritz RE, Korf BR, eds, *Principles and Practice of Medical Genetics*. Edinburgh, Churchill Livingstone, pp. 1659–1692.

Maher ER, Yates RW (1991). Familial renal cell carcinoma: clinical and molecular genetic aspects. *Br J Cancer* **63**, 176–179.

Ravine D, Walker RG, Gibson RN (1994). Phenotype and genotype heterogeneity in autosomal dominant polycystic kidney disease. *Lancet* **340**, 1330–1333.

Sessa A (ed.) (1997). *Hereditary Kidney Diseases*. Basel, Karger.

Tryggvason K (ed.) (1996). *Molecular Pathology and Genetics of Alport Syndrome*. Basel, Karger.

CHAPTER 22

Endocrine and reproductive disorders

DIABETES MELLITUS

The genetics of diabetes mellitus provides a paradigm for the role of genetic factors in common disorders of complex determination. The following summary is an over-simplification of a difficult subject, but several recent reviews are available that give more detail.`

Diabetes can be divided broadly into three main groups:

- type I (insulin-dependent or juvenile) diabetes
- type II (non-insulin-dependent or maturity onset) diabetes
- diabetes of varying types associated with specific primary genetic disorders (Table 22.1).

TYPE I DIABETES

Type I diabetes affects around 1 in 300 individuals in most of Europe and a moderate familial tendency has long been recognized. Approximate risks to different categories of relative are given in Table 22.2. Autoimmune destruction of the insulin-producing beta cells of the pancreas, associated with T-cell dysfunction, results in low or absent insulin production. Viral infections may be an important environmental trigger. The HLA region

Table 22.1 Specific genetic disorders frequently associated with diabetes

Disorder	Type of diabetes	Inheritance
Cystic fibrosis	I	AR (see Chapter 19)
Haemochromatosis	II	AR (but see Chapter 20)
Myotonic dystrophy	II	AD (trinucleotide repeat, see Chapter 11)
Seip syndrome (lipoatrophic diabetes)	II	AR
Kobberling partial lipodystrophy	II	X-linked
Alstrom syndrome (with deafness, retinal degeneration)	II	AR (see Chapter 18)
Werner syndrome	II	AR
Prader–Willi syndrome	II	15q microdeletion
Bardet–Biedl syndrome	II	AR
DIDMOAD syndrome (diabetes insipidus, diabetes mellitus and optic atrophy)	I	AR or mitochondrial
Friedreich's ataxia	Variable	AR (trinucleotide repeat, see Chapter 12)
Leprechaunism (Donohue syndrome)	II	AR (insulin receptor receptor defect)
Ataxia telangiectasia	II	AR (see Chapter 25)

AR, autosomal recessive; AD; autosomal dominant.

Table 22.2 Approximate genetic risks in diabetes mellitus

Risk category	Type I	Type II
General population	1 in 300	Very variable (commonly 1–5%)
Sib of isolated case	1 in 14	1 in 10
Sib, no shared HLA haplotype	1 in 100	–
Sib, two or more shared HLA haplotypes	1 in 6	–
Sib and another first-degree relative affected	1 in 6	1 in 5
Offspring of isolated case	1 in 25	1 in 10
Monozygous co-twin affected	1 in 3	1 in 2

of chromosome 6 is one of the principal determinants of genetic susceptibility. Sibs with an identical HLA haplotype have around double the usual sib risk, while those with a completely different haplotype have only a 1 per cent risk; it is uncertain how useful such modest risk modifications are in genetic counselling. The focus of research is now the genes of the HLA region themselves and the primary structure of the proteins they determine. The HLA-DQ region appears to be particularly important, with some alleles giving susceptibility and other alleles conferring protection, the findings applying in a number of races.

Outside the HLA system, a series of other susceptibility loci have been proposed, including the region of the insulin gene on chromosome 11. Despite much research, no associations have proved to be sufficiently consistent or strong to alter the empiric estimates in Table 22.2.

TYPE II DIABETES

Type II diabetes is an exceptionally common and increasing disorder which shows extreme geographical variation, probably due to genetic as well as environmental factors. Attempts to replace Neel's 'thrifty genotype' hypothesis by a 'thrifty phenotype' based on intra-uterine nutrition to explain the increase shown by certain populations have not, in the author's view, been convincing. Insulin levels are initially increased and insulin resistance is present, but the specific genetic determinants are currently even less clear than in type I diabetes. Risks to relatives are high (see Table 22.2), especially for monozygotic twins, but are mainly for the same form of diabetes, not for severe type I disease.

With insulin resistance a feature of the disorder, molecular defects in the insulin mol-ecule or its receptor might have been expected, but these have been found only in a few individuals. The rare MODY (maturity-onset diabetes in youth) form with juvenile onset, which appears to follow autosomal dominant inheritance (although with incomplete penetrance), has been linked to the glucokinase gene locus in some families, with specific mutations found in this gene and also in the hepatocyte nuclear factor-1 alpha gene. This appears to make up about 1 per cent of all type II diabetes. Other susceptibility loci have so far proved too inconsistent to use in practice. Mitochondrial mutations have also been found in some families showing maternal transmission.

The risk of developing diabetes is not the only factor to be considered in giving genetic counselling to diabetic families. The offspring of a diabetic mother face special hazards, although these appear to be declining markedly with better diabetic control during preg-nancy. The perinatal mortality has been shown to correlate with the severity of maternal diabetes; one large early study gave an overall perinatal mortality of 20 per cent, rising to almost 40 per cent in the most severely affected group. Although risks have declined since these data were collected, they are far from negligible.

There is also an increase in the incidence of congenital malformations in the offspring of the diabetic mother, with a threefold excess over the general population. Recent Scandinavian data show a clear relation to control of the diabetes. There is no detectable increase in malformations when the mother has preclinical or gestational diabetes.

A few rare specific malformations seem to occur particularly in the offspring of dia-betic mothers, including sacral agenesis, proximal femoral deficiency and related caudal regression syndromes. The recurrence risk of these is small in relation to the other mal-formations, which do not follow any specific pattern.

PITUITARY GLAND DISORDERS

Although the pituitary gland may be involved in a variety of generalized syndromes, (see the review by Mosely *et al.*, Further reading, for a full list) most of the genetic counselling

Table 22.3 Genetic disorders involving pituitary hormone deficiency

Disorder	Inheritance
Anterior pituitary	
Familial panhypopituitarism	Autosomal recessive or X-linked recessive
Isolated growth hormone deficiency	All types of inheritance (see text)
Laron pituitary dwarfism	Autosomal recessive (HGH receptor defect)
Pituitary unresponsiveness	Uncertain
(African pygmy type)	
Septo-optic dysplasia	Usually sporadic
Holoprosencephaly group	See Chapter 12; mainly sporadic
	(but heterogeneous)
Posterior pituitary	
Familial diabetes insipidus	Autosomal dominant
(vasopressin sensitive)	
Familial nephrogenic diabetes insipidus	X-linked semidominant
DIDMOAD syndrome (diabetes insipidus,	Autosomal recessive
diabetes mellitus, optic atrophy)	

problems arise in relation to specific hormonal deficiencies, many of which follow mendelian inheritance, as indicated in Table 22.3. Molecular defects in the hormones or their receptors are now being detected in some of these conditions (e.g. Laron dwarfism), which should help to resolve heterogeneity, as well as providing tests for family members.

Isolated growth hormone deficiency may follow autosomal recessive, autosomal dominant or X-linked inheritance. In the autosomal recessive Laron dwarfism, growth hormone levels are high but receptor function is deficient, with a specific molecular defect in some patients. It is possible that molecular variations in growth hormone may also play a more general role in short stature.

Among the posterior pituitary deficiencies, the DIDMOAD (Wolfram) syndrome has already been noted in Chapter 17. Isolated vasopressin deficiency causing diabetes insipidus is usually autosomal dominant, whereas most cases of primary nephrogenic diabetes insipidus are X-linked, with variable manifestation in females.

Acromegaly and related disorders of pituitary hypersecretion are mostly sporadic, but may form part of the autosomal dominant type 1 multiple endocrine neoplasia (see below). Apart from specific pituitary defects, there are numerous disorders of growth whose basis is not clearly understood, both of increased and of decreased growth. Many represent primary genetic syndromes.

THYROID GLAND DISORDERS

CONGENITAL HYPOTHYROIDISM

Most cases of congenital hypothyroidism are due to failure of thyroid gland development and are sporadic. Occasional occurrence in sibs may indicate recessively inherited forms which cannot at present be distinguished. Recessively inherited cases of thyroid-stimulating hormone deficiency have also been recorded. Newborn screening is now universal in developed countries and has led to the recognition of hypothyroidism being part of several unusual malformation syndromes. No satisfactory data on offspring risks exist at present.

The presence of a goitre in a non-endemic region indicates that an inborn error of thyroxine synthesis is likely. The various types all follow autosomal recessive inheritance, including Pendred syndrome, in which defective iodine organification is associated with nerve deafness (see Chapter 18) and due to defects in a specific ion transport gene.

Absence of thyroxine-binding globulin may be X-linked recessive or autosomal dominant. It is usually harmless, but may be confused with hypothyroidism biochemically.

AUTOIMMUNE THYROID DISEASE

Autoimmune thyroid disease may frequently form part of a broader autoimmune disorder, with other endocrine glands and also different systems affected (e.g. myasthenia gravis, pernicious anaemia), something which must be borne in mind when investigating families. An autosomal dominant susceptibility gene is likely to be involved in many such families.

Both Graves' disease and Hashimoto's thyroiditis show strong familial aggregation, with both disorders commonly seen in the same family. A common autoimmune basis is now recognized, association with antigens HLA-Dw3 and HLA-B5 being seen in addition to other abnormalities. About 50 per cent of monozygotic twins are concordant (compared with 5 per cent of dizygotic twins). Clinical thyroid disease in other relatives is much less frequent than the incidence of thyroid antibodies. The lifetime risk probably does not exceed 10 per cent, except in a small number of families where a pattern strongly suggestive of autosomal dominant inheritance is seen. Transient neonatal hyperthyroidism may occur in infants of affected mothers with Graves' disease.

A distinct, recessively inherited, autoimmune polyglandular syndrome (APECED), which involves parathyroid and pancreas as well as thyroid, is due to mutations in a specific gene isolated on chromosome 21.

PARATHYROID GLAND DISORDERS

Most, but not all, familial cases of hyperparathyroidism are part of multiple endocrine neoplasia type 1 (see below), but the great majority of parathyroid tumours are non-mendelian, with a low recurrence risk for relatives; the same applies to Cushing's syndrome and to pituitary tumours.

A dominantly inherited, benign entity of hypercalcaemia with hypocalciuria has been recognized which can mimic hyperparathyroidism.

Hypoparathyroidism is commonly sporadic, but a rare X-linked recessive type has been recognized, as has an autosomal recessive syndrome with adrenal failure and candidiasis. Absent parathyroid glands are a feature of DiGeorge syndrome, part of the broader microdeletion syndrome involving chromosome 22q (see Chapter 19).

Albright's hereditary osteodystrophy (encompassing pseudohypoparathyroidism and pseudopseudohypoparathyroidism) is now understood in molecular terms as being due to receptor defects in the adenyl cyclase system. Formerly considered to be X-linked, it is now recognized as autosomal dominant, with most fully expressed cases being maternally transmitted, probably due to an imprinting effect.

MULTIPLE ENDOCRINE NEOPLASIA

Multiple endocrine neoplasia comprises two major types:

- *Type 1* - parathyroid, anterior pituitary and pancreatic endocrine tumours are the most frequent. Inheritance is autosomal dominant, with the gene on chromosome 11 isolated
- *Type 2* - medullary carcinoma of the thyroid may occur alone or coexist with phaeochromocytoma and with mucosal neuromas (type 2b). Some patients may be 'marfanoid' in appearance. Inheritance is usually autosomal dominant. The *RET* oncogene has proved to be the gene responsible, with a small number of specific mutations responsible for most cases of both 2a and 2b types.

Both major forms are important examples of high-risk neoplastic disorders, where recognition of the mendelian inheritance and the existence of a genetic register can prevent fatal disease in relatives, quite apart from the importance of genetic counselling (see Chapter 25).

CONGENITAL ADRENAL HYPERPLASIA (ADRENOGENITAL SYNDROME)

At least eight types of congenital adrenal hyperplasia exist, resulting from different disorders of steroid hormone biosynthesis; all follow autosomal recessive inheritance. The most important type, 21-hydroxylase deficiency, is closely linked to the HLA system. The gene has been isolated and a variety of deletions and other mutations identified, correlating with phenotype to some extent and allowing accurate prenatal diagnosis and carrier detection.

Direct prenatal diagnosis from amniotic fluid is also possible, and could allow neonatal treatment to avoid a salt-losing crisis. Whether termination of an affected pregnancy is required may be strongly influenced by the severity of effects, particularly virilization of a female, in the first affected child, some families opting for first trimester prenatal diagnosis and termination, and others for steroid therapy.

HYPOGONADISM AND ALLIED STATES

Recent advances in understanding the molecular basis of sex determination have considerable relevance to the classification and pathogenesis of the different forms of hypogonadism and intersex. The principal points of relevance are as follows:

- A specific gene on the Y chromosome (*Sry*) has been identified that commits the undifferentiated gonad to become a testis. If this is absent or defective, the gonadal phenotype will be female.

- Male phenotype is dependent on the presence of and sensitivity to androgen, which is itself dependent on a differentiated testis.
- Two functioning X chromosomes are needed for formation of a fully developed ovary with ova.
- Other hormonal influences (e.g. adrenal steroid precursors) may modify genital development and result in ambiguous genitalia.

Genetic counselling in this area must rest on a well-defined clinical and endocrinological diagnosis, with cytogenetic and (increasingly) molecular analysis as appropriate. Recognition of X-linked and autosomal recessive disorders, along with translocations involving X and Y chromosome material, is especially important, as it is these groups where recurrence in the family is most likely.

The following broad groups are important to distinguish for genetic counselling.

PRIMARY SEX CHROMOSOME DISORDERS

In particular, these include XXY (Klinefelter) and 45,X (Turner) syndromes, which have been discussed in Chapter 4. Recurrence in a family is exceptional, except where there is mosaicism.

DISORDERS WHERE CHROMOSOMAL AND PHENOTYPIC SEX DO NOT CORRESPOND, INCLUDING XX MALES AND XY FEMALES

This complex group is becoming resolved with isolation of the specific genes on the Y and X chromosomes involved with sex determination. A careful endocrine, cytogenetic and molecular assessment is essential before genetic counselling can be given. The main disorders include:

- *XX males* – usually sporadic and resulting from Y chromosome material translocated on to an X chromosome and often detectable by molecular tests
- *XY females* – the most frequent cause is the androgen insensitivity syndrome (formerly known as testicular feminization) where a normal female phenotype is associated with presence of a testis. In XY gonadal dysgenesis, due to molecular defects in the Y-linked sex-determining *Sry* gene, or to corresponding X-linked defects, there may be a normal phenotype or varying degrees of intersex. The dysgenetic gonad is at risk of malignant change and should be removed. Both these disorders may follow X-linked recessive inheritance with phenotypic and chromosomally normal female relatives at risk of having an affected XY daughter.

Genetic counselling in these conditions needs to be especially sensitive to the true sexual identity of those affected and to link closely with overall management. In general, it will be the phenotypic and psychological sexual identity that is more relevant than chromosomal sex. Great care must be taken not to confuse or upset affected individuals by inappropriately assuming that sex chromosomal status must necessarily determine actual sexual identity.

Table 22.4 Genetic causes of infertility and hypogonadism

Phenotypic male
Sex chromosome anomalies and reversal
Y chromosome microdeletions
Androgen insensitivity (partial)
Kennedy's disease (spinobulbar muscular atrophy)
Kallmann syndrome
Pituitary hormone defects (various)
Dysmorphic syndromes with hypogonadism
(e.g. Bardet–Biedel, Prader–Willi)
Myotonic dystrophy
Cystic fibrosis
Primary ciliary dyskinesia

Phenotypic female
Sex chromosome anomalies and reversal
Androgen insensitivity (complete)
Fragile-X pre-mutation (premature ovarian failure)
Congenital adrenal hyperplasia (some types)
Pituitary hormone defects (various)
Sry gene defects (Y chromosome)
Galactosaemia (premature ovarian failure)

HYPOGONADISM DUE TO SPECIFIC GENETIC DISORDERS

Here the recurrence risk will be that of the underlying disorder, while the hypogonadism itself may be of gonadal, pituitary or hypothalamic origin (see Table 22.4).

INFERTILITY

Genetic counselling in cases of infertility may seem a contradiction in terms, because the problem is only discovered when a couple is actively trying to conceive. However, two important questions that need to be asked (but frequently are not) by those attempting to investigate and treat infertility are as follows:

• Is the infertility one aspect of a genetic disorder that might be transmitted?
• Will correction of infertility give an increased risk of malformations in the offspring?

The genetic causes of both female and male infertility are numerous and in part overlap with those of hypogonadism already mentioned (see Table 22.4). As with these, it is only X-linked or autosomal recessive disorders that are of practical importance for genetic counselling, because only in these will unaffected people be at risk of having an affected child.

Premature ovarian failure has been shown to result in some cases from an X chromosome gene mutation already known to cause sterility in *Drosophila*, but it may also be associated with pre-mutations in the fragile-X (*FMR*) gene.

Disorders of sperm production include primary sex chromosome disorders such as XXY (Klinefelter) syndrome, other disorders affecting the testis (e.g. myotonic dystrophy), balanced chromosomal translocations causing abnormalities of chromosome pairing in meiosis, clinical defects affecting motility and a variety of poorly defined biochemical disorders. Blockage or aplasia of the vas deferens causes infertility in most male cases of cystic fibrosis. A mild form of this may be responsible for some apparently primary cases of such obstruction.

The question of increased risk to offspring arises principally in those patients in whom apparent infertility is really a reflection of early unrecognized fetal loss as a result of abnormal gamete production. The most important group to detect is where one parent carries a balanced translocation, where the risk of an unbalanced chromosome abnormality in a pregnancy that goes to term is considerable, especially when the defect is carried by a female (see Chapter 4). This problem is closely related to that of recurrent abortion, considered below.

Artificial insemination by donor (AID) and *in vitro* fertilization have already been mentioned in Chapter 10 as increasingly used modes of treating infertility. There has now been sufficient experience with AID to make it clear that there is no increase in abnormalities. The same is probably true of *in vitro* fertilization from preliminary studies of children conceived in this way, but there are doubts remaining about the safety of intracytoplasmic sperm injection (ICSI).

GENETIC COUNSELLING AND RECURRENT ABORTIONS

Most women with a history of recurrent abortions will be under the care of a gynaecologist, who will have already searched for a gynaecological cause and will have excluded most serious maternal disorders. Rhesus haemolytic disease is now usually prevented as a cause of later pregnancy loss. Factors such as lupus anticoagulant or maternal thrombotic disorders may be relevant in a small proportion, but numerous proposed factors and corresponding remedies have failed to be confirmed and the cause of most recurrent abortions remains unknown.

The main question to be answered is not so much whether another abortion will occur, but what are the chances of having a healthy child, together with the risk that a pregnancy reaching term will result in an abnormality. The question of amniocentesis may also arise: clearly one does not want to expose a pregnancy to any added risk of abortion unless there is a likelihood of an abnormality detectable by this.

There will be many women in whom careful search reveals no genetic or other factors involved, but with care considerable help can be given by the following measures:

- pathological examination of the abortus where possible – this may identify major structural malformations
- cytogenetic study of parents – this is especially important where a translocation is a possibility and should always be done. In general the finding of a chromosome

abnormality in the abortus but not in a parent is not likely to be relevant or to affect the genetic risks (see Chapter 4)

- a search for possible lethal mendelian causes, e.g. consanguinity (which increases the risk of autosomal recessive lethals), X-linked dominant disorders lethal in the male, and myotonic dystrophy, which gives heavy fetal loss in the offspring of mildly affected women.

The most important group to detect are the autosomal translocations, where one parent is a balanced translocation carrier. As stated in Chapter 4, these carry a significant risk of an abnormal live-born offspring, probably around 12 per cent where the carrier is female, but nearer 5 per cent where the male is the carrier, the precise risk depending on the type of translocation. Amniocentesis or chorion biopsy is clearly indicated in any such pregnancy, and there is no evidence that it is accompanied by a greater risk of abortion in such a situation.

It is important for couples to realize that spontaneous abortion is an exceedingly common event, occurring in at least 1 in 8 recognized pregnancies. Thus 1 in 64 women might be expected to have two consecutive abortions on the grounds of chance alone, and unless there are other reasons, it is probably not worth undertaking investigations unless they have had at least three spontaneous abortions, when around 5 per cent of couples will be found to carry a balanced translocation.

OTHER REPRODUCTIVE PROBLEMS

HYDATIDIFORM MOLES

Hydatidiform moles are masses of trophoblastic tissue that are rarely familial but show unusual chromosomal features. The complete hydatidiform mole has a normal chromosome number that is of entirely paternal origin, while the partial mole is a complete triploid, with two paternal complements. These structures represent perhaps the most extreme examples of genomic imprinting (see p. 26). A 1 per cent recurrence risk in future pregnancies is likely for the complete mole and may represent persistence of the original mole with the risk of malignant change; the recurrence risk is probably less than this for the partial form, which is not associated with malignancy.

TOXAEMIA OF PREGNANCY (PRE-ECLAMPSIA)

Toxaemia of pregnancy may be associated with genetic disorders affecting placental development (e.g. trisomy 18), but in the absence of a specific cause it is frequently familial, possibly determined by a common autosomal recessive gene giving toxaemia when both mother and fetus are homozygous for this. Recurrence risks are around 20 per cent for a pregnancy in a woman whose own mother had toxaemia in the pregnancy leading to that woman's birth; and about 15 per cent where a sister has had toxaemia in pregnancy, figures rather less than suggested in earlier studies (the population risk is around 10 per cent).

FURTHER READING

Arngrimson R (2002). Preeclampsia. In: Rimoin DL, Connor JM, Pyeritz RE, Korf BR, eds. *Emery and Rimoin's Principles and Practice of Medical Genetics*. Edinburgh, Churchill Livingstone, pp. 1496–1518.

Elliot DJ, Cooke HJ (1997). The molecular genetics of male infertility. *Bioessays* **19**, 801–809.

Froguel P (1997). Genetics of type 1 insulin-dependent diabetes mellitus. *Horm Res* **48**, 55–57.

Gardner RJM, Sutherland GR (2003). *Chromosome Abnormalities and Genetic Counselling*. Oxford, Oxford University Press – helpful sections on reproductive failure, intersex and on sex chromosome anomalies.

Jameson JL (1996). Inherited disorders of the gonadotrophin hormones. *Mol Cell Endocrinol* **125**, 143–149.

Kahn CR, Vicent D, Doria A (1996). Genetics of non-insulin-dependent (type-II) diabetes mellitus. *Annu Rev Med* **47**, 509–531.

Layman LC (2002). Human gene mutations causing infertility. *J Med Genet* **39**, 153–161.

Medeiros-Neto G, Stanbury JB (1994). *Inherited Disorders of the Thyroid System*. London, CRC Press.

Mosely CT, Phillips JA, Rimoin DL (2002). Genetic disorders of the pituitary gland. In: Rimoin DL, Connor JM, Pyeritz RE, Korf BR, eds. *Emery and Rimoin's Principles and Practice of Medical Genetics*. Edinburgh, Churchill Livingstone, pp. 2135–2182.

Newfield RS, New MI (1997). 21-hydroxylase deficiency. *Ann NY Acad Sci* **816**, 219–229.

Rotig A, Bonnefont JP, Munnich A (1996). Mitochondrial diabetes mellitus. *Diabetes Metab* **22**, 291–298.

Scriver CK, Beaudet AL, Sly WS, Valle D (eds) (2001). *The Metabolic and Molecular Bases of Inherited Disease*. New York, McGraw-Hill – a series of chapters give valuable details on individual disorders.

Inborn errors of metabolism

Since almost all mendelian disorders will eventually prove to be the result of a deficient or defective specific gene product, there is no absolute distinction between inborn errors of metabolism and other genetic disorders. Indeed, the concept of 'inborn errors of development' has now become a reality, as discussed in Chapter 6 (and as foreseen by Garrod himself). For this chapter it seems wise to restrict the term to those conditions where some form of metabolic basis, usually enzymatic, has been clearly identified, but each year more diseases are added to the group. In many cases, the discovery of a specific metabolic basis radically changes the concept of a disease. Thus, Tay–Sachs disease is no longer thought of as purely a brain degeneration but as a generalized metabolic disorder, and the preventive measures of carrier detection and prenatal diagnosis involve biochemical and genetic techniques far removed from those generally associated with neurology. Xeroderma pigmentosum and allied disorders of DNA repair are further examples of disorders entering the inborn error category, while the positional cloning approach has been responsible for isolation of the genes for important metabolic disorders such as Batten's disease, Menkes syndrome and Lowe syndrome, whose primary protein defect was previously unknown.

The development of specific tests for direct identification of gene mutations (see Chapter 5) is causing rapid changes in our understanding of many inherited metabolic diseases. In particular, heterogeneity in the types of mutation involved is becoming apparent; in some cases it is becoming possible to predict the form or severity of phenotype from the type of mutation.

From the viewpoint of genetic counselling, inborn errors of metabolism have several characteristics which must be taken into account:

- Almost all follow mendelian recessive inheritance, the great majority being autosomal.
- Precise biochemical and molecular techniques for early recognition, carrier detection and prenatal diagnosis are often available, although sometimes they are confined to a very few expert centres.

Table 23.1 X-linked inborn errors of metabolism

Disorder	Enzyme defect (where relevant)
Angiokeratoma (Fabry's disease)	Alpha-galactosidase
Chronic granulomatous disease	β cytochrome subunit
Glucose-6-phosphate dehydrogenase deficiency	Glucose-6-phosphate dehydrogenase
Glycogenosis type VIII	Liver phosphorylase kinase
Haemophilia A	Factor VIII (procoagulant subunit)
Haemophilia B	Factor IX
Hyperammonaemia type I	Ornithine carbamyl transferase
Hypophosphataemic rickets	Renal tubule phosphate transport defect
Ichthyosis, X-linked	Steroid sulphatase
Lesch–Nyhan syndrome	Hypoxanthine–guanidine phosphoribosyl transferase
Menkes syndrome	Defective copper transport protein
Mucopolysaccharidosis II (Hunter syndrome)	Iduronate sulphatase
Lowe syndrome	Inositol phosphate phosphatase

- Genetic heterogeneity in terms of multiple loci is frequent, but can usually be detected biochemically if not clinically. Further redefining of apparently well-defined disorders will undoubtedly continue.

No attempt is made here to describe or even list the large number of inborn errors, mostly very rare, that have been documented. *The Metabolic and Molecular Bases of Inherited Disease* (see 'Further reading') is a definitive source of information. Some disorders are covered in the specific system chapters. Peroxisomal disorders are mentioned in Chapter 6. For the great majority of disorders where the inheritance is autosomal recessive, this means that a high genetic risk (1 in 4) is usually confined to sibs of the affected individual. Unless consanguinity exists, or the gene is especially common in a particular population, the risks to the offspring of healthy sibs or more distant relatives are extremely low, and carrier detection or prenatal diagnosis is not likely to be required in such situations. Indeed, it may be unwise to embark upon tests whose margin of error may be considerably greater than the individual's prior risk of having an affected child (see Chapter 7), unless there are particular reasons in the individual situation.

Tables 23.1 and 23.2 give some important disorders known to follow X-linked or autosomal dominant inheritance. The X-linked group is especially important for carrier detection, because the female carrier will have a 50 per cent risk of transmitting the condition to her sons (see Chapter 7). Prenatal diagnosis is feasible in almost all serious inherited metabolic disorders, although rarity often means it is restricted to one or two centres worldwide. Further discussion of this area is given in Chapter 8. The recent rapid increase in the number of disorders where the gene has been cloned is producing a marked shift towards DNA analysis in both prenatal diagnosis and carrier detection, but there remain many situations where an enzyme-based approach may be preferable or where a combination of both is needed.

Table 23.2 Inborn errors of metabolism following autosomal dominant inheritance

Porphyrias
  Acute intermittent
  Variegate
  Coproporphyria
  Protoporphyria
Familial hypercholesterolaemia (rarely homozygous)
Hereditary angioedema

The following notes deal with some of the situations particularly relevant to genetic counselling in individual conditions. Some other inherited metabolic disorders are dealt with in the specific chapters.

AMINO ACID DISORDERS

PHENYLKETONURIA

With a mean frequency of around 1 in 10 000 births in the UK (carrier frequency 1 in 50), this is one of the more common inborn errors, although it is geographically variable. Successful dietary treatment and newborn screening (see Chapter 27) have resulted in a generation of young adults who are, in most cases, mentally normal and are living healthy, active lives, although it has become clear that treatment needs to be strictly controlled and prolonged, at least in some degree, into adult life to achieve optimal results. This undoubted success story has largely transferred the burden of genetic risks on to the adult females who were identified in the newborn period. Here, although the risk of transmitting phenylketonuria is low (around 1 per cent), there is a high risk of brain damage in all offspring of affected women due to phenylalanine crossing the placenta. It is now clear that only strict dietary treatment started prior to conception offers the likelihood of a normal child, and that even therapy started as soon as pregnancy is recognized is likely to be associated with mental handicap.

There is no evidence that such problems occur among the offspring of asymptomatic individuals with moderately raised blood phenylalanine detected by screening.

Prenatal diagnosis is rarely requested except for the very rare and usually fatal form of phenylketonuria, due to dihydropteridine reductase deficiency, which does not respond to the usual dietary treatment and where the gene has now been cloned. In the classic form due to phenylalanine hydroxylase deficiency, the enzyme is confined to the liver. Different mutations are proving to be correlated with severity and need for dietary control. Carrier detection is feasible by DNA analysis of polymorphisms within the gene or by specific mutation analysis, and so is prenatal diagnosis for the minority of families likely to opt for it. It should be borne in mind that the great majority of treated phenylketonuria patients are now entirely normal. Prenatal diagnosis is only finding significant application in countries without effective dietary treatment.

HISTIDINAEMIA

Most cases of histidinaemia appear to be asymptomatic and the original association thought to exist with speech problems and mental retardation seems doubtful. There is no evidence of a significant maternal effect in the heterozygous offspring of affected women.

CYSTINURIA

Renal calculi are the only significant clinical features in cystinuria. Heterozygotes in one of the two types may excrete small amounts of amino acids in the urine, but are symptomless and must not be confused with the affected homozygotes, where large quantities of cystine and other dibasic amino acids are excreted. The disorder is quite distinct from cystinosis (also autosomal recessive), which is a generalized storage disease of cystine, with much more serious clinical effects, including renal failure (see Chapter 21 for other causes of renal calculi).

BARTTER'S SYNDROME

This disorder of electrolyte metabolism, causing hypertension and hypokalaemia, is proving to be heterogeneous, with several different ion channel genes responsible in different families.

GALACTOSAEMIA

Recognition of galactosaemia, a rapidly fatal disorder, is important not only because effective treatment exists, but also to allow immediate diagnosis from cord blood in a subsequent pregnancy. Distinction of classic galactosaemia must also be made from the form due to galactokinase deficiency in which cataract is the only abnormality, and from harmless enzyme variants that may be picked up by screening programmes.

Prenatal diagnosis is feasible but not widely requested in view of the relatively good outcome of treatment in most cases, although long-term prognosis is less clear than for well-treated phenylketonuria. The various options and their consequences must be fully discussed with the couple concerned before a decision is made. Pituitary–ovarian dysfunction may result in infertility in treated women.

SPHINGOLIPIDOSES

Specific lysosomal enzyme defects have been identified for most disorders in the clinically confusing group of sphingolipidoses, and prenatal diagnosis is feasible in these.

Carrier detection is only of major significance for Tay–Sachs disease, where the gene is at high frequency in Ashkenazi Jewish populations. Screening for adult carriers, with prenatal diagnosis offered to couples who both carry the gene, has been successfully applied in some American Jewish communities, in which 1 in 30 individuals are carriers. Other important sphingolipidoses, all autosomal recessive in inheritance, include Gaucher's disease, Niemann–Pick disease, metachromatic leucodystrophy and generalized gangliosidosis. Batten's disease, also autosomal recessive, has had no specific enzyme defect known until positional cloning identified one form on chromosome 16, with one particularly frequent mutation, allowing, for the first time, prenatal diagnosis for some families with this devastating disorder (see also p. 191).

Fabry's disease is X-linked, with minor signs and biochemical changes often detectable in female carriers. The alpha-galactosidase gene has been cloned. The **mucopolysaccharidoses** are mentioned in Chapter 14.

The importance of obtaining a precise enzymatic (and where possible DNA) diagnosis in inborn errors of metabolism has already been stressed, but it is probably more important in the group of lysosomal enzyme deficiencies than in any other, since clinical differentiation is often extremely difficult and the prognosis poor, but prenatal diagnosis is feasible if one knows which enzyme is defective (see Chapter 8). Bone marrow transplantation is proving effective in some members of this group, while in Gaucher disease, direct enzyme replacement therapy is feasible.

GLYCOGEN STORAGE DISEASES

All members of the heterogeneous group of glycogen storage diseases are autosomal recessive in inheritance, apart from the exceedingly rare type VIII (X-linked recessive). Type II (Pompe's disease), caused by lysosomal acid maltase deficiency, can be prenatally diagnosed and exists in two distinct forms:

- an infantile type with severe cardiomyopathy and cerebral involvement
- a later neuromuscular type that may mimic a muscular dystrophy.

The classic type I (von Gierke) glucose-6-phosphatase deficiency has the enzyme confined to the liver, but identification of the gene should now permit prenatal diagnosis.

HYPERLIPIDAEMIAS

The classification of the hyperlipidaemias is still in a state of flux, but is beginning to be clarified by recognition of specific molecular defects. Most hyperlipidaemias, even with multiple affected family members are likely to be secondary to diet and other external factors. Type I hyperlipidaemia (hyperchylomicronaemia) and type V are autosomal recessive. The relatively common type II (familial hypercholesterolaemia), especially important because of its association with early coronary heart disease, is discussed in Chapter 19.

THE PORPHYRIAS

The acute porphyrias form the most striking exception to the rule of recessive inheritance for most inborn errors due to enzyme defects. Acute intermittent porphyria, porphyria variegata, hereditary coproporphyria and protoporphyria all follow autosomal dominant inheritance. Careful investigation of urine and faecal porphyrins, enzyme studies and, where possible, molecular analysis are needed to exclude subclinical disease. Now that specific enzyme and gene defects are known, prenatal diagnosis may be possible but is rarely requested. The severe congenital erythropoietic porphyria follows autosomal recessive inheritance. Porphyria cutanea tarda, much the most common of the group, is usually sporadic, with low recurrence risk for family members. It appears to result from a combination of homozygosity for mutation in the iron storage haemochromatosis susceptibility gene with adverse environmental factors such as alcoholic liver damage. A rare familial type can be distinguished enzymatically.

PSEUDOCHOLINESTERASE DEFICIENCY

Pseudocholinesterase deficiency – an important cause of apnoea following muscle relaxants (notably suxamethonium) – follows autosomal recessive inheritance. Sibs are thus the principal relatives at risk, although, because the gene is relatively common, it may also be worth testing the parents. Heterozygotes (4 per cent of the population) are not at significant risk of clinical problems, and in testing relatives it is most important not to confuse them with affected homozygotes. Since heterozygotes commonly show a moderate reduction in pseudocholinesterase level, the dibucaine number, which measures the degree of inhibition of the enzyme by dibucaine, should be measured. This will be under 25 in affected homozygotes, 50–70 in heterozygotes, and over 75 for normal homozygotes. Other rare genetic variants exist; their nomenclature is most confusing, but the subject is clearly discussed by Whittaker (see 'Further reading'). Molecular analysis has not yet come into regular clinical use.

PHARMACOGENETICS

Inherited differences in metabolism of and response to drugs has been recognized for over 50 years, but the possibility of finding simple DNA-based tests that will predict response or avoid serious adverse reactions has attracted recent attention. It is not clear at present whether such inherited variation might also be predictive for disease risk, nor whether it will really lead to individually tailored therapy. As with all common disease genetics, the underlying basis seems likely to require a considerable amount of more basic research before it reaches practical applications, including genetic counselling.

FATTY ACID METABOLIC DEFECTS AND SUDDEN INFANT DEATH

Several previously unrecognized defects in fatty acid and organic acid metabolism (e.g. MCAD deficiency) have been shown to be responsible for some cases of unexplained sudden infant death, and for some cases of Reye's syndrome with rapidly developing hypoglycaemia and encephalopathy. The proportion that are genetic has probably risen since the removal of likely environmental factors such as aspirin in infancy. The forensic implications in this field are exceptionally serious and provide a striking example of how essential it is to use and integrate all available information in a statistically appropriate manner before attempting to estimate the chance that an underlying metabolic defect may be responsible for a particular case. Since effective therapy appears possible by dietary modification, recognition of a possible metabolic basis in such situations is most important; autosomal recessive inheritance seems likely and prenatal diagnosis theoretically possible. The frequency of most such disorders appears to be very low in the general population, although the predominance of one specific MCAD mutation, with frequency of homozygotes 1 in 18 000, makes molecular diagnosis of this condition feasible. Population newborn screening using tandem mass spectrometry is also now technically feasible, but it is not yet clear that it will be beneficial.

FURTHER READING

Public Health Genetics Unit (2003). *My Very Own Medicine. What Must I Know? Information Policy for Pharmacogenetics*. Cambridge, Public Health Genetics Unit.

Scriver CR, Beaudet AL, Sly W, Valle D (eds) (2001). *The Metabolic and Molecular Bases of Inherited Disease*. New York, McGraw-Hill – this is the definitive source of information on all inborn errors of metabolism and related metabolic disorders.

Whittaker M (1986). *Cholinesterase*. Basel, Karger.

Disorders of blood and immune function

DISORDERS OF HAEMOGLOBIN STRUCTURE AND SYNTHESIS

The large group of haemoglobin disorders, of great importance in many parts of the world, contains perhaps the best understood disorders (in molecular terms) that exist. Most are autosomal recessive in inheritance, and only a few points will be mentioned here. The works listed in the 'Further reading' section, particularly those by Weatherall (1991, 1997), give full details.

SICKLE-CELL DISEASE

Sickle-cell disease, caused by a glutamic acid to valine mutation at a specific site in beta-globin, is exceptionally common in some regions, and the heterozygote frequency approaches 1 in 8 in some parts of Africa. Thus, carrier testing is of great importance, but fortunately it is readily feasible using a sickling test screen on the red cells, with haemoglobin electrophoresis as a confirmatory measure. Only couples who are both carriers will be at risk of having an affected child. Heterozygotes are essentially healthy and have partial protection against malaria in endemic areas. It is important for them not to be given the erroneous impression that they have a mild form of the disease. Severity in homozygotes can vary greatly according to geographical region.

Prenatal diagnosis, originally using fetal blood but now normally based on DNA analysis of chorionic villi or amniotic cells, has been feasible for some years but has not found wide application, in part because of the variation in clinical severity. The early screening programmes for carriers also met with little success, partly because of their hasty and ill-judged introduction, partly because of the stigmatization of carriers that resulted. Recent, more sensitively approached programmes are proving more acceptable, as is newborn screening in high-risk groups to allow early treatment of complications.

Numerous other beta-globin chain abnormalities are known, some of which, such as haemoglobin C, may be encountered in combination with haemoglobin S. This may result in complex genetic situations, emphasizing the need for expert haematological – and increasingly molecular – diagnosis to be available to those undertaking genetic counselling for haemoglobinopathies.

THALASSAEMIAS

Thalassaemias, characterized by a failure of globin chain synthesis due to a variety of underlying causes, are another disease group that is exceedingly common in some regions of the world, as well as in immigrant populations in Europe and America. All the thalassaemias are recessively inherited, and various compounds with different abnormal alleles may occur. Beta-thalassaemia major is an important problem in parts of the Mediterranean, the Middle East and Asia, whilst in South-east Asia forms of alpha-thalassaemia make a large contribution to intrauterine and neonatal deaths. Carrier detection of most forms is feasible, and so is prenatal diagnosis, particularly for beta-thalassaemia major, for which there is now considerable experience. Molecular techniques had their first diagnostic applications in this group, and identified a wealth of different defects at the DNA level (see Weatherall, 1997). The advent of first-trimester prenatal diagnosis based on DNA makes it particularly important to establish the precise molecular nature of the disorder. In planning prenatal diagnosis, it is important to recognize that the great majority of cases in any particular population will result from a few specific mutations and that the programme must be adjusted to this. Deletions may be frequent in some situations (especially for alpha-thalassaemias), whilst DNA polymorphisms, especially when used in combination as a haplotype, may still be used for cases of beta-thalassaemia where the specific mutation is unknown. Carrier detection and prenatal diagnosis have been taken up on a large scale by many populations, notably in Mediterranean countries. Population and screening aspects are discussed further in Chapter 27. The uncommon but important alpha-thalassaemia mental retardation syndromes, due to defects on chromosome 16 and the X chromosome, have been mentioned in Chapter 13.

OTHER RED BLOOD CELL DISORDERS

HEREDITARY SPHEROCYTOSIS AND ELLIPTOCYTOSIS

Hereditary spherocytosis is a disorder of the red cell membrane which usually follows autosomal dominant inheritance, but haemolysis is often mild, requiring red cell fragility tests to be sure that an individual is not affected. Numerous other causes of spherocytosis must be excluded before this diagnosis is made. Specific forms of hereditary spherocytosis have been identified as due to defects in several different red cell membrane proteins, including spectrin and ankyrin.

Hereditary elliptocytosis is also autosomal dominant. Several forms exist, several due to defects in glycophorin C and other membrane proteins.

GLUCOSE-6-PHOSPHATE DEHYDROGENASE DEFICIENCY

This important red-cell enzyme defect is particularly common in parts of the Middle East, the Mediterranean and South-east Asia and in people of African descent, but is not unknown in others. Numerous enzyme variants exist, with varying loss of activity which determines the haemolytic severity of the disease. The disorder is X-linked recessive, but alterations in the gene (which has been cloned) are so common in some areas (e.g. the Arabian peninsula) that homozygous affected females are frequent. Carrier detection is often feasible, but this depends on the type of the abnormality.

OTHER RED-CELL ENZYME DEFECTS

Other red-cell enzyme defects are mostly autosomal recessive, with the exception of phosphoglycerate kinase deficiency, which is X-linked. Some are confined to the red cell, others have generalized clinical effects (e.g. triose phosphate isomerase deficiency). Prenatal diagnosis from fetal blood is a possibility for this group, but as the genes are cloned, DNA analysis will be preferable.

SIDEROBLASTIC ANAEMIA

Most cases, especially in later life, are acquired, but an X-linked recessive form, though rare, is important to recognize.

PERNICIOUS ANAEMIA

Pernicious anaemia has already been mentioned in connection with atrophic gastritis (see Chapter 20). Congenital vitamin B_{12} deficiency is an exceptionally rare disorder caused by intrinsic factor deficiency, following autosomal recessive inheritance.

RHESUS INCOMPATIBILITY

The prevention of haemolytic disease of the newborn due to rhesus incompatibility has been so successful that there is a danger of overlooking the problem completely.

It certainly ranks as one of the major contributions of genetics to medicine. Although the genetics of the rhesus system is complex (its molecular basis has now been established) and is not discussed here, in essence the problem arises when a homozygous rhesus-negative woman with a rhesus-positive partner (heterozygous or homozygous) develops antibodies that will react with the red cells of a rhesus-positive fetus. Sensitization may be the result of a previous pregnancy or abortion, prenatal diagnostic procedures or transfusion, and is now usually prevented by giving anti-RhD antibody at the appropriate time.

Once sensitization has occurred, any rhesus-positive fetus will be at risk. This relates to 50 per cent of pregnancies where the father is heterozygous, and 100 per cent where he is homozygous for the RhD antigen.

HYDROPS FETALIS

The control of rhesus haemolytic disease means that other causes must now be sought for hydrops. These are often genetic and include various haemoglobinopathies, red-cell enzyme defects and congenital heart defects (some associated with Down's syndrome and other chromosome abnormalities), as well as non-genetic causes such as fetal infections.

OTHER BLOOD GROUP SYSTEMS

In the past, these were relevant to paternity and zygosity testing (see Chapter 9). Most blood group systems do not cause regular clinical problems, although haemolytic disease of the newborn may occur, particularly with the ABO and Kell systems. Most blood group antigens are co-dominant, expressing themselves without interfering with the action of other alleles that may be present. The specific genes have now mostly been identified.

A variety of disease associations have been described with the ABO blood group system, but are too weak to be of use in genetic counselling. Similarly, although blood groups have been useful genetic markers in the study of genetic linkage, it is rare to be able to apply this form of information in risk prediction. DNA markers have superseded blood groups in these areas.

WHITE BLOOD CELLS AND PLATELETS

A number of rare genetic disorders of white blood cells and platelets exist and information is summarized in Table 24.1. There is some overlap with the immune deficiency disorders considered below.

A number of syndromal associations with skeletal dysplasias also exist and should be carefully looked for.

Leukaemias are considered in Chapter 25.

Table 24.1 Hereditary disorders of blood cell production

Disorder	Inheritance
Blackfan–Diamond red cell hypoplasia	Autosomal recessive
Fanconi pancytopenia	Autosomal recessive
Infantile hereditary agranulocytosis	Autosomal recessive
Cyclic neutropenia	Autosomal recessive or dominant
Chediak–Higashi syndrome	Autosomal recessive
Chronic granulomatous disease	X-linked recessive (rarely autosomal recessive)
Hereditary isolated thrombocytopenia	X-linked recessive (may be autosomal recessive or autosomal dominant)
Thrombocytopenia–absent radius (TAR) syndrome	Autosomal recessive
Familial lymphohistiocytosis	Autosomal recessive

IMMUNE DEFICIENCY DISEASE

Numerous forms of immune deficiency exist, mostly mendelian in inheritance (Table 24.2). The X-linked types, probably involving at least five distinct loci, are particularly important to recognize in view of the high risk to offspring of female carriers. Some carriers can be recognized by lowered immunoglobulin levels in their blood, but levels are

Table 24.2 Immunological deficiency disorders

Disorder	Inheritance
Hypogammaglobulinaemia	
Bruton type	X-linked recessive
Swiss type	Autosomal recessive and X-linked recessive
Combined immunodeficiency due to:	
Adenosine deaminase deficiency	Autosomal recessive
Nucleoside phosphorylase deficiency	Autosomal recessive
Other types	X-linked and autosomal recessive
Pure thymic dysplasia	Autosomal recessive
Thymic and parathyroid aplasia (DiGeorge syndrome)	Small chromosome 22 deletion; most cases sporadic (see Chapter 19)
Ataxia telangiectasia	Autosomal recessive
Wiskott–Aldrich syndrome	X-linked recessive
Chronic granulomatous disease	X-linked recessive (rarely autosomal recessive)
Complement factor deficiencies (various types)	Autosomal recessive
Hereditary angioedema (C1 inhibitor)	Autosomal dominant

frequently normal. Study of the clonal origin of lymphocytes may allow more definitive recognition of the carrier state. Fetal blood sampling will often allow prenatal detection of both immune deficiencies and blood cell disorders but is progressively being replaced by molecular analysis of chorion villus samples, as the specific genes are identified. Bone marrow transplantation is proving valuable in some situations, but the possible role of gene therapy is still uncertain in terms of long-term safety.

The autosomal recessive, severe combined immunodeficiency due to adenosine deaminase deficiency can be recognized prenatally in chorionic villi or cultured amniotic cells. The X-linked chronic granulomatous disease is located close to the gene for Duchenne muscular dystrophy at Xp2l and may be associated with it due to deletions in the region.

Disorders of the complement system form a sequence of recessively inherited defects, some characterized by immune deficiency, others of which are symptomless. An exception is the dominantly inherited C1 esterase inhibitor deficiency, responsible for hereditary angioedema. In view of the potentially lethal laryngeal problems and the success of preventive and acute therapy, it is important for all close relatives of a patient with this disorder to be carefully checked for the deficiency.

GENETIC ASPECTS OF INFECTIOUS DISEASE

Susceptibility and resistance to major infectious diseases have a strong genetic basis, something that has been recognized for many years, especially when the environmental agent was close to universal (e.g. tuberculosis, rheumatic fever). The underlying basis is beginning to be understood and may involve both rare genetic changes in the immune system and also more common population variants (e.g. susceptibility to meningitis).

So far these developments have not impacted on genetic counselling, but this could well change. It should be remembered also that past major infections are likely to have played an important role in the population distribution of a number of common polymorphisms, not just those related to malaria where the relationship can still be seen today.

HAEMOPHILIA

Haemophilia represents a major genetic counselling problem, particularly since most haemophilic males now reach adult life with only moderate disability, and frequently reproduce. Both major forms of haemophilia are X-linked; haemophilia A results from a deficiency of factor VIII, while haemophilia B (Christmas disease) results from a deficiency of factor IX. It is now recognized that factor VIII occurs in association with its carrier molecule, von Willebrand factor (VWF). Factor VIII is encoded by the X-linked locus defective in haemophilia A, whilst von Willebrand factor is encoded by an autosomal locus, defective in the disorder von Willebrand's disease (VWD).

Occasional forms of 'autosomal haemophilia A' occur owing to defects in the FVIII-binding site of VWF.

Genetic advice for men affected with haemophilia (A or B) is straightforward, although mistakes are often made. As with any X-linked recessive disorder, all sons will be healthy, as will their descendants; all daughters will be carriers. It is unnecessary and often misleading for such daughters to have tests of carrier detection, because whatever results these give, the daughter of an affected male must be a carrier. A daughter can only be fully affected (though expression in heterozygotes is variable) if her father is affected and her mother is a carrier (an exceptionally rare event), or if there is a sex chromosome abnormality, such as Turner (45,X) syndrome.

Risks for the offspring of definite carriers are also clear, there being a 50 per cent risk of sons being affected and of daughters being carriers (see Chapter 2). The main problems in genetic counselling lie in determining how great is the chance of women at risk being carriers, and this is of particular importance if decisions are to be made regarding fetal sexing and prenatal diagnosis. The risk of being a carrier will depend on:

- the prior genetic risk
- other genetic information
- the results of carrier detection studies.

The general approach to the subject for X-linked diseases has been discussed in Chapters 2 and 7. Although specific molecular defects can now identify most carriers, it remains extremely important to identify the genetic risks appropriately from pedigree information if molecular investigations are to be interpreted accurately and not used wastefully.

The factor VIII gene, located at Xq28, is a large gene which shows relatively few polymorphisms and is only deleted in 4 per cent of affected males, but an inversion within the gene is responsible for around 40 per cent of severe cases. Point mutations differ widely between families so prediction is still sometimes dependent on DNA polymorphisms. The factor IX gene, located more proximally at Xq26, is more informative. In both disorders, the identification of a mutation in one family member will usually allow much simpler prediction for any relative, so it is important for this information to be recorded and to be available. The concept of a 'mutational register' has been established for both haemophilia A and B.

The shift to first-trimester DNA testing makes it imperative for carrier status to be established before a pregnancy occurs. This anticipatory approach is greatly enhanced if there is close communication regarding testing and counselling between the haemophilia and genetics services within a region, which unfortunately is still not always the case.

The use of immunological and coagulation assays is now largely ancillary to DNA analysis in carrier testing, but should not be ignored. In prenatal diagnosis, DNA analysis from chorion biopsy samples is now the approach of choice, but where the family is not informative or presents too late, fetal blood sampling and analysis of the appropriate factor is still a reliable test.

These striking advances in the haemophilias have tragically been overshadowed by the catastrophe of HIV infection and AIDS in these families. Not only must HIV infection be especially considered in the handling of samples, but it has to be recognized that this disaster has radically affected attitudes to haemophilia, both within families and in the community at large. Many families now opt for prenatal diagnosis and termination who would not have done so before, and the stigmatization of families that has occurred gives reason for profound concern in relation to the attitudes of society towards those with presymptomatic tests proving positive for other serious disorders.

Table 24.3 Inherited coagulation disorders

Deficiency/disorder	Inheritance
Deficiency resulting mainly in bleeding	
Factor VIII (haemophilia A)	XR
Factor IX (haemophilia B)	XR
Von Willebrand disease	See text
Other coagulation factor deficiencies (V, VII, X, XI, XII, XIII)	AR
Deficiency resulting mainly in thrombosis	
Antithrombin III deficiency	AD
Protein C deficiency	AD
Protein S deficiency	AD
Factor V (Leiden variant)	See text
Plasminogen deficiency	AD
Dysfibrinogenaemias	AD

OTHER COAGULATION DISORDERS

Von Willebrand's disease, determined by the autosomal portion of the factor VIII molecule, is usually mild in heterozygotes, although a very rare, severe homozygous form also exists. Deficiencies of numerous other coagulation factors have been recognized (see Table 24.3). All are autosomal recessive. A variety of forms of thrombocytopenia have also been identified, showing various modes of inheritance, but an X-linked recessive form is the best recognized. Prenatal diagnosis from a fetal blood sample or by molecular analysis is becoming possible for most of these disorders.

An increased risk of venous thrombosis is now known to result in some families from coagulation factor alterations. In some instances (e.g. factor V), deficiency may cause bleeding, whereas other alterations may predispose to thrombosis. Table 24.3 lists some of this group. In general, the thrombotic tendency (which may be very variable) is shown by heterozygotes, i.e. the inheritance is autosomal dominant. The relatively common population 'Leiden' variant of factor V deserves note since here it occurs at a frequency of around 5 per cent of northern European populations; those carrying it have a two- to threefold increase in thrombotic risk, which may be higher in relation to oral contraceptive use. This should be regarded as a susceptibility risk factor, rather than a genetic disorder, and it is not clear that widespread screening or testing of family members is of value, since the risk of venous thrombosis for heterozygotes is less than 0.1 per cent per year.

Unfortunately, because results on patients are reported as genotypes, inappropriate testing of relatives has become widespread, usually without adequate information, so that genetic counselling referrals are mainly occupied with attempting to reduce problems already created.

FURTHER READING

Arya R, Layton DM, Bellingham AJ (1995). Hereditary red cell enzymopathies. *Blood Rev* **9**, 165–175.

Beutler E (1996). G6PD: population genetics and clinical manifestations. *Blood Rev* **10**, 45–52.

Bloom AL, Thomas DP (1993). *Haemostasis and Thrombosis*. Edinburgh, Churchill Livingstone.

Bossi D, Russo M (1996). Hemolytic anemias due to disorders of red cell membrane skeleton. *Mol Aspects Med* **17**, 171–188.

Cooper DN, Krawczak M (1997). *Venous Thrombosis: from Genes to Clinical Medicine*. Oxford, BIOS.

George JN, Nurden AT, Phillips DR (1984). Molecular defects in interactions of platelets with the vessel wall. *N Engl J Med* **311**, 1084–1098.

Machin GA (1981). Differential diagnosis of hydrops fetalis. *Am J Med Genet* **9**, 341–350.

Modell B (1983). Prevention of the haemoglobinopathies. *Br Med Bull* **39**, 386–391.

Serjeant GR (1997). Sickle-cell disease. *Lancet* **350**, 725–730.

Tuddenham EGD, Cooper DN (1994). *The Molecular Genetics of Haemostasis and its Inherited Disorders*. Oxford, Oxford University Press.

Weatherall DJ (1991). *The New Genetics and Clinical Practice*. Oxford, Oxford University Press.

Weatherall DJ (1997). The thalassaemias. *Br Med J* **314**, 1675–1678.

Weatherall DJ, Clegg JB (1981). *The Thalassaemia Syndromes*. Oxford, Blackwell Scientific.

Genetic risks in cancer

Cancer genetics now forms a major part of genetic services, a striking contrast to only a decade ago, when there was little practical help that could be offered to most families at risk for cancer. The change has largely resulted from recognition of the fact that genetic risks for cancer are rather sharply partitioned. The great majority (~95 per cent) of cases show only weak inherited influences, while a small proportion (~5 per cent) show mendelian inheritance, with very high risks.

Alongside this has come the possibility of recognizing many of the high-risk forms through identifying the genes involved, allowing specialist genetic services, including molecular testing, to be concentrated on these rather than spread diffusely across a much larger number that mostly do not need such applications. Again, the end result is a further partitioning into those where high risk is excluded (the majority), and the smaller number of individuals known or likely to carry mutations conferring high cancer risk, who can benefit from surveillance and early therapy.

These advances have become a paradigm for common disorders showing a mendelian or high-risk subset, and it is likely that genetic services in other fields (e.g. cardiac disorders) will reflect this. The advances also create two considerable challenges:

- How can one accurately distinguish those families with a high-risk genetic situation from the great majority for whom risks are low?
- How can one ensure that scarce resources and specialist services are appropriately targeted at those who need them?

In terms of the first challenge, there are helpful clinical and genetic pointers for identifying high-risk situations. The first is to recognize the numerous rare clinical syndromes that show mendelian inheritance by careful clinical and pedigree assessment. Secondly, other risk factors can be used, such as young age at onset and multiple tumours, as well as the presence of close relatives. These can be turned into useful guidelines, as in the 'Amsterdam criteria' for familial colorectal cancer (see below). The properties of the tumour itself may give indications (e.g. microsatellite instability in colorectal cancer).

The second challenge, of providing a systematic service to patients and families appropriate to the level of risk, is also beginning to be met, at least in those countries with planned rather than consumer-led health services. For this, a partnership between specialist genetics services, the relevant clinical specialities, including oncologists and surgeons, and, most importantly, primary care workers is essential, with guidelines for their relevant roles. Such programmes are becoming established for familial breast and colorectal cancer and will follow for other forms as their genetic basis becomes better understood and molecular analysis becomes possible.

Genetic counselling problems in cancer fall into several major groups, listed below, which will be considered in turn (although many of the individual disorders are covered in other chapters):

- familial tumour syndromes following mendelian (usually but not always autosomal dominant) inheritance
- common cancers of later life and their genetic subsets
- genetic disorders giving a general predisposition to malignancy (commonly autosomal recessive)
- embryonal and childhood cancer.

Before these groups are considered, it is essential to give a brief background to some of the key scientific advances that have so radically affected possibilities for genetic counselling.

THE MOLECULAR GENETIC BASIS OF CANCER

It has long been recognized that chromosomal changes are seen in many cancers, and that while not completely specific in most cases, they are not random. Molecular analysis has now given added precision to these changes, with the result that a number of tumour types can now be associated with somatic cell changes in specific chromosomal regions. Loss of heterozygosity is the most important finding, as measured by comparing the DNA of the tumour with DNA of blood from the same individual.

In parallel with this work, genetic linkage studies on rare mendelian tumours have shown that the same loci (or at least the same chromosome regions) are often involved as in the tumours themselves, indicating a direct relationship between the familial and non-familial forms of the same tumour type.

This research has validated a long-standing concept, the two-hit hypothesis. This proposes that for a tumour to occur, the gene defect must be homozygous. Normally this will be the result of two independent somatic mutations, but if an individual has inherited one defect germinally, only a single somatic event will be required to initiate a tumour. This readily explains why, in inherited forms of cancer, the tumours tend to be earlier and multiple. Retinoblastoma and Wilms' tumour provided the initial examples of these changes being directly identified. This concept also explains the previously puzzling examples of 'lack of penetrance' in retinoblastoma (see Chapter 17).

The genes involved in this process are mostly tumour suppressor genes, with an important normal function in growth, development and cell signalling pathways, which

Table 25.1 Familial tumour syndromes following autosomal dominant inheritance

Disorder	Gene locus	Gene identified
Retinoblastoma (inherited and syndromal)	13q	+
Wilm's tumour (syndromal form)	11p	+
Neurofibromatosis (type 1)	17q	+
Bilateral acoustic (type 2) neurofibromatosis	22q	+
Von Hippel–Lindau syndrome	3q	+
Basal cell naevus syndrome	9q	+ (PATCH)
Familial glomus tumours	14q	+ (imprinting; only affected if paternally transmitted)
Familial melanoma	1,19	+ (some types)
Multiple self-healing keratoacanthoma	9q	+ (? also PATCH)
Multiple endocrine neoplasia type 1	11q	+
Multiple endocrine neoplasia type 2	10	+ (RET oncogene)
Li–Fraumeni syndrome	17p	+ (P53)
Oesophageal cancer with tylosis	17q	−
Polyposis coli	5q	+
Ovarian dysgerminoma	17q	−
Cowden disease	10q	+ (PTEN)

is progressively becoming better understood. Most of the disorders listed in Table 25.1 are due to inherited defects in tumour suppressor genes. The 'second hit' or somatic event is often a more extensive loss of the relevant chromosome region in the cell.

A second major category of genes involved in cancer is that of the **oncogenes**, whose activation may predispose to tumour formation. The structure of these oncogenes is homologous to that of particular RNA retroviral sequences. Their normal counterparts, the cellular or proto-oncogenes, present in all individuals, are proving to be the site of somatic point mutations or chromosomal rearrangements characteristic of a number of tumour types, especially leukaemias and lymphomas. Thus the 9/22 translocation characteristic of chronic myeloid leukaemia (the 'Philadelphia' chromosome) occurs at the site of the *c-abl* oncogene locus on chromosome 9.

Numerous oncogene loci are now recognized, and those so far characterized are proving to represent important growth factors or receptors involved in cell regulation. These loci may also be important in early development and some (e.g. the *RET* oncogene) are proving to be involved in developmental malformations as well as tumours, linking the two important areas of cancer and developmental genetics.

TUMOUR SYNDROMES FOLLOWING MENDELIAN INHERITANCE

Although individually rare, the number of mendelian tumours is considerable (Table 25.1) and there is little doubt that many cases are missed from lack of careful history-taking in what initially may appear to be an ordinary 'common or garden variety' of non-familial neoplasm. It can be seen that almost all these conditions follow autosomal dominant inheritance and the recognition of specific loci for a number of them has been one of the major contributions of molecular genetics. Not only is it now possible to provide practical tests for relatives at risk, but, as outlined above, these loci are also proving to be involved in the somatic mutations producing common non-inherited tumours of the same organs. More than any other group of genetic disorders, the familial cancers are proving the value of systematic genetic register systems. The combination of early ascertainment, molecular diagnosis and effective therapy provides direct benefits to the health of those who are affected or at risk, as well as allowing risks to be reduced or excluded for many family members. Familial adenomatous polyposis (FAP) provides an excellent example of this, and is likely to form a prototype of how genetic services can be delivered in the rare dominantly inherited cancers.

FAMILIAL ADENOMATOUS POLYPOSIS

This is an important autosomal dominant disorder which shows around 90 per cent penetrance for polyps by early adult life and carries a very high risk of colonic malignancy if left untreated. It is thus a prime candidate for a genetic register, which can facilitate the direct management of those at risk and those affected, as well as allowing genetic counselling. The gene (*APC* on chromosome 5q) has been cloned, with mutations detectable in some patients and accurate prediction from either mutation analysis or RFLPs possible for almost all families. DNA analysis allows avoidance of invasive procedures in those shown to be at low risk, while giving extra motivation for these procedures where the risk is confirmed to be high. The occurrence of bony and soft tissue desmoid tumours, previously considered to be a separate disorder (Gardner's syndrome), is now known to be part of regular polyposis coli; a rare but fatal complication is hepatoblastoma in infancy.

The occurrence of eye lesions representing congenital hypertrophy of the retinal pigment epithelium (CHRPE) is a further systemic feature, but it is too inconsistent for use in clinical or presymptomatic detection.

Familial aspects of colorectal cancer without polyposis are considered on page 335.

OTHER FORMS OF POLYPOSIS

Other forms of polyposis include the following:

- *Peutz–Jeghers syndrome (autosomal dominant).* Characterized externally by circumoral pigment spots, polyps and neoplasms may occur throughout the gastrointestinal tract. The risk of malignancy is lower than in polyposis coli but is considerable and less preventable owing to the wider distribution of lesions. The gene has been mapped to chromosome 19p and recently isolated.
- *Discrete solitary colonic polyps.* A few families following autosomal dominant inheritance have been reported.
- *Juvenile polyposis.* This appears to be histologically distinct and to follow autosomal dominant inheritance. Whether the genetic locus is the same as for FAP is not yet clear.

- *Recessively inherited attenuated polyposis and colorectal cancer due to defects in the DNA repair gene* MYH. This newly recognized disorder is of considerable significance, since it means that one can no longer assume that all familial colorectal cancer and polyposis are dominantly inherited. It is likely that a number of apparently isolated cases will prove to be due to this.

GENETIC COUNSELLING AND THE COMMON CANCERS

Until recently, it was considered that genetic factors in most common cancers were relatively subsidiary to environmental influences, such as diet and viral factors. Family studies had shown some risk increase to close relatives, but these were rather non-specific and genetic counselling requests were few, reflecting the public perception that most cancer was not genetic in nature. The striking change in recent years has resulted from two related advances:

- The recognition that, while most cases do indeed probably not involve major heritable factors, an important minority of cases follow mendelian inheritance. Although this minority is only around 5 per cent of all cases, where this can be determined accurately, for common conditions this makes up a large number of families at high risk by comparison with most other inherited disorders, considerably exceeding all the rare tumour syndromes mentioned above.
- The specific genes involved are progressively being identified, most notably for colorectal and breast cancer, discussed below. This has not only produced practical implications for genetic counselling and testing, but has radically altered the general attitude to genetic services of those with a family history of cancer.

These developments make it extremely important for clinicians to recognize the familial subsets among the much larger number of cancers likely to be largely non-genetic. Some relevant factors applying generally to different forms of cancer that might suggest a mendelian basis include:

- any evidence of one of the rare tumour syndromes (listed in Table 25.1)
- particularly young age at onset
- multiple cancers in a single individual
- strong family history of a single form of cancer.

Awareness of these risk factors will not only prevent many high genetic risk cases being overlooked, but will also help to avoid indiscriminate referral or genetic testing of those (the great majority) who, while worried, do not have a significantly increased risk.

COLORECTAL CANCER

This has provided a most important development in terms of both practical applications and increase in our fundamental understanding of the disease. It has long been recognized that, apart from FAP, there are rare families with dominantly inherited colorectal cancer without polyps (hereditary non-polyposis colon cancer, HNPCC). Also previously recognized were dominantly inherited families where colon cancer occurred along with other adenocarcinomas, such as stomach, pancreas and breast, a condition variably termed adenocarcinomatosis, cancer family syndrome or Lynch syndrome. It is now clear that these are essentially the same disorder, probably best considered as HNPCC, provided that the less frequent occurrence of these other tumours is not forgotten.

The discovery of the genes involved stemmed from the recognition that the tumours themselves show genetic instability of a characteristic type, also seen in a series of genetic defects in yeast and bacteria. When the human equivalents of these genes were isolated, they were found to map to precisely the same chromosome regions as the loci defined by studying HNPCC families, and were rapidly found to show specific mutations. Four gene loci are involved (the phenotypes appear similar), and molecular testing is now able to provide presymptomatic testing where a defect has been identified in an affected member. As with FAP, this will allow regular clinical surveillance to be specifically targeted at those who are definite gene carriers, rather than all those at risk. It should be emphasized that this is only appropriate for those fulfilling strict criteria for this category (the 'Amsterdam criteria'), with at least three relatives with colorectal cancer, one or more diagnosed at under 50 years, and not for the great majority of colorectal cancers. Wider testing is less likely to be helpful, particularly in the absence of a confirmed gene defect in an affected family member. The use of microsatellite instability testing on tumour samples in conjunction with mutation analysis is likely to help in the recognition of mendelian cases.

The discovery of a recessively inherited form of colorectal cancer (see p. 335) means that genetic risks and genetic counselling will need reassessing where the condition is present in a sibship rather than in two or more generations.

In giving genetic risks for non-mendelian colorectal cancer, one has to rely on the older empiric data, as given in Table 25.2. Computer programs have been developed to individualize risk estimates, as for breast cancer, but it must be remembered that there will be a considerable number of patients with mendelian cancer whose family history does not suggest this, while the true risks for most patients may be smaller than current data suggest once all mendelian cases have been recognized and excluded from the calculations.

Table 25.2 Genetic risks in colorectal cancer

Lifetime risks of colorectal cancer for relatives (excluding **HNPCC and FAP**)	**Risk**	**% (approx.)**
Population risk	1 in 50	2
One first-degree relative affected	1 in 17	6
One first- and one second-degree relative affected	1 in 12	8
One first-degree relative with onset under 45 affected	1 in 10	10
Two first-degree relatives affected	1 in 6	15
Clear dominant inheritance pattern; first-degree relative affected	1 in 2	50

Based on Houlston RS et al. (1990), Br Med J **301**, 366–368.

BREAST CANCER

Around 5 per cent of breast cancers are now recognized as being the result of specific mutations in major genes, and as following autosomal dominant inheritance. Apart from family history, factors pointing to this group include young age at onset and bilateral breast involvement. Two specific tumour suppressor genes (*BRCA1* and *BRCA2*) have been isolated. Their large size and the wide range of different mutations make clinical use difficult, as have unwarranted and currently disputed attempts to restrict use on commercial grounds, but the advances have had a powerful effect on public awareness of the genetic aspects of breast cancer.

Breast cancer is a common disorder (lifetime risk for women is 1 in 10), and therefore multiple affected members may occur by chance. Table 25.3 summarizes the overall risks, which are strongly age-related, in terms of both the affected patient and the individual at risk. If the family history is typical of autosomal dominant inheritance, or if a specific mutation has been identified, then risk estimates should be given accordingly.

Several points need consideration for *BRCA1* and *BRCA2* gene carriers. First, penetrance is not complete, i.e. a woman who is a definite gene carrier has only an 85–90 per cent chance of developing breast cancer. In each case males only rarely show clinical features, but male *BRCA1* carriers may have an increased risk of prostate cancer, while *BRCA2* is associated with male breast cancer (again only rarely). Clearly it is important for male relatives to recognize that they are as likely to transmit the disorder to their daughters as are female gene carriers. *BRCA1* is also associated with increased risk of ovarian cancer (dependent on the site of the mutation in the gene).

Most women concerned by a family history of breast cancer will prove to have little increased risk, and genetic testing in such low-risk situations will give only a low yield of abnormal results. A normal result in such a situation will have little meaning and may well lead to false reassurance, given the high general population incidence.

Likewise, the benefits for those women detected as being *BRCA1* or *BRCA2* gene carriers are less clear-cut in terms of reducing mortality than is the case in colorectal cancer, as evidence on the value of early (or prophylactic) surgery is still limited, while there have

Table 25.3 Genetic risks in breast cancer

	Lifetime risk	% (approx.)	Increase relative to population
General population*	1 in 12	8	1
First-degree relative with diagnosis at over 55	1 in 8	12	1.6
First-degree relative with diagnosis at under 55	1 in 6	18	2.3
First-degree relative with diagnosis under 45	1 in 3	30	3.8
First-degree relative with bilateral breast cancer	1 in 2	50	6.4

*North Europe, North America.

been suggestions that these individuals may be unduly radiosensitive and thus have their breast cancer risk increased by frequent mammography. All of these factors support a cautious approach to the use of genetic tests in breast cancer until more evidence becomes available.

The prevalence of breast cancer and the high level of media attention given recently to genetic aspects have created serious logistical problems in providing genetic counselling for women concerned because of their family history. The large numbers and the fact that most are at low risk make it both impractical and inappropriate for specialist genetic services to be involved in all instances, but those in primary care are often unhappy to give risk estimates, while surgical family history clinics are more suited to give reassurance that a person is currently unaffected than to advise on genetic aspects. Current UK policy has developed towards a 'tripartite' system of management. Genetics centres, increasingly containing a specialist cancer geneticist, are concentrating on the small, high-risk group where presymptomatic genetic testing is most relevant; the intermediate group is being handled by staff in specialist breast clinics, usually having links with clinical genetics services and by genetic counsellors; while attempts are being made to educate those in primary care and give them sufficient information to allow the majority of concerned but low-risk individuals to be dealt with at this level. The success of this approach makes it likely that it will prove to be a prototype for handling the genetic aspects of other common cancers (e.g. colorectal) and be more widely adopted by genetic services for common disorders.

Presymptomatic genetic testing in breast cancer, like presymptomatic genetic testing in general for late-onset disorders, needs to be undertaken within a framework of full information, preparation and consent, and not purely as a laboratory procedure (see Chapter 5). Identification of a specific mutation in an affected relative is currently a prerequisite. It should be borne in mind that, as with other serious late-onset disorders where treatment is unsatisfactory, not all those at risk wish to be tested; only 50 per cent of high-risk women taking part in one research study wished to know their result, even when they knew it was already available.

OTHER COMMON CANCERS

After the impressive genetic developments in colorectal and breast cancer, it is not surprising that both clinical and basic research workers have been looking closely at other common cancers to see if comparable mendelian subsets exist. The current situation is fluid, but the evidence for most common cancers suggests that it will be possible to identify families with a mendelian pattern, but that these will mostly be fewer in number and less easy to define. From the viewpoint of clinicians asked about genetic risks, accurate documentation of family history is the most important task. If this looks clearly mendelian, then it is probably wise to consider the risks high, especially if the affected members show the same specific tumour type, if age at onset is unusually young, or if there are multiple tumour types or tumour sites in a single individual.

Ovarian cancer represents a particular problem, partly because BRCA1 gene carriers are at increased risk of this, especially with some specific mutations, but also because methods of screening and prevention are of uncertain value. Other gene loci are likely to be identified in high-risk families without breast cancer. The proportion of definitely mendelian cases seems to be very low; for other families the empiric risk for first-degree relations is around 5 per cent with one affected relative, and 7 per cent with two (population risk around 1.5 per cent).

Prostate cancer, a relatively neglected field, shows a susceptibility locus on chromosome 1 in some families; an X-linked locus has also been identified. Problems are created by the late age at onset, making recognition of a mendelian pattern difficult, and by the high proportion of tumours that do not progress significantly. Male *BRCA1* gene carriers appear to be at increased risk for relatively early onset prostate cancer.

Uterine endometrial cancer can occur as part of HNPCC, but a separate locus on chromosome 10q seems to account for a few rare dominant families. Cervical cancer, like lung cancer, is mainly due to external agents, in this case viral ones.

For those attempting to ensure that an efficient system of service delivery is developed for cancer genetics, it is perhaps fortunate that scientific discoveries in this field should be sequential rather than simultaneous. Hopefully, the evolution of a system such as that outlined for breast cancer, using the combined resources of primary care, cancer clinicians and geneticists, should allow genetic counselling and testing guidelines to be drawn up that can be applied to the entire area of common cancers. This should help to avoid wasteful use of scarce resources and needless worry for many patients and their relatives. It should also be useful when future population screening programmes for cancer (see Chapter 27) begin to incorporate genetic approaches, as is beginning to happen in relation to breast cancer screening.

GENETIC SYNDROMES PREDISPOSING TO MALIGNANCY

In contrast to the dominantly inherited specific tumour syndromes, the majority of mendelian disorders showing a generalized tendency to malignancy, especially in early life, follow autosomal recessive inheritance (Table 25.4). Some of these have already been shown to be inborn errors of DNA repair and it is likely that others will prove to have a comparable basis. Others are immune deficiencies (see p. 325).

Table 25.4 Mendelian syndromes predisposing to malignancy

Syndrome	Inheritance	Type of neoplasm
Xeroderma pigmentosum	Autosomal recessive	Various skin tumours
Fanconi pancytopenia	Autosomal recessive	Leukaemias
Ataxia telangiectasia	Autosomal recessive	Leukaemias and carcinomas
Bloom syndrome	Autosomal recessive	Leukaemias
Chediak–Higashi syndrome	Autosomal recessive	Lymphomas
Werner syndrome	Autosomal recessive	Various
Dyskeratosis congenita	X-linked recessive	Pharyngeal and oesophageal cancer
Wiskott–Aldrich syndrome	X-linked recessive	Leukaemias, lymphomas
Lymphoproliferative disease	X-linked recessive	Lymphomas

The syndromes in this group are progressively proving amenable to prenatal diagnosis as more specific molecular tests are becoming available. This is already feasible for xeroderma pigmentosum, for which several of the underlying DNA repair genes have been isolated, and for ataxia telangiectasia. The earlier use of cytogenetic studies on fetal blood samples is being superseded by DNA analysis.

A potentially important early suggestion was that heterozygotes for these rare recessive disorders might be at increased risk of developing malignancy. The evidence for this was never convincing, and now seems to be disproved, particularly in relation to ataxia telangiectasia and breast cancer.

EMBRYONAL AND CHILDHOOD CANCER

When known genetic syndromes are excluded, the overall risk of malignancy in childhood is around 1 in 600. The risk of malignancy occurring in sibs is approximately doubled (1 in 300), with most cases concordant for the same neoplasm. The relative increases in risk divided into the major groups of leukaemias, lymphomas and other malignancies are given in Table 25.5, although for some of these, the familial factors may prove to be environmental rather than genetic.

It would seem reasonable to use this estimate for the various rare forms of childhood cancer where individual data are not yet available, where no other cases of childhood cancer have occurred and where a clear genetic basis for the neoplasm is not known to exist. Cytogenetic and molecular analysis of the tumours is becoming increasingly important in defining, distinguishing and planning treatment of these disorders. Retinoblastoma is considered more fully in Chapter 17.

WILMS' TUMOUR (NEPHROBLASTOMA)

The incidence of Wilms' tumour is 1 in 10 000. Survival into adult life has only recently become usual, but it is now clear that the situation is comparable to that seen in retinoblastoma (see p. 252) and that a proportion of cases follow mendelian dominant

Table 25.5 Increase in risk for sibs of a proband with childhood cancer

Sib	Proband		
	Leukaemia	Lymphoma	Other malignancy
Leukaemia	×2.3	×2.3	×1.3
Lymphoma	×2.9	×5.4	×0.7
Other malignancy	×1.2	×0.6	×2.7
Total	×1.7	×1.7	×2.0

After Draper GJ, Heaf MM, Wilson LMK (1977), *J Med Genet* **14**, 81–90.

Table 25.6 Risks for relatives in Wilm's tumour

Affected member	Risk for subsequent children (%)
Parent with bilateral tumours	30
Parent with unilateral tumour; affected relative	30
Parent unaffected: two affected children	30
Parent with unilateral tumour	10
Sib with bilateral tumours	10
Sib with unilateral tumour; no chromosome defect or associated malformations	1

inheritance, including most of those with bilateral tumours. Unfortunately, it is often impossible to separate this group from the other cases, and as with retinoblastoma, penetrance is incomplete (around 60 per cent). Empiric risks for relatives of patients with Wilms' tumour are given in Table 25.6. Other estimates of the sib risk for isolated cases are much lower than the 5 per cent estimate given here; an upper limit of 1 per cent seems likely for cases where high-risk factors have been carefully excluded. These risk estimates will require reassessment as molecular studies become more precise.

In addition, Wilms' tumour may occur in syndromal association with aniridia, genital defects and mental retardation, as well as with hemihypertrophy and Beckwith–Wiedemann syndrome. A series of overlapping microdeletions, involving a tumour suppressor gene on the short arm of chromosome 11, is responsible for these syndromal cases. Molecular studies have shown that, as with retinoblastoma, the tumour may be homozygous for a defect present in heterozygous state throughout the body, i.e. the tumour-predisposing gene is 'recessive' even though the trait is 'dominant' in its transmission. Most cases of familial but non-syndromal Wilms' tumour are determined by a separate locus.

NEUROBLASTOMA

In contrast to Wilms' tumour, the great majority of cases of neuroblastoma are sporadic, but poorer survival means that adequate data are not available for the offspring of affected patients. In the few two-generation families known, the parent has usually had spontaneous maturation of the tumour. The risk for further sibs of an isolated case is unlikely to exceed 1 per cent and is probably nearer the 1 in 300 risk found overall for sibs in childhood cancer. Where two sibs, or a parent and child, are affected, the risk for further sibs is much greater, probably that of an incompletely penetrant dominant gene, about 30 per cent, as for Wilms' tumour. No specific gene locus is yet definite, although chromosome rearrangements suggest chromosome 1. The case for regular screening of sibs, or for general population screening of infants using urine, has not yet been proved.

LEUKAEMIAS AND RELATED DISORDERS

The great majority of cases of all types of leukaemia do not seem to have a significant hereditary basis, but specific oncogenes and somatic mutations appear to be involved.

ACUTE LEUKAEMIA

Acute leukaemia is most commonly seen in childhood, where it accounts for a major proportion of all malignancies. The risks for sibs have been given above and amount only to a doubling of risk for leukaemia with a 1 in 300 chance of childhood malignancy overall. Monozygotic twins appear to carry a risk of around 25 per cent for concordance of childhood leukaemia, a finding that might seem to suggest a strong genetic influence, but probably results from shared circulation of precursor cells. Whatever the case, the high risk has important implications for the careful surveillance and early therapy of such co-twins. The various chromosomal abnormalities described in blood cells appear to be the result of somatic genetic changes, some involving particular oncogenes. The well-recognized relationship between leukaemias and irradiation has led to concern about the possible epidemiology and association of childhood leukaemia clusters with radiation sources such as nuclear power stations. It was suggested that such cases may be related to occupational exposure of the father, implying that a germ-line rather than somatic mutational mechanism might be operating, but this now seems unlikely.

Leukaemia may also be a complication of a number of primary genetic disorders, including immune deficiencies, DNA repair defects and Down's syndrome. No data are yet available for the offspring of the increasing number of survivors. Risks of leukaemia are likely to be small, but an increase in other abnormalities as a result of therapy cannot be excluded.

CHRONIC MYELOID LEUKAEMIA

Chronic myeloid leukaemia carries little risk to relatives, although the 'Philadelphia' chromosome abnormality – a partial deletion of chromosome 22 resulting from translocation of part of it on to chromosome 9 – is a constant finding in most cases. This is a somatic event, not affecting the germ line, and involves the *c-abl* locus on chromosome 9.

CHRONIC LYMPHATIC LEUKAEMIA

Chronic lymphatic leukaemia rarely recurs in a family, but a small number of multi-generation families makes it possible that a dominantly inherited form exists among the much more common non-genetic cases.

LYMPHOMAS

As with leukaemias, most cases of lymphoma are sporadic; clustering is suggestive of an infective or immunosuppressive agent and may well not be genetic. Burkitt's lymphoma shows a characteristic translocation at the site of the immunoglobulin genes on chromosome 14. The same primary genetic diseases as predispose to leukaemias (except for Down's syndrome) may also be responsible for lymphomas, and the same reservations about the offspring of 'cured' patients apply. Lymphomas may also occur in the X-linked immune deficiencies, notably in X-linked lymphoproliferative disease.

Study of the sibs of childhood lymphoma cases shows a fivefold increase in risk for lymphomas, but the overall risk of childhood malignancy is still only around 1 in 300.

HISTIOCYTOSIS

Histiocytosis comprises a confused and heterogeneous group including several mendelian disorders presenting in childhood – adult cases appear to be non-genetic. The group includes:

- familial erythrophagocytic lymphohistiocytosis (autosomal recessive) – rapidly progressive and fatal
- familial reticuloendotheliosis with eosinophilia (Omenn syndrome) – autosomal recessive.

FURTHER READING

Eeles RA, Ponder BAJ, Easton DF, Horwich A (eds) (1996). *Genetic Predisposition to Cancer*. London, Chapman & Hall.

Hodgson SV, Maher ER (1993). *A Practical Guide to Human Cancer Genetics*. Cambridge, Cambridge University Press.

Lalloo F (2002). *Genetics for Oncologists*. London, Remedica.

Mitelman P (1998). *Catalog of Chromosome Aberrations in Cancer*. New York, Wiley (CD-Rom also available).

Morrison PJ, Hodgson SV, Haites NE (2003). *Familial Breast and Ovarian Cancer: Genetics, Screening and Management*. Cambridge, Cambridge University Press.

Phillips RKS, Spigelman AD, Thomson JPS (1994). *Familial Adenomatous Polyposis*. London, Arnold.

Sampson JR, Dolwani S, Jones S *et al.* (2003). Autosomal recessive colorectal adenomatous polyposis due to inherited mutations of MYH. *Lancet* **362**, 39–41.

Vogelstein B, Kinzler KW (1998). *The Genetic Basis of Human Cancer*. New York, McGraw-Hill.

Environmental hazards

At first sight, the subject of environmental hazards might seem to bear little relation to genetic counselling, but in practice there are several reasons why environmental agents and their risks need consideration. First, they may come into the differential diagnosis of malformation syndromes, e.g. congenital rubella must be considered among the possible causes of congenital cataract, and the recurrence risks will be greatly affected if such an agent can be confirmed or firmly excluded. Congenital infections share a number of features, including growth retardation, microcephaly and liver involvement, that may easily be confused with a primary development or metabolic cause. Secondly, many agents causing fetal damage in pregnancy may also cause harmful mutations; radiation is a prime example. Thirdly, enquiry may be made as to whether cytogenetic or prenatal diagnostic tests may be of help in confirming or excluding fetal damage.

Three groups of agents are briefly discussed here:

- congenital infections damaging the fetus
- drugs believed to be teratogenic
- radiation and other potential mutagenic agents.

The role of genetic factors in susceptibility to infectious diseases is also considered briefly.

CONGENITAL INFECTIONS

Table 26.1 lists the major types of congenital infection. Of these, congenital syphilis is rarely seen now in Western populations; overwhelmingly the most important is congenital rubella. Systematic immunization is reducing the frequency of this in some populations, but it remains a major problem.

CONGENITAL RUBELLA

The principal malformations seen in congenital rubella include cataracts, nerve deafness, congenital heart defects (commonly patent ductus arteriosus) and microcephaly with

Table 26.1 Congenital infections

Agent	Common defects
Rubella	Cataract, deafness, congenital heart disease
Cytomegalovirus	Microcephaly, chorioretinitis, hepatosplenomegaly
Varicella	Microcephaly, chorioretinitis, scarring limb defects
Hepatitis virus	Biliary atresia(?), hepatic damage
HIV (AIDS)	Immune deficiency; possibly minor dysmorphic features
Other viruses	See text
Toxoplasma	Chorioretinitis, microcephaly, hepatosplenomegaly
Syphilis	Facial and other bony abnormalities, keratitis

mental retardation. Since congenital rubella may occur in the absence of overt maternal infection, it is a condition that must be considered seriously in the differential diagnosis of any syndrome where these abnormalities occur.

The risk to a subsequent pregnancy after a child with congenital rubella has been born is negligible. The critical information usually required is the risk to a current pregnancy in which the mother has developed or has been exposed to the infection. When the mother is already known to have immunity, on the basis of immunization or previous serological tests, the risk to the fetus is exceedingly low. When this information is not available, it is extremely difficult to obtain rapid direct evidence for fetal infection or lack of it. Tests on amniotic fluid are not reliable, but preliminary evidence suggests that IgM-specific anti-bodies on a fetal blood sample may be an accurate indicator of infection. Techniques for detecting viral antigens or nucleic acids are available, but these have not yet been fully evaluated for the diagnosis of congenital infection.

General information that can currently be used to predict risks is that infection in the first month of pregnancy carries an extremely high risk of abnormality (around 60 per cent), which falls to about 25 per cent for infection in the second month and about 8 per cent in the third month. Risks are small for serious abnormality after infection in the second trimester, and negligible after this. Indications for termination of pregnancy are clearly strong in the early stages, but the decision may be difficult around the third month, or if dates are uncertain. More specific tests will be of great help. Careful examination of an apparently normal infant at risk (especially audiometry) is important to exclude minor degrees of damage.

CYTOMEGALOVIRUS INFECTION

Microcephaly with mental retardation, cerebral palsy, chorioretinitis, deafness, hepatosplenomegaly and purpuric rash are common features of cytomegalovirus infection. MRI brain scan has helpful distinguishing features, although only around 5 per cent of cases have serious neurological problems. Maternal infection is often asymptomatic, and no preventive measures – apart from avoidance of known or potential sources of infection – are available. Child care and health care workers may be at increased risk of acquiring CMV infection. Good hygiene, particularly washing hands after changing nappies, regular cleaning of toys and surfaces, and care with food preparation, may reduce this risk.

VARICELLA ZOSTER VIRUS

Varicella in pregnancy poses a risk to the fetus. If acquired during the first 5 months of pregnancy, maternal varicella can occasionally result in the congenital varicella syndrome. Varicella-induced defects include areas of skin scarring with a clear dermatomal distribution, hypoplasia of the bone and muscle of a limb, microcephaly, mental retardation, cataract, microphthalmia and chorioretinitis.

PARVOVIRUS B19

Infections are common in childhood. Infection in pregnancy, particularly the second trimester, may not be apparent clinically but may present as hydrops fetalis with severe anaemia, congestive heart failure, generalized oedema and fetal death. A prospective study of symptomatic and asymptomatic maternal infection found an overall fetal loss rate of 16 per cent. There is no convincing evidence that B19 is teratogenic. Animal parvoviruses are not known to be transmissible to humans.

HIV INFECTION

Congenital HIV infection is a growing problem among the offspring of women carrying the virus. It seems unlikely that it produces significant dysmorphic features in affected infants, but it may need consideration in the context of immune deficiencies and of unusual infections.

OTHER VIRAL INFECTIONS

Although there have been many suggested associations, evidence for the teratogenicity of other viruses is not well established. It is possible that hepatitis virus may be involved in at least some cases of biliary atresia. Maternal transmission of this virus, especially hepatitis C, gives a high risk for chronic liver disease, including liver cancer in later life in susceptible individuals. Congenital herpes simplex virus infection is extremely rare but may cause fetal death – mainly after primary infection in the first trimester.

Influenza virus has been claimed to be responsible for some of the cyclical peaks of malformations such as neural tube defects. Live viral vaccines, while obviously undesirable in pregnancy, have in fact only occasionally produced any evidence of fetal damage.

TOXOPLASMOSIS

Chorioretinitis (which may be progressive and not always present at birth), central nervous system involvement with convulsions, hepatosplenomegaly, pneumonia, myocarditis and rash are the main features of *Toxoplasma gondii* infection. The incidence of severe fetal infection falls from 75 per cent associated with first trimester maternal infection to under 5 per cent when the woman is exposed to *T. gondii* in the third trimester. Children born infected but symptom-free will develop retinal disease in over 85 per cent of cases. Late development of mental retardation and hearing defects can occur. Maternal infection is often asymptomatic and is usually from domestic animals, cats in particular.

DRUGS AND MALFORMATIONS

Since the epidemic of limb defects due to thalidomide, not only has there been stringent testing of new drugs for teratogenicity, but many studies have investigated possible associations. In fact, the number of specific malformation syndromes clearly related to individual drugs is extremely small (Table 26.2); much more difficult to assess are situations in which a commonly used drug (e.g. an anticonvulsant) appears to be associated with an increased incidence of certain malformations, and where the type of malformation is either variable or commonly seen in the absence of the agent. It is likely that most of the associations still to be discovered are in this latter group, where proof of a causal relationship is exceedingly difficult to obtain.

Despite the small number of firm teratogenic syndromes due to drugs, it is clearly prudent for all drugs that are not strictly essential to be avoided in pregnancy, and indeed avoided by all women who are at risk of conceiving. Avoidance of cigarette smoking and the taking of a nutritious, balanced diet with folate supplementation are additional common-sense factors that are desirable even in the absence of specific evidence. General advice of this type can often be given as part of more general pre-conception advice because most couples known to be at increased risk for abnormality in the offspring will be anxious to do anything possible to reduce this risk (see Chapter 27).

Table 26.2 Drugs with teratogenic effect

Definite
Thalidomide
Warfarin
Alcohol
Retinoids
Aminopterin and methotrexate
Probable
Anticonvulsants (in particular phenytoin, trimethadione, valproate)
Lithium
Possible
Sex hormones
Antiemetics
Anaesthetic gases
Industrial chemicals

THALIDOMIDE

A generation of children with thalidomide-induced limb defects and other abnormalities has now grown up, particularly in continental Europe, but also in the UK. Those used to seeing malformations in younger children may not think of thalidomide as a possible cause; a useful clinical review by Smithells and Newman (1992; see 'Further reading') gives the range of features.

Where the relationship with thalidomide is clear-cut, there should, of course, be no increased risk of abnormalities in the offspring of these patients, but it seems likely that some dominantly inherited limb reduction defects, including Holt–Oram syndrome, may have mistakenly been attributed to thalidomide, in which case affected children may well be born. The recessively inherited pseudothalidomide or Roberts' syndrome should not be confused if full radiographs are available.

WARFARIN

Warfarin has been clearly associated with a syndrome identical to the severe form of chondrodysplasia punctata. Although occurring only in a small proportion of exposed pregnancies, there is a high fetal and perinatal loss overall, so it seems clear that warfarin and related anticoagulants are undesirable in women who are pregnant or at risk of becoming so. In one case known to the author, the pregnancy resulted from stopping oral contraceptives which had produced a venous thrombosis, warfarin then being used for therapy in a double iatrogenic misfortune.

ALCOHOL

There seems no doubt as to the existence of a syndrome of abnormal facies, reduced somatic and brain growth, mental retardation and congenital heart disease in children of mothers with a high alcohol intake during pregnancy. There is, however, real doubt as to how common this fetal alcohol syndrome disorder is and whether lesser degrees of alcohol consumption are teratogenic.

Recent studies suggest that the full syndrome only occurs when alcohol intake exceeds 80 g per day, but that low birthweight is seen at lower intake levels, with an effect from very early in the pregnancy.

ANTIEPILEPTIC DRUGS (see also Chapter 12)

There is now little doubt that there is an overall increase in the incidence of malformations in the offspring of epileptic mothers (around 6–7 per cent compared with 2–3 per cent in controls), and that this is related to therapy rather than to the epilepsy *per se*. The spectrum of defects is broad, including congenital heart disease, clefting and neural tube defects. The risks may be dose-related.

It is difficult to blame or to exonerate specific drugs since multiple therapy is frequent, but it is essential that all epileptic women of child-bearing age receiving therapy should be told of the potential risks, as well as the parents of young girls who may remain on drugs initially prescribed in childhood. Before embarking on child-bearing, there should be a reassessment of the need for therapy and, if possible, a trial period on no drugs or a minimal dose, with careful blood level measurements. Neurologists may protest that this is unnecessary, but they do not generally see the resulting problems. The author's personal view is that this is probably the major avoidable source of teratogenic agents at present.

Specific syndromes related to antiepileptic drugs exist but are much less common than the overall effects.

Phenytoin

Phenytoin is associated with a moderately specific syndrome of low birthweight, mental retardation, unusual facies with hypertelorism, congenital heart defects and hypoplastic digits, which appear to occur rarely. There is an overall increase in the incidence of cleft lip and palate and the overall malformation rate is doubled in comparison with the general population.

Trimethadione

Again, after trimethadione administration there appears to be an occasional specific combination of congenital heart defects, genitourinary abnormalities, unusual facies with V-shaped configuration of eyebrows, and mental retardation, with a considerable increase (possibly as high as 20 per cent) of congenital heart disease in isolation.

Valproate

An increased incidence of neural tube defects is likely with the use of sodium valproate, and a characteristic craniofacial appearance has been suggested. Overall the malformation rate is increased around fourfold (6.6 vs. 1.6 per cent for controls in one study).

Lithium

Lithium, a frequently used agent in affective disorders, has now been convincingly associated with the occurrence of congenital heart disease, in particular Ebstein's anomaly.

VITAMIN A ANALOGUES

A relatively characteristic pattern of defects with some similarities to DiGeorge syndrome is associated with the administration of vitamin A analogues in early pregnancy, and with vitamin A excess for other reasons. Agents such as isotretinoin and etretinate are used increasingly for various skin disorders, while an increasing use of high-dose vitamin A supplements in some areas has caused concern.

SEX HORMONES

The use of female sex hormones in early pregnancy for prevention of threatened abortion and for treatment of infertility is now rare, partly due to concern regarding fetal abnormalities. Doubt still exists as to whether conception while on oral contraceptives is harmful. An increased malformation rate has been seen following ovulation-inducing drugs, but whether this is a direct effect, or related to the frequently associated twinning or the underlying cause of the infertility, is unknown.

An important example of delayed teratogenicity is the occurrence of vaginal adenocarcinoma in the daughters of women treated with diethyl-stilboestrol during pregnancy because of threatened abortion.

IMMUNOSUPPRESSIVE AND CYTOTOXIC DRUGS

Increasing numbers of women are reproducing while taking immunosuppressive or cytotoxic drugs for previously lethal diseases or following renal transplantation. So far, few obvious abnormalities have been found in pregnancies going to term. Aminopterin and its derivative methotrexate have been associated with specific craniofacial anomalies, mental retardation and limb reduction defects. Problems in this group are perhaps more likely to arise from their mutagenic properties (see below).

INDUSTRIAL AND OTHER CHEMICALS

Despite widespread and reasonable concern, actual evidence for human teratogenic effects is scanty. Claims for increased abnormalities after deliberate mass spraying or industrial accidents involving the herbicide 2,4,5-T are circumstantial, as is the case for other chemicals such as hair dyes. An effect of anaesthetic gases inhaled by pregnant operating theatre staff and anaesthetists seems more soundly based; an increase in spontaneous abortions and in a variety of common malformations was seen, rather than any particular combination.

GENETIC EFFECTS OF RADIATION

The genetic effects of radiation are of much concern in view of the very real possibility of a localized accident involving a civil or military nuclear installation. While the genetic effects of nuclear conflict would be overshadowed by the scale of the immediate catastrophe, the consequences of an isolated disaster or near-disaster should be anticipated. Although reactions to such an event are likely to be largely based on fear, the Chernobyl disaster, which exposed large parts of Europe to radioactive contamination and which resulted in large numbers of probably unnecessary terminations of pregnancy, has emphasized how ill-prepared are the radiation protection services of most countries. The great majority of individuals exposed are likely to receive a low or even insignificant dose of irradiation, but it may be difficult to be certain of this at the time. Provided that the dose is approximately known, information on the possible genetic effects can be given with a reasonable degree of confidence, because of the very large amount of work that has been done on the topic.

Much of the biological information available on the effects of radiation relates to population effects (see below), but first the risks for a particular conception or pregnancy must be dealt with. Two separate situations must be considered, which are often confused by those requesting information:

- mutagenic effects, resulting in damage to germ cells before fertilization
- teratogenesis, i.e. damage to the developing embryo.

Mutagenesis must be considered separately for the two parents, because the method of germ cell formation in each sex is entirely different. In males, animal experiments have shown two major classes of abnormality:

- major chromosomal abnormalities, occurring mainly in the offspring conceived a few days or weeks after irradiation
- an increased incidence of point mutations, persisting in offspring conceived long after irradiation has been given.

For the human male, some direct evidence is now available from the study of human sperm chromosomes; the incidence of abnormalities more than doubles after radiotherapy and changes may persist for at least 3 years. One can probably draw the following conclusions regarding risks to offspring:

- Diagnostic and similar low-level irradiation does not significantly increase the risk to an individual offspring.
- Conception in the few months after therapeutic or other high-dose irradiation (especially of the gonads) is unwise; amniocentesis is advisable should pregnancy occur in order to detect chromosomal defects. The same probably applies when a man is, or has recently been, taking cytotoxic drugs or other known chemical mutagens.
- A variable period of infertility is common after gonadal irradiation (and with cytotoxic drugs), but should not be relied upon.
- Long-term risks for a pregnancy conceived many months or years after irradiation are small, and result mainly from increased dominant mutations, which are unlikely to be detected by amniocentesis. However, the incidence of such abnormalities is low (not more than 1 per cent).

In women the oocyte is especially radiation-sensitive around the time of fertilization. Outside this period, the risk is likely to be similar to or less than that for males. Diagnostic radiation is unlikely to be a significant risk factor for future children of an individual woman, although unnecessary exposure clearly should be avoided to prevent even a small population increase in point mutations and chromosome defects.

Irradiation during pregnancy is a somewhat different problem and is the most common cause of referral for genetic counselling in this context. Such irradiation is almost always diagnostic, with a dose of 0.01 Gray (Gy) or less; it is usually inadvertent and given in the earliest weeks of pregnancy before a pregnancy has been recognized. It is not uncommon for such irradiation to be given during the course of investigation for infertility, and the combination of a wanted pregnancy with the feelings of guilt shared by patient and doctor that radiation exposure should have occurred may produce considerable anxiety.

Until recently, termination of pregnancy has been frequently advised in such a situation, but it is likely that the risks to the fetus have been considerably overestimated and are in fact very small for diagnostic levels of radiation. A valuable review by Mole (see 'Further reading') concludes that after 0.01 Gy (the upper limit for most diagnostic radiation) the total added risk to the fetus is unlikely to exceed 1 in 1000, this risk being partly for malformations, partly for mental retardation and possibly childhood cancer. In such circumstances, neither termination nor amniocentesis seems warranted, although it is probably wise to stress the relatively frequent occurrence of abnormalities in the general population, because there is a real danger that any such occurrence will be attributed to the radiation.

Information on the risks of heavy doses of radiation (see UNSCEAR reports in 'Further reading') has come mainly from follow-up of Japanese atomic bomb casualties. At levels over 0.6 Gy there is a clear and dose-related increase in mental retardation and microcephaly in such exposed pregnancies (10 per cent at 2 Gy). Because amniocentesis or other prenatal procedures are unlikely to exclude this, there is a strong indication for termination of pregnancy. Such an exposure is rare in peacetime and would probably be associated with severe maternal illness anyway if therapeutic irradiation were involved. No clear increase in the incidence of malformations or other genetic disorders in children conceived after exposure has been shown, despite much concern and publicity. Leukaemia and other malignancies involving somatic cells currently seem to be a greater short-term hazard, but the hidden load of recessive mutations will take many generations to show itself and may ultimately prove to be the more serious aspect. Neel (1993) provides interesting background information and more recent evaluation of this important study. Evidence from direct studies of DNA mutations is now beginning to be available and so far supports the older studies.

Similarly, there is no clear evidence to support any increase in malformations or genetic disorders in the offspring of military personnel exposed to nuclear test explosions, despite considerable publicity.

IRRADIATION AND THE POPULATION

The generally low risks to future offspring and to radiation-exposed individuals themselves have been emphasized. The population and long-term effects stand in contrast to this, but are difficult to consider because they are so spread out in both space and time. Even a slight increase in background radiation will be likely to cause a significant increase in both point mutations and chromosome disorders, although in the case of recessive mutations, the full effects will not be noticed for many generations. Thus the exposure of a population of 1 million to an increased level of radiation of 1 Gy per generation has been estimated as likely to result in an extra 2000 genetic disorders per million births in the first generation; the eventual total, including the effect on subsequent generations, would be considerably higher. Because these cases are indistinguishable from 'naturally' arising mutations, they tend to be overlooked; were such an occurrence to be concentrated in a single town it would be considered a disaster.

At present, most gonadal radiation received over the background level comes from medical diagnostic X-rays. Responsibility for this is shared by all physicians, who should help to reduce this load to the minimum necessary. In the author's view, the profession has an equal social duty to help to ensure that this load is not further increased by the avoidable exposure from other sources, notably nuclear weapons or accidents in the future. The widespread nuclear contamination resulting from the disaster at Chernobyl and a series of lesser accidents are examples of the potential danger of nuclear power, and have resulted in greatly increased awareness of the problems in the population as a whole. Whether action will be taken is a different matter.

FURTHER READING

Congenital infections

Berrebi A, Kobuch WE, Bessieres MH *et al.* (1994). Termination of pregnancy for maternal toxoplasmosis. *Lancet* **344**, 36–39.

Friedman JM, Polifka JE (1994). *Teratogenic Effects of Drugs. A Resource for Clinicians.* Baltimore, MD, Johns Hopkins University Press.

Greenough A, Osborne J, Sutherland S (eds) (1992). *Congenital Perinatal and Neonatal Infections.* Edinburgh, Churchill Livingstone.

Teratogens

Briggs GG, Freeman KK, Yaffe SJ (1990). *Drugs in Pregnancy and Lactation. A Reference Guide to Fetal and Neonatal Risk.* Baltimore, MD, Williams & Wilkins.

Sever JM, Brent RL (1986). *Teratogen Update: Environmentally Induced Birth Defects.* New York, Alan Liss.

Shephard TH (1995). *Catalog of Teratogenic Agents,* 8th edn. Baltimore, MD, Johns Hopkins University Press – an electronic database, TERIS, derived from this work is available.

Radiation

Doll R (1993). Epidemiological evidence of effects of small doses of ionising radiation with a note on the causation of clusters of childhood leukaemia. *J Radiol Prot* **13**, 233–241.

International Atomic Energy Authority (1991). *International Chernobyl Project. An Overview.* Vienna, United Nations.

Mole H (1979). Radiation effects on prenatal development and their radiological significance. *Br J Radiol* **52**, 89–101.

Neel JV (1993). *Physician to the Gene Pool.* New York, Wiley.

Searle A (1987). Radiation – the genetic risk. *Trends Genet* **3**, 152–157.

Smithells RW, Newman CGH (1992). Recognition of thalidomide defects. *J Med Genet* **29**, 716–723.

UNSCEAR report (1982). *Ionizing Radiation. Sources and Biological Effects. Annex 1: Genetic Effects of Radiation.* New York, United Nations.

PART III

Genetic counselling: the wider picture

Population aspects of genetic counselling

The primary aim of this book has been to provide information that will help particular families in which a genetic disorder exists or is at risk of occurring. Throughout the book, the family, at times nuclear, at times extended, has been the unit under consideration, and it is hoped that both the general discussions and the more specific information in the later chapters will have helped readers deal with most of the problems they are likely to meet, as well as alerting them to some of the pitfalls and unsolved problems that exist.

Most people, however, will not be fully satisfied dealing with these individual problems in isolation, but will wish to place them in the more general context of the disorder overall – and to know how far they can relate these individual instances of genetic counselling to the wider prevention of inherited disorders in the population they serve.

These wider population aspects have so far received very little emphasis in this book, in part because the author's view is that the primary duty of a physician is to individuals and their immediate families, and in part because the general aspects can usually only be approached through study of the specific conditions. However, it would be entirely wrong to suggest, as is sometimes done, that these wider aspects are not the concern of those involved with genetic disorders. In the author's opinion, to take such a view would be as short-sighted as it would have been for the 19th-century physician to insist that only the individual case of typhoid fever was his concern, not the broader epidemiology or prevention of the disease.

The increasing application of prenatal and other screening programmes has highlighted the differences in approach and potential for conflict between population-based and individual family approaches and has in some instances resulted in considerable disagreement. The debate has been helpful in clarifying both the issues and the thoughts of those involved. The author's principal conclusions are as follows:

- Genetic counselling is an activity whose goals and processes relate to individuals and families, and will thus inevitably and appropriately vary according to the nature, attitudes and wishes of different families, as well as the society in which they live.
- Success or failure in genetic counselling (extremely difficult to evaluate) must be gauged by the extent to which it has helped the problems of individual families, not

by any effect on the frequency of a genetic disorder or by a particular type of outcome (e.g. termination of affected pregnancies).

- Prevention or avoidance of a genetic disorder in an individual family is a valid goal provided that it is also the goal of the family. For most severe genetic disorders, this will commonly be the case, but with milder or more variable conditions it may well not be so in a variable proportion of families.
- Population prevention of serious genetic disorders is also a valid goal, provided that it does not conflict with the individual aims of families, and provided that it is clearly recognized as something separate from genetic counselling. The potential for conflict will depend partly on the nature of the disorder, but also on the degree to which those introducing any population-based programme are aware of and sensitive to the wishes and needs of individual families.

For those responsible for the delivery and development of genetic services to particular regions and populations, it is clearly important to know the extent to which a genetic counselling service is reaching the families that need it, and whether it is having beneficial effects. It is also important to be aware of changes in the overall frequency of the commoner disorders. Equally, though, it is essential to resist pressure to establish or extend programmes on 'economic' grounds, where the primary aims could be of a 'public health' or 'eugenic' nature in terms of reducing disease frequency. There may be a considerable temptation to use economic arguments when attempting to obtain funding for programmes, but the author's strong view is that any possible short-term benefit from such an approach would be greatly outweighed by longer-term loss of trust and respect for the field of medical genetics by families and professionals alike. Increasingly, medical geneticists are to be found arguing against population-based programmes that are inappropriate or not fully considered.

The wider population aspects considered in the rest of this chapter fall into two main groups:

- extensions of 'family-based' services to ensure equity of and full access to services – the wider aspects of genetic counselling
- population screening for genetic disorders.

WIDER ASPECTS OF GENETIC COUNSELLING

WHOM DOES GENETIC COUNSELLING REACH?

Anyone regularly involved in genetic counselling will be under no illusions that their advice is reaching all the individuals who wish for or need it. In general, one will be seeing a small segment of the community which is both sufficiently motivated and sufficiently articulate to ask for referral or to ask the type of question that makes their own doctor either answer them or arrange for referral. Inevitably, this means that the less privileged, generally with the greatest need, are less well served. Even in a system like the UK's National Health Service, where no direct payment is required, the same situation applies, and at present it seems likely that genetic counselling is still only dealing with the 'tip of the iceberg', even in those situations where it could have a profound effect on people's options and decisions.

Improved awareness of genetic problems among medical and paramedical staff in primary care and hospital-based specialities will undoubtedly help, and is the principal aim of this book. This alone, however, is unlikely to have more than a minor effect unless there is a comparable change in the awareness and motivation of the population as a whole. Genetic counselling given to those who do not wish it or who are unaware of the underlying problem is often an unrewarding procedure for professional and patient alike.

The author's view is that genetic counselling will only have its full impact when an awareness of its importance and availability is built into the general education of young people, especially around school-leaving age, and when the population is much more scientifically literate in general. At a time when small families are the rule, it seems essential for those having children to be given every opportunity to ensure that their children will be healthy and to avoid known risk factors if they so wish. At present, public awareness of the subject, largely the result of television, is often focused on problems and diagnostic techniques during pregnancy itself – quite the worst time for a rational appreciation of the situation. As a result, there is a real danger at present of increasing the general level of anxiety without any corresponding increase in the overall level of people's knowledge.

A shift of emphasis is already occurring to the preconceptual phase, with genetic counselling increasingly requested prior to reproduction. Should this continue, it will markedly increase the demand for genetic counselling both from primary clinicians and from the specialist genetics services. This is another reason why the author feels strongly that all interested clinicians should be involved in the process for families that they see, and that it should not be seen purely as an isolated specialist activity.

THE PRECONCEPTION CLINIC

A logical extension of the ideas expressed in the previous paragraph is the development of 'preconception clinics' where couples planning a pregnancy or school-leavers considering their future families could receive information on a wide range of subjects relating to the health and well-being of a future child. Genetic aspects could be included along with other factors such as diet (notably folic acid), avoidance of smoking and medications, and the need for rubella immunization; rather than formal genetic counselling being directly associated with such a venture, it should be reserved for the small minority where a clear problem is identified by the taking of a simple family history.

A well-organized and motivated family practice would make an excellent setting for a preconception clinic and could allow contact with the less educated and motivated parts of the population who, as already mentioned, are the least likely to request advice although the most in need. If our health services are indeed to be 'primary care led', this seems an important and appropriate field in which primary care can indeed take the lead. So far, there are few signs of this happening on a wide scale and this remains an unmet challenge for all those involved.

THE PREVENTION OF GENETIC DISEASE

Even with the most complete ascertainment and cooperation from the population, the prevention of inherited disorders has to rest on the basic facts of the genetic situation. Thus, in such dominantly inherited disorders as the familial cancers, where the proportion of cases due to new mutation is low, the prospect for prevention is ultimately good, certainly for preventing disease in those genetically at risk, and possibly also (but much less certainly) for reducing the numbers born with the harmful mutation. For many other more severe and early-onset conditions, such as those many congenital malformations where almost all cases are new mutations, or even in a more common disorder such as achondroplasia (where mutations account for 80 per cent of cases), genetic counselling and application of genetic tests will have little impact on the population incidence of the disorder, since most cases will arise 'out of the blue' into a family that is not known to be at risk.

In previous editions of this book, Huntington's disease was cited as an example of a dominant disorder with very few new mutations, where a genetic register and systematic genetic counselling might be expected to result in a marked long-term decline in disease prevalence. Recognition of the molecular basis has shown that, for this and other trinucleotide repeat disorders, such a suggestion is an over-simplification. The unstable nature of the mutation means that most apparent new mutations are arising from a pool of healthy individuals carrying 'intermediate alleles', which can expand and cause overt disease in later generations. This does not in any way invalidate the systematic approach to genetic counselling for such conditions, nor the value of genetic registers, but it reinforces the need for careful consideration of what the goals for such efforts should be.

The same lack of population effects will apply to most rare autosomal recessive disorders, since the overwhelming majority of the abnormal genes are in healthy heterozygotes, who will not be aware of this unless they marry someone carrying the same harmful gene and have an affected child. Only the small number of second or subsequent cases in a sibship are likely to be preventable unless population screening of heterozygotes is feasible and appropriate, as discussed below.

X-linked disorders seem at first sight to be a suitable area for prevention in the population, and certainly the testing of the extended family for carrier status is probably one of the most valuable parts of genetic counselling. Even here, however, new mutations may account for a considerable proportion of cases, and efforts at prevention have to be seen in perspective. However, the experience of centres that have maintained a genetic register of Duchenne muscular dystrophy patients and carriers has shown a progressive decrease in recurrent cases within a family, alongside an increase in healthy births to couples at risk, while new mutations are still as common as before.

For chromosome disorders, the benefits of the 'extended genetic counselling' approach are of great value where a translocation is identified that could be carried in balanced form by healthy relatives (see Chapter 4). Prevention of the great majority of serious chromosome disorders (including Down's syndrome) is only feasible through prenatal screening programmes (see below), implying the acceptance of termination of affected pregnancies.

PREVENTION OF DISEASE IN THOSE AT RISK

While the reduction of serious genetic disorders by prenatal diagnosis and termination of pregnancy can be a valid goal when treatment is absent or unsatisfactory, there are numerous situations where the application of genetic approaches may result in the avoidance of serious morbidity or death for those who are at risk or affected, as discussed in Chapter 10. A combination of systematic ascertainment, maintenance of a genetic register and the offer of genetic testing to those at risk is forming the basis of many preventive programmes. Examples that have already been discussed include the familial cancers, drug-induced disease (e.g. the porphyrias and malignant hyperpyrexia), and other chronic diseases such as adult polycystic kidney disease, where control of blood pressure and infection is facilitated by early detection. The most common disorder in this category, familial hypercholesterolaemia, has been relatively ignored until very recently (see Chapter 19), reflecting perhaps inadequate awareness of genetic approaches by the clinicians and epidemiologists involved.

Common, 'multifactorial' disorders such as diabetes, hypertension and certain cancers are often raised as examples where the widespread identification of those at increased genetic susceptibility might be of benefit through allowing subsequent prevention of disease (see also Chapter 3). 'Changes in lifestyle' and 'targeted drug therapy' are arguments given in favour of this, but it has to be said that, at present, the evidence of benefit is almost wholly lacking. 'Lifestyles', whether in relation to diet or other aspects, are often remarkably resistant to change unless this involves the entire population, while selective drug therapy based on genetic differences is equally speculative at present, however attractive to pharmaceutical manufacturers.

WILL GENETIC COUNSELLING INCREASE THE LOAD OF DELETERIOUS GENES?

The pessimist predicting harmful effects of genetic advances is likely to be as wrong as the optimist who hopes to 'wipe out genetic disease', if generalizations are made. We have already seen that genetic counselling may result in a reduction in frequency of serious disease in certain dominantly inherited disorders, but with other disorders there is little effect. Influences increasing gene frequency are likely to be equally diverse.

Successful treatment of previously fatal or disabling dominant disorders might certainly allow a rapid rise in frequency if accompanied by unrestrained reproduction, although it would be the treatment, rather than genetic counselling, that would tend to produce this. If treatment of a disorder really proves successful, then the problem will probably have disappeared anyway.

X-linked disorders where fetal sexing is employed without a direct prenatal diagnosis might probably have provided the major example where genetic measures could increase the population frequency. By allowing female carriers to have daughters (half of whom will themselves carry the gene) without the risk of having an affected son, it is likely that a steady (though at present undefined) increase would be seen. Direct prenatal diagnosis of affected males, increasingly feasible for most X-linked disorders, will reduce this trend because, by avoiding abortion of healthy male fetuses, fewer pregnancies would be needed to reach the desired family size.

A more important potential source of increase in deleterious genes might be expected to arise with the numerous polygenic malformations which in the past were generally fatal but for which treatment (usually surgical) now allows a near-normal lifespan and fertility. Congenital heart disease, pyloric stenosis, Hirschsprung's disease and hydrocephalus are but a few examples. Although the risks for offspring of such individuals are relatively low (usually under 5 per cent), there is no doubt that reproduction of such individuals will produce a slow but eventually appreciable rise in the overall level of genetic liability in the population. Again, genetic counselling is not likely to be a significant factor in any such change.

MARRIAGE BETWEEN AFFECTED INDIVIDUALS

Marriage between affected individuals is common in some groups of disorders, such as congenital deafness and blindness, and dwarfism. It may well be increasing as a result of the social activities of 'disease-specific' lay societies. The genetic risks for couples in particular situations have already been discussed, but worry is sometimes expressed as to the overall effects of such assortative matings on the population level of the particular harmful genes. In fact, such effects are negligible in the case of rare mendelian disorders and usually also for the more common polygenic disorders (e.g. diabetes). The general effect is a redistribution of affected children so that more are likely to be born to affected parents and fewer to unaffected parents. Thus, although genetic counselling is of great importance for these high-risk couples, their reproduction will have little overall effect on the population frequency of the disease or the genes.

INBREEDING AND OUTBREEDING

Many inbred populations are characterized by high levels of autosomal recessive disorders and, where this is the case, there is no doubt that outbreeding would greatly reduce the frequency of the disease. Thus, a marked increase in the proportion of marriages between Ashkenazi Jews and gentiles would sharply decrease the incidence of Tay–Sachs disease, especially common in the former. The gene frequency would not be decreased, but a greater proportion of the genes would be present in healthy heterozygotes.

Conversely, fragmentation and isolation of populations combined with inbreeding, as seen in some immigrant minority populations, are likely to increase the incidence of autosomal recessive disorders, even when the parent population does not have a particularly high frequency of deleterious genes. Again, it is not the gene frequency but the frequency of affected homozygotes that is increased. Prolonged inbreeding over many generations might in theory actually 'breed out' harmful recessive genes by progressively eliminating them as homozygotes. However, this is not a helpful course to recommend prospectively and there is no evidence that it has actually occurred in inbred populations. The precise effects on gene and phenotype frequencies are thoroughly analysed in a number of books on population genetics; the moral for the clinician is to be wary of generalizations, and to realize that in the great majority of situations the advice given to individual couples may have a profound effect on them and their offspring, but will rarely alter the population structure to a significant extent. The social aspects of consanguineous marriage have already been discussed in Chapter 9.

CULTURAL ASPECTS OF GENETIC COUNSELLING

Genetic counselling cannot be carried out in a vacuum, and the way it is practised inevitably reflects and interacts with the attitudes and structure of the society in which one works. In most Western countries, this society is now heterogeneous, containing a variety of ethnic, cultural and religious groups whose views on medicine, genetics and life in general may differ considerably. The author, trained in a 'Western' milieu like most medical geneticists, has become increasingly aware that the approaches to genetic counselling outlined in this book cannot always be applied easily to families coming from different societies.

A comparable recognition has led to the involvement of workers from specific minority groups, especially when population programmes are involved, as with the haemoglobin disorders. The issue of consanguinity, already discussed, is another major area of societal difference, while the importance of using a language familiar to those seeking advice is a further obvious, though often overlooked, point.

Some differences are difficult to reconcile with accepted concepts of genetic counselling, but need to be recognized and perhaps confronted. The attitude to women in many more traditional societies may result in stigma and even divorce if a particular genetic defect is found to come from the female partner, even if this is only implied or construed. One may have to be extremely careful in divulging information to a husband or male relative. Not infrequently, a woman may understand little English, and information filtered through the husband may be different from that given originally. In other communities (including much of the author's own south Wales population), men are traditionally peripheral to reproductive decisions, women frequently attending with their own mother, while the husband is left at work, or parking the car!

The traditional pattern of the extended family often runs contrary to the concept of privacy regarded as so important in modern Western society. In such a situation everyone in a family may want to know the result of someone's test, while requests for testing (including decisions on prenatal diagnosis) may be determined by older patriarchs or matriarchs, who may well not have been seen by those giving genetic counselling. Marriages may be arranged in childhood, leading to requests for testing on children that would otherwise have been postponed until adult life.

These are only a few of the complex issues about which anyone giving genetic counselling needs to be aware. However, awareness does not necessarily mean that genetic counselling should always try to fit in with the accepted practices of society. Thus in eastern Europe, genetic counselling was traditionally directive, and colleagues in these countries frequently assured the author that this was what people expected and wanted. I long suspected that this was largely a reflection of people being faced with authoritarian rules and attitudes in all fields of life, and it has been interesting to see that recent changes in these countries have been accompanied by a trend towards non-directive genetic counselling.

POPULATION SCREENING FOR GENETIC DISORDERS

The term 'screening' is one that is used widely but often misleadingly in relation to various aspects of medical genetics. It should be confined to those programmes that aim to identify genetic disorders or gene carriers by studying broad groups, either entire populations or large subgroups (e.g. pregnant older women and the mentally handicapped), rather than specific individuals or families. Thus genetic testing for Huntington's disease, or indeed most genetic testing, is not a screening activity.

Screening for genetic disorders may in principle be a clinical activity or involve any form of testing, not just those using genetic technologies. For this reason, the term genetic screening needs to be used cautiously and specifically, since DNA-based tests can also be used to screen for non-genetic disorders (e.g. viral infections), while most primary screening tests for genetic disorders do not use genetic technology.

Despite this, screening for genetic disorders does raise important issues over and above the more general ones common to all forms of screening. It is most important that these are not ignored when programmes are being planned and implemented, and there is a real danger of this happening since most of those involved with screening have an epidemiology and public health medicine background and are largely unfamiliar with genetic issues. Points of fundamental importance include the aim of the screening programme: is it primarily to eliminate a disorder or to help individual families and to allow choice? The impact on other family members must be taken into account, while the issues arising from detection of healthy carriers in a programme primarily designed to detect affected homozygotes must also be considered. Most important of all is that, in a screening programme, those tested will mostly have no personal experience of the particular disorder and will not usually have actively requested the test, while the numbers involved may preclude the provision of adequate information and personally delivered genetic counselling.

All these factors point to major differences between the ethos and practice of screening for genetic disorders and those of genetic counselling. They also help to explain why so many workers in clinical genetics are reluctant to see screening programmes introduced without very careful thought and planning.

Table 27.1 summarizes the main categories of screening programmes that have been introduced or considered in relation to genetic disorders. Although the three main categories of newborn, prenatal and adult screening cannot be separated completely, this provides a reasonable framework for discussing the main issues.

Table 27.1 Population screening for genetic disorders – current and proposed examples

Newborn	Phenylketonuria
	Sickle cell disease
	Cystic fibrosis
	Duchenne dystrophy (?)
Prenatal	Down's syndrome
	Neural tube defects
	Cystic fibrosis (?)
Adult (presymptomatic)	Familial cancers (?)
	Familial hypercholesterolaemia (?)
	Haemochromatosis (?)
Adult (carrier detection)	Haemoglobinopathies
	Tay–Sachs disease
	Cystic fibrosis (?)

(?) indicates situations where the case for screening is not proven or where serious reservations apply.

NEWBORN SCREENING

Newborn screening in the population is principally established for treatable genetic disorders such as phenylketonuria, along with less clearly genetic disorders such as congenital hypothyroidism, both of which amply fulfil the traditional criteria of severity if untreated, good response to early treatment, simple and satisfactory screening and confirmatory tests, and a relatively high frequency. A case can similarly be made for including screening for sickle cell disease in high-risk populations, in order to provide prompt recognition and treatment of clinical problems. The genetic aspects are not the most important ones in such screening programmes.

More recently, newborn screening has been suggested for genetic disorders that are not fully treatable but where recurrence in sibs could be avoided by early diagnosis in the first child. Duchenne muscular dystrophy is a notable example, currently under evaluation, while in cystic fibrosis a case can be made to some extent on grounds of therapy as well. It is clear that to justify screening for disorders on genetic grounds requires a detailed and prolonged analysis of the effects on families in addition to the criteria already mentioned.

PRENATAL SCREENING FOR GENETIC DISORDERS

There has been a succession of developments in screening for genetic disorders in pregnancy which have collectively had a major impact on the way in which pregnancy is managed and perceived. Whether these have been a success or not depends largely on what the appropriate aims and outcomes of such programmes have been considered to be. If the primary aim is to reduce the birth frequency of a serious disorder, then some have certainly been successful; if, on the other hand, the aim is to give maximum choice, information and support to women and their families, then the outcomes have been much more questionable, and in most cases the relevant issues have not been adequately examined.

Almost all prenatal screening programmes have assumed the termination of an affected pregnancy, with one notable exception – rhesus haemolytic disease detection and immunization – which stands alone as an example of successful true prevention of a genetic disorder by prenatal screening.

Down's syndrome – the commonest single cause of mental handicap – has been the focus of prenatal screening for many years (see Chapters 4 and 8). Initially based on increased maternal age and amniocentesis, and now utilizing maternal serum for the main preliminary screening test, this has certainly reduced the birth frequency of Down's syndrome in many populations. There have been some concerns about inequity of availability and information to women concerning this service, but equally there have been concerns in relation to quality of information, pressure to be tested, proper consent and choice, and subsequent support. These latter issues were inadequately considered in the setting up of most programmes and are only now receiving proper evaluation, reflecting the fact that the primary aims have not so much been orientated to the choice and benefit of individual women as to the 'public health' goal of reducing the birth frequency of Down's syndrome in the population.

Exactly the same concerns apply to screening for neural tube defects using serum alpha-fetoprotein (see Chapter 8) and to the more general screening for structural malformations using ultrasound. The lack of prior information and experience concerning a disorder can cause particular difficulties when coming at such a sensitive time as pregnancy.

So far, most prenatal screening approaches have not used genetic technology, but this could change in future (e.g. maternal blood screening for fetal cells with trisomy 21). Suggestions that cystic fibrosis and fragile-X syndrome might be screened for prenatally have not given sufficient weight to the incidental detection of carriers or to other family aspects. It is probably fair to say that the entire development of prenatal genetic screening has been unbalanced, based almost exclusively on the aim of eradicating particular disorders and giving inadequate consideration to the wishes and potential effects of the programme on individuals. It is important that this field is radically and critically reassessed from a wider perspective.

GENETIC SCREENING IN ADULTS

Population screening in later life for genetic disorders is infrequent at present. Indeed, the potential for identifying a common and serious genetic disorder, familial hypercholesterolaemia, has been largely ignored in cholesterol screening, one of the most common and controversial adult screening tests. This is a pity, since it could be argued that the high frequency and treatable nature of familial hypercholesterolaemia make it perhaps the only subgroup of disorders with raised cholesterol levels that everyone would agree is worth detecting.

Detection of the genetic subset of common cancers is an area under considerable discussion in relation to screening, although at present this is entirely confined to family-based testing for the high-risk mutations. The term 'screening' is especially open to confusion here since those at high genetic risk may be offered screening for overt disease (e.g. mammography, ovarian ultrasound) while non-genetic screening may be the first line in general population detection (e.g. cervical cancer screening). At present, it seems unlikely that detection of heritable mutations giving a high cancer risk will be used as a screening tool, although it has been proposed where a single specific mutation occurs at high frequency (e.g. for BRCA1 in Ashkenazi Jewish people).

A disorder for which screening was recently suggested is haemochromatosis, where recognition of a genotype giving increased susceptibility is now feasible (see Chapter 20). This provides an excellent example of the potential pitfalls and lack of clear thinking that abound in the screening field. In contrast to the testing of high-risk sibs, the great majority of individuals detected would not be likely to develop disease and would not require treatment, while even larger numbers of heterozygotes would be detected where issues would arise as to what (if anything) they should be told.

This example shows how screening for an apparently definite mendelian disorder can merge into the more general area of susceptibility testing (Chapter 3), where at present even family-based testing is rarely helpful and wider screening is most likely to be positively harmful.

Screening of particular subgroups, rather than of entire populations, may be appropriate for certain genetic disorders. A case can be made for this in screening the mentally handicapped for fragile-X syndrome, allowing a high genetic risk situation to be recognized which may give options for families avoiding recurrence of the disorder. Clear information and proper consent, with access to fuller genetic counselling, are essential factors that must be built into any such programmes (and properly resourced), which should be carefully distinguished from more general population and prenatal screening.

CARRIER SCREENING FOR AUTOSOMAL RECESSIVE DISORDERS

Most of our experience with carrier screening has come from work on the haemoglobin disorders, in particular beta-thalassaemia, which represents a serious and extremely common problem in many Mediterranean and Asian countries. It is notable that carrier screening only became widely accepted once the option of prenatal diagnosis was available, in particular first-trimester DNA diagnosis. The remarkable degree of acceptance of carrier screening with prenatal diagnosis in widely different countries, many with a traditional society not previously accepting termination, is an indication of how screening programmes can be successful, provided that they are carried out in sympathy with the attitudes of ordinary people. Such programmes must be accompanied by education and full information and must have a tangible result to offer – in this case the possibility of having healthy children without the risk of a severely disabling disease.

A comparably successful programme has been the introduction of carrier screening for Tay–Sachs disease in people of Ashkenazi Jewish origin. By contrast, sickle-cell carrier screening was not successful in early programmes, partly because of the more variable nature of the disorder, partly because of the defects in the necessary educational and information aspects of the programmes.

The identification of the gene for cystic fibrosis, the most common autosomal recessive disorder in northern Europe, has given the possibility of DNA-based screening for the carrier state. Over 90 per cent of mutations can be identified in countries such as Britain, while the use of PCR-based assays employing DNA from a mouthwash can even remove the need for blood sampling. A series of pilot projects has been carried out in Britain and the USA to assess the feasibility and desirability of screening. Aspects studied include the timing and location of carrier screening (antenatal clinic and primary care settings); the psychological effects on those screened; the attitudes of professionals and families; and the costs of testing and counselling.

The results of these pilot programmes have been interesting and not entirely expected. Essentially they show a high degree of compliance with a thorough and sensitively handled screening programme, but only a low uptake when the initiative is left to individuals or when they are given a time interval to make a decision. The launch of 'over the counter' carrier testing for cystic fibrosis carrier status, introduced in the UK to meet the supposed 'unmet demand' for this, has likewise had minimal uptake. Thus the conclusion must be that such carrier testing is a low priority for most people and has not made a strong case for carrier screening outside families at risk, whether during pregnancy or before, becoming an established part of health services.

Cascade screening is worth noting in relation to cystic fibrosis carrier screening and other autosomal recessive disorders. Essentially, this is extended family testing, radiating outwards from an affected individual. It has the advantage that a much higher proportion of individuals tested will be carriers and also that many of them will be aware of the disorder because of its occurrence in the family.

CONCLUSION

When genetic counselling is dealing with the individual family, it is often capable of being precise and helpful, and of profoundly affecting the decisions of individual couples. This is rarely true at the population level, and here the clinician should be sceptical about whether genetic counselling is having any significant effect, either beneficial or adverse, save in a few specific situations. This is perhaps fortunate, for it means that there is rarely any ethical conflict for either physician or patient between the course that is most beneficial for an individual or a family and that which is beneficial for society as a whole.

Finally, it should be borne in mind that variation is the basis of life and of human evolution, and that genetic characteristics today considered harmful may not always remain so. The 'thrifty genotype' of the diabetic patient may once have been associated with advantageous factors and may yet be again in a world with shrinking food resources. The phenylketonuric genotype, recently genetically lethal, is now almost of neutral effect, at least for males, and the advent of successful treatment will undoubtedly ameliorate many other genetic diseases.

FURTHER READING

Bekker H, Modell M, Denniss G *et al.* (1993). Carrier screening for cystic fibrosis in primary care: supply push or demand pull? *Br Med J* **306**, 1584–1586.

Clarke A (1997). Newborn screening. In: Harper PS, Clarke A, eds. *Genetics, Society and Clinical Practice*. Oxford, Bios, pp. 107–118.

Clarke A, Parsons E (eds) (1997). *Culture, Kinship and Genes. Towards Cross-Cultural Genetics*. Basingstoke, St Martin's Press.

Darr A (1999). *Access to Genetic Services by Minority Ethnic Populations*. London, Genetic Interest Group.

Middleton A, Hewison J, Mueller RF (1998). Attitudes of deaf adults towards genetic testing for hereditary deafness. *Am J Hum Genet* **63**, 1175–1180.

Mitchell J, Cupua A, Clow C, Scriver CR (1996). Twenty-year outcome analysis of genetic screening programs for Tay-Sachs and beta-thalassaemia disease carriers in high schools. *Am J Hum Genet* **59**, 793–798.

Modell B, Darr A (2002). Genetic counselling and customary consanguineous marriage. *Nat Rev Genet* **3**, 225–229.

Nuffield Council on Bioethics (1993). *Genetic Screening – Ethical Issues*. London, Nuffield Council.

Super M, Schwarz MJ, Malone G *et al.* (1994). Active cascade screening for carriers of the cystic fibrosis gene. *Br Med J* **308**, 1462–1468.

Genetics and society

The previous chapter examined some of the ways by which new genetic advances can be delivered more generally to the population, rather than just to those who are already aware of their own need. It also addressed the advances that may occur in genetic screening and some of the problems. In this final chapter, the broader issues involving society itself are considered.

These new advances are having powerful effects on our social attitudes, widely disseminated through media publicity and often resulting in concern and controversy. This process is also affecting how genetics as a whole, including medical genetics, is perceived by the general population, a perception that is often ambivalent, even at times antagonistic, and which will have powerful effects on whether and how people use medical genetics services.

It may be argued that these wider issues are not directly relevant to genetic counselling, but this is not the case. The services we try to offer, at both individual family and population levels, are strongly influenced by the societal background and attitudes of the community involved, and need to be adapted to those particular factors. One need look no further than such topics as prenatal diagnosis and consanguineous marriage to see how this has affected the development of genetic services in different populations. Many of these issues have already been raised in the specific chapters of this book, but it is useful to bring them together here. No attempt is made to cover general ethical and philosophical topics, but rather those that impinge directly on clinical genetic practice, whether carried out by a specialist or by other clinicians in their particular field.

GENETIC TESTING ISSUES

Although genetic testing has been in practice for many years in the form of chromosome and protein analyses, the large-scale development of DNA-based testing and its progressive use outside specialist centres have created important issues that are largely new in practice, if not in concept. Some of these are raised here to promote further thinking and debate.

WHAT DO WE MEAN BY GENETIC TESTING?

The author has offered the following working definition:

> Genetic testing is the analysis of a specific gene, its product or function, or other DNA and chromosome analysis, to detect or exclude an alteration likely to be associated with a genetic disorder.

Although most genetic testing is DNA-based, it is the aim of the test, rather than the technology, that is important. Thus phenotypic tests such as ultrasound or electrophysiology can be regarded in principle as genetic tests when used to detect asymptomatic gene carriers (see Chapter 7), while DNA-based tests used for diagnosing infectious diseases are clearly not. Despite this lack of absolute distinction, though, it is principally the analysis of specific genes, especially in healthy individuals, that we are concerned with.

PRESYMPTOMATIC TESTING FOR LATE-ONSET DISORDERS

This important topic has been largely covered in Chapter 5, but here the broader societal impact needs consideration. Experience from Huntington's disease and familial cancers has shown the need for the cautious handling of such testing, with proper consent, information and support. The perception of those tested and found to have an abnormal result that they consider themselves already 'affected' is often mirrored by professionals and society in general, and may powerfully affect society's attitude towards those carrying genes for serious late-onset disorders.

As such presymptomatic testing becomes more widespread, there is likely to develop a population of asymptomatic gene carriers destined to develop serious genetic disorders. The situation is not unlike that for HIV carriers, and the potential for stigmatization and discrimination is comparable, whether this be for employment, insurance or general relationships. One could argue that the way in which a society treats such individuals is an indicator of its maturity and humanity; experience with HIV carriers leads me to be far from optimistic in this respect.

GENETIC TESTING OF CHILDREN

The age independence of DNA testing makes it possible to test for a disorder at any age, regardless of the usual time of onset. To test young children for a late-onset disorder that is not likely to have effects until adult life, and which is untreatable, poses serious problems. The author first encountered this in relation to Huntington's disease and was surprised to receive requests to test children from parents and social workers. Testing was refused on the grounds that it would not benefit the child and would remove any later choice, and subsequently guidelines from both the UK and USA have supported the view that testing for late-onset disorders should normally be postponed until the individual can give full consent. Clearly the situation may vary according to whether treatment exists or if the condition may also have childhood onset; individual circumstances need careful consideration, but the general principle remains valid.

Different issues arise when adolescents themselves request genetic testing (although the two situations are often confused). Again, general guidelines suggest postponement of testing until an individual becomes an adult, but the topic will need full discussion with the individual, and the maturity of the adolescent will be an important factor – often a request for testing is a mask for a more general need for information and support, making it all the more important that sensitive discussion precedes any decision on actual testing.

Most paediatricians, and other clinicians, have given little thought to this important topic until recently but, in the UK at least, there has been a marked shift in views towards those outlined above, already held by most clinical geneticists.

USE OF RESEARCH SAMPLES

Most research on genetic disorders requires samples from patients and many workers have large series of stored DNA samples from both affected and at-risk family members. When the gene is discovered for the particular disease, what should one do – or not do – with these samples? Using the samples from affected individuals does not pose serious problems, but to test samples from those at risk carries grave consequences, since it is likely that some will show the mutation. The research worker is then in the serious situation of having important information on people without their knowledge, often not knowing whether they would have wished to be tested or what they originally gave consent for. Such samples should not have been used in the first place; if the person requests testing, it is better to take a separate sample specifically for this. Comparable issues can arise when genetic tests are incorporated into a more general research study, identifying individuals with a genetic basis among a larger group (e.g. studies of cancer).

INSURANCE AND GENETIC TESTING

The past decade has seen a continuing battle between the insurance industry, unwilling to accept any regulation and insisting that genetic tests on healthy individuals are 'no different from other medical information', and professionals in genetics, supported by a series of independent government reports in several countries, who have pointed out the dangers of individuals being forced to disclose information on genetic tests that they have had for entirely different purposes. Detailed actuarial studies have now confirmed the author's view that, at least for life insurance, the industry would suffer little from not demanding such results except for very large sums. The continuing obstructive attitude of the insurance industry is now likely to be overtaken by legislation in both Europe and the USA, which will restrict the use of genetic test results and quite possibly the use of more general genetic information such as family history data. Fortunately, a 5-year moratorium has now been agreed in the UK, while the field is analysed objectively. The adverse publicity that this issue generated for the insurance industry is an indication of how society is becoming reluctant to see new advances used to harm, rather than to benefit, its members.

'OVER THE COUNTER' GENETIC TESTING

The concept of having a test without any medical or professional information or involvement has raised widespread concern, but would probably not have been considered a serious possibility until it was introduced in 1994 without warning for cystic fibrosis carrier testing by a UK commercial company. Since then, a government report has advised strict limits for such testing, but interestingly, the demand for it has proved minimal and the prospect of widespread 'over the counter' testing in relation to serious genetic disorders has receded. More recently, attempts have been made to market tests for genetic variants claimed to be of significance to diet. Although evidence of benefit is non-existent, there will probably always be those gullible enough to believe the claims. DNA testing for paternity, which carries no direct medical implications, will probably continue to be the most useful test delivered in this way, although the very real issues of consent and interpretation make a full framework of information important.

REGULATION OF GENETIC TESTING

Few existing laws were drafted with new developments in genetics in mind, so the rapid spread of genetic testing has led to fears that the total lack of regulation could result in abuse, or at least inappropriate applications and poor standards. After a long lag period, this situation has been rectified. The UK now has a well established regulatory committee, the Human Genetics Commission, which deals with broad social and ethical issues in genetics and has already produced statements and reports on genetic testing and insurance, genetic privacy, 'over the counter' testing and genetic testing for late-onset disorders. It is a broad-based body with only a minority of expert professionals.

In the USA, despite a series of professional and government reports, there is little sign of effective regulation, but in various continental European countries valuable reports and, in some cases, specific laws have been produced.

AIMS AND OUTCOME MEASURES IN GENETIC COUNSELLING

Any professional activity, especially if it is being supported by public funding, needs to be able to produce clear goals as to what it is trying to achieve and objective evidence that it is being successful in meeting those goals. In relation to genetic counselling, the whole area of aims and outcome measures is extremely complex and it is as well to recognize that there are no simple answers. It is somewhat easier to indicate which aims and outcome measures are inappropriate, especially since some of these have already been, and continue to be, used.

Thus the reduction or elimination of genetic disorders is not (at least in the view of the author and most professionals in the field) an aim of genetic counselling, even though it could, under some circumstances, be a valid aim of a broader population programme. Correspondingly, outcome measures such as number of pregnancies terminated or estimated financial savings from abnormal births avoided are not appropriate for genetic counselling.

Recent reports (see 'Further reading') have tried to take initial steps in providing satisfactory alternatives. Such areas as understanding of information given, reproductive plans and behaviour, client satisfaction and quality of process are all relevant, although all also have drawbacks. Perhaps the most important point is that much thought is now going into the difficult process of defining satisfactory aims and outcomes.

PRIVACY AND CONFIDENTIALITY

Genetic counselling raises some extremely difficult issues in this important area, something that is inevitable since the process so often depends on having accurate information on family members and since its implications may extend far beyond those individuals seeking advice.

It should be stressed that, in practice, most difficulties can be resolved provided that time and trouble are taken to ask people's permission, to explain why information is being requested and, in the case of risks to the extended family, to ascertain as far as possible whether they wish for information to be given.

Given such a careful and sensitive approach, most family members will prove helpful and reasonable, although the process may take a considerable time. The temptation to 'cut corners' and assume consent when it has not been specifically given must be strongly resisted. Written permission is increasingly the rule, and is a valuable safeguard if problems arise at a later stage.

In the very few situations where relatives still refuse to give access to their records or test results after appropriate approaches have been made, this usually reflects family conflict or sometimes fear and denial of a genetic disorder. It has been suggested that the need of relatives may in some circumstances override the basic principles of confidentiality, but the author's view is that such situations are exceptional and must be based on clear evidence of the harm that would result if the information were not available. Against such abandonment of confidentiality must be set the effects of a general loss of trust if individuals were to feel that their personal genetic data could be divulged in situations other than dire need.

Much more common, in the author's experience, are requests for information from third parties which can and should be firmly denied unless specific permission is given. These include requests from insurers, employers, social services, adoption agencies and various other bodies. There is no case for 'public health interest' disclosure of information as may be present for infectious diseases.

At a practical level, difficulty may arise when one is seeing several members of a family separately and is unaware of what information they have shared. It is best to assume that nothing has been shared and to keep information compartmentalized unless one has clear permission to the contrary. Sometimes it can be preferable for a colleague to see the other part of the family if it becomes too complicated to keep things separate.

General issues of privacy, confidentiality and consent have become of increasing concern in medicine overall and the consequences of ignoring this have been shown in a series of high-profile cases involving pathology (see Chapter 10). Legislation is increasingly being introduced, but in the practical situations involving genetic counselling one is currently rarely in serious difficulty if one follows the broad lines indicated above.

EUGENICS AND THE ABUSE OF GENETICS

Everyone working in medicine, whether clinician or scientist, likes to believe that their own field is making a special contribution to human health and well-being. Those of us in medical genetics are no exception, and indeed the advances of recent years have helped families in ways that were unthought of only a generation ago. There is a darker side, though, which needs to be recognized, not ignored. This relates to what is generally known as eugenics, in which the principles of genetics (as understood in the past) were applied to changing the genetic make-up of the population in general, rather than to individual families.

Eugenics had its origins in 19th-century Britain, but later became widespread in other European countries and in the USA. It was closely bound up with the social systems of the time, notably the rigidities of class and the deprivation of much of the population. It was convenient to find a biological explanation in terms of genetic inferiority for these deep-seated problems, with solutions that justified the maintenance of the social status quo. The newly emerging patterns of quantitative and mendelian inheritance were enthusiastically applied to a whole series of diseases and characteristics that today would be regarded as heterogeneous and complex in their basis, such as mental impairment, epilepsy and criminality.

These and other studies, enthusiastic but largely uncritical in nature, provided the scientific justification for a series of coercive measures, including the segregation, institutionalization and (particularly in the USA) sterilization of mentally impaired people and other groups. Restrictive legislation on proposed immigrants was another aspect in the USA and Australia. While politicians were responsible for the implementation of these measures, they were enthusiastically supported by scientists (notably Charles Davenport, director of the Cold Spring Harbor Laboratory).

The lowest point in the history of eugenics was reached in Nazi Germany in 1933, where a national eugenics law was one of the first measures introduced, and where compulsory sterilization of those with mental illness or impairment, along with people suffering from disorders such as Huntington's disease, was followed by active killing of such individuals, together with those with congenital malformations. Again it is tempting to regard this terrible chapter in history as an aberration and to blame the politicians, but this would be wrong. The entire basis for these policies was provided by scientists, including some of the most eminent geneticists of the time, and by clinicians, notably psychiatrists. It should not be forgotten that Josef Mengele was himself a human geneticist.

Eugenics is now a largely discredited field, but it has recently, to the great concern of many people, re-emerged in China, where a frankly eugenic law has been introduced under the guise of 'maternal and child health'. If serious abuses of new genetic developments are not to occur again, everyone – especially those working in medical genetics – must be aware of the past and its potential threat to the future. The increase in the power of technology, especially in computing and molecular genetics, makes it especially necessary to ensure that safeguards are introduced as these techniques are applied.

CONCLUSION

The range and depth of the many societal issues arising in genetic counselling, including those outlined above, may seem daunting for the professionals involved and it is easy to feel at times that one's own concepts of 'good practice' are likely to be submerged beneath an avalanche of inappropriate or even harmful developments. My own view, however, is a more optimistic one; it is remarkable to see how issues recognized and views held by a very small number of practising clinical geneticists have gradually permeated not only the medical genetics community, but also the work of clinicians and laboratory colleagues more generally, until they have eventually become standard good practice.

Working in the field of medical genetics, and being involved in genetic counselling in one's own particular area, offers remarkable opportunities for being in the forefront of, and helping to shape, new patterns of medical practice. It provides challenges, too, in trying to ensure that one's own practice can set an example to others, and in one's efforts to educate colleagues more generally to adopt comparable standards. Medical genetics in general, and genetic counselling in particular, is now an activity which extends far beyond the boundaries of medical genetics as a speciality, and how families are best helped is increasingly dependent on those whose main background and training lie outside this field. This book has been written in the hope that such workers can recognize the facts, problems and issues that arise in relation to genetic disorders, and can use them wisely and sensitively in genetic counselling to help the families with whom they are involved.

FURTHER READING

Adams MB (1990). *The Wellborn Science*. Oxford, Oxford University Press.

Advisory Committee on Genetic Testing (1997). *Code of Practice and Guidance on Human Genetic Testing Services Supplied Direct to the Public*. London, UK Health Departments (see Appendix for internet address).

Advisory Committee on Genetic Testing (1998). *Genetic Testing for Late-onset Disorders*. London, UK Health Departments.

American Society of Human Genetics Social Issues Subcommittee on Familial Disclosure (1998). ASHG statement. Professional disclosure of familial genetic information. *Am J Hum Genet* **62**, 474–483.

Anderson RM (ed.) (1997). Human genetics – uncertainties and the financial implications ahead. *Phil Trans R Soc B* **352**, 1035–1114 – a valuable symposium report on genetic testing and insurance.

Harper PS, Clarke AJ (1997). *Genetics, Society and Clinical Practice*. Oxford, Bios – topics covered include genetic testing of children, insurance, genetic privacy, ethical aspects of genetic screening, China's 'eugenics' law and the abuse of genetics in Nazi Germany.

Holtzman NA, Watson MS (1997). *Promoting Safe and Effective Genetic Testing in the United States*. Washington, DC, NIH.

Human Fertilisation and Embryology Authority (2003). *Sex Selection: Options for Regulation. Human Fertilisation: Options for Regulation*. London, Human Fertilisation and Embryology Authority.

Human Genetics Commission (2002). *Inside Information. Balancing Interests in the Use of Personal Genetic Data*. London, Department of Health.

Human Genetics Commission (2003). *Genes Direct. Ensuring the Effective Oversight of Genetic Tests Delivered Direct to the Public*. London, Department of Health.

Kevles DJ (1986). *In the Name of Eugenics*. New York, Knopf.

Mao X (1994). China's misconception of eugenics. *Nature* **367**, 1–2.

Marteau T, Richards M (eds) (1996). *The Troubled Helix: Social and Psychological Implications of the New Genetics*. Cambridge, Cambridge University Press.

Müller-Hill B (1998). *Murderous Science*. New York, Cold Spring Harbor Laboratory Press – a re-issue of the English translation of this important and disturbing book; even more relevant now than when first published (and should be compulsory reading for all those involved in medical genetics).

Nuffield Council on Bioethics (1993). *Genetic Screening – Ethical Issues*. London, Nuffield Council on Bioethics.

Working Party of the Clinical Genetics Society (1994). Report on the genetic testing of children. *J Med Genet* **31**, 785–797.

Useful information in connection with genetic counselling

Various items of information which it is hoped will be of practical use are listed below. Since this type of information is particularly liable to change, any amended or supplementary details will be welcomed for inclusion in future editions of this book. The internet now provides a wealth of information (see also Chapter 10) available directly to patients and families but also often very useful for professionals.

REGIONAL GENETIC CENTRES

All parts of the UK now have specialist genetic counselling centres, usually working in close association with genetics laboratories. These are not listed here, partly to save space, but also because any interested clinician should find out personally the best channels of referral. Most regional services provide a network of genetics clinics outside teaching hospitals, reducing the need for families to travel, while still giving access to centralized laboratory services. Most other European countries, Australia and Canada have a comparable service network.

In the USA, the number of centres involved in genetic counselling is much greater and many do not have a clearly defined and secure service basis.

LAY SOCIETIES INVOLVED WITH INHERITED DISORDERS

Few genetic disorders now seem to be without their own society, and these organizations often produce helpful information for patients and their families (and their doctors), which is increasingly web-based and which may be extremely useful in conjunction with genetic counselling. Many families find the support given by such lay groups valuable, while raising money for research and pressing for adequate services are also valuable functions. On the other hand, it has to be remembered that many families do not wish to be associated with lay groups, and it is important that clinicians involved in providing genetic counselling do not become so closely identified with such groups that they fail to provide an equal service to those families not involved with them.

The number of such societies is now too large to list comprehensively, and addresses change frequently. Fortunately, in both the UK and USA, 'umbrella' groups have been formed to coordinate the activities of the different societies, and in particular to lobby governments and other bodies for improved services, a role that is effectively performed by these groups and which is much more appropriately undertaken by them than by doctors or scientists. The addresses are given below.

Genetic Interest Group (GIG) (UK)

Unit 4d, Leroy House, 436 Essex Road, London N1 3QP, UK. Tel: 020 7704 3141; fax: 020 7359 1447; e-mail: post@gig.org.uk; website: *www.gig.org.uk*

Genetic Alliance (formerly Alliance of Genetic Support Groups) (USA)

4301 Connecticut Ave. NW, Suite 404, Washington, DC 20008-2369, USA. Tel: (202) 966-5557; fax: (202) 966-8553; e-mail: info@geneticalliance.org; website: *www.geneticalliance.org*

European Alliance of Genetic Support Groups (EAGS)

Current address and e-mail is via GIG (see above).

Contact a Family (UK)

209–211 City Road, London, EC1V 1JN, UK. Tel: 020 7608 8700/020 7608 8701; e-mail: info@cafamily.org.uk; website: *www.cafamily.org.uk*

This is a UK-based charity for families with disabled children, providing them with support and advice whatever the medical condition of their child.

CLIMB (Children Living with Inherited Metabolic Diseases)

Climb Building, 176 Nantwich Road, Crewe, CW2 6BG, UK. Tel: 0800 652 3181; fax: 0870 7700 327; e-mail: steve@climb.org.uk; website: *www.climb.org.uk*

Climb provides advice, information and support on all metabolic diseases to children, young adults, families, carers and professionals.

ADOPTION

Specialist agencies that may be helpful in case of difficulty, both for the potential adoptive parent and for the child for adoption with a disability, are listed below.

British Agencies for Adoption and Fostering (BAAF)

Skyline House, 200 Union Street, London, SE1 0LX, UK. Tel: 020 7593 2000; fax: 020 7593 2001; e-mail: mail@baaf.org.uk; website: *www.baaf.org.uk*

Adoption UK (PPIAS)

Manor Farm, Appletree Road, Chipping Warden, Banbury, OX17 1LH, UK. Tel: 01295 6601221; fax: 01295 660123; e-mail: helpdesk@adoptionuk.org.uk; website: *www.adoptionuk.org.uk*

Little People of America (USA)

Little People of America, Inc., 5289 NE Elam young Parkway, Suite F-700, Hillsboro, OR 97124, USA. Tel: (503) 846-1562; fax: (503) 846-1590; e-mail: info@lpaonline.org; website: *www.lpaonline.org*

Restricted Growth Association (UK) (formerly Association for Research into Restricted Growth)

PO Box 4744, Dorchester, DT2 9FA, UK. Tel: 01308 898445; e-mail: rga1@talk21.com; website: *www.rgaonline.org.uk*

Both Little People of America and the Restricted Growth Association offer information and help for people with dwarfing conditions wishing to adopt a child with a similar problem.

INTERNET ADDRESSES

The list given below is a sample of useful sources of information. It is increasing very rapidly and it is often not apparent from the title how much clinically useful information the site contains. Frequently one will encounter cross-links to other addresses which may prove more useful than the original site. The best course is to try out the different websites and this list may be a useful starting point.

An increasing number of genetics journals are also available on the internet, while official reports are often now available in this way. As well as specific disease organizations, many medical genetics units have their own website, giving a useful picture of services and research interests, e.g. the Institute of Medical Genetics, Cardiff (*http://www.uwcm.ac.uk/medical_genetics/*).

American Journal of Human Genetics
http://www.journals.uchicago.edu/AJHG/

American Society of Gene Therapy
http://www.asgt.org

American Society of Human Genetics
http://www.faseb.org/genetics/ashg/

British Society for Human Genetics
http://www.bshg.org.uk

Directory of National Genetic Voluntary Organizations (in the USA)
http://www.geneticalliance.org/diseaseinfo/search.html

European Directory of DNA Diagnostic Laboratories
http://www.eddnal.com

European Society of Human Genetics
http://www.eshg.org

Geneclinics
http://www.geneclinics.org

GeneTests (International directory of genetic laboratories)
http://www.genetests.org

Hereditary Hearing Loss homepage
http://www.uia.ac.be/dnalab/hhh

Human Gene Mutation Database
http://www.hgmd.org/

Human Genome Organisation
http://www.gene.ucl.ac.uk/hugo/

National Society of Genetic Counselors, Inc (in the USA)
http://www.nsgc.org

NORD (National Organization for Rare Disorders)
http://www.rarediseases.org

On-line Mendelian Inheritance in Man (OMIM)
http://www3.ncbi.nlm.nih.gov/omim/

Research Program on Ethical, Legal and Social Implications of Human Genome Project
http://www.genome.gov/10001618

UK Department of Health genetics information and documents
http://www.doh.gov.uk/genetics

The following list covers only those genetic terms used in this book that may be unfamiliar. A fuller list can be found in King RC, Stansfield WD (1996). *A Dictionary of Genetics*. Oxford, Oxford University Press.

allele	One of several alternative forms of a gene sequence at a given locus
amniocentesis	The procedure of taking a sample of amniotic fluid from the pregnant uterus
aneuploidy	The occurrence of an additional or missing chromosome to give an unbalanced chromosome complement
anticipation	The occurrence of a genetic disorder at earlier age of onset and/or at greater severity in successive generations
autosomal	Determined by a gene on one of the chromosomes other than the sex chromosomes
Barr body	The sex chromatin body visible beneath the nuclear membrane of a cell from a female, representing the inactive X chromosome
candidate gene	A gene suspected as being the gene mutated in a given disorder
cDNA (complementary DNA)	A DNA sequence corresponding to the messenger RNA produced by a gene, and lacking the non-coding regions (introns) of the gene
C. elegans	A simple nematode worm, used as a model organism, whose genome has been completely sequenced
centromere	The portion of the chromosome joining the two chromatids and separating the long and short arms of the chromosome
chimaera	An individual containing cells of more than a single genetic origin
chorion biopsy (chorionic villus sampling)	The sampling of tissue from the chorionic membrane of the embryo
chromatid	A single DNA strand of a dividing chromosome, joined to its 'sister chromatid' at the centromere
chromatin	The proteins and other materials composing the structure of the chromosomes in conjunction with the DNA itself
chromosome	A structure within the nucleus (normally 46 in humans), consisting of a long molecule of double-stranded DNA, bearing a linear arrangement of genes, which is associated with nucleoproteins and RNA; it condenses to become visible under the microscope at cell division and it is able to reproduce its molecular structure with great fidelity through successive cell divisions and in transmission from generation to generation
clone	An identical copy of a DNA sequence, cell or whole organism; 'to clone' also means to isolate a specific DNA sequence or gene

congenital	Present from birth
consanguinity	Marriage between close relatives
consultand	The individual (not always affected) through whom a family with a genetic disorder comes to clinical attention
cytogenetics	The study of chromosomes, their structure, function and abnormalities
deletion	Loss of genetic material (may be applied to a chromosome or a gene)
disomy, uniparental	The transmission of both copies of a chromosome from a single parent, instead of one from each parent
dizygotic twins	Twins originating from two fertilized eggs
DNA	Deoxyribonucleic acid, the molecule whose sequence and replication determine the genetic information present in genes and chromosomes
dominant	A characteristic or disorder expressed in the heterozygote, i.e. requiring only one altered copy to show itself
Drosophila	A fruit fly, a classical experimental organism for genetic studies, whose genome has been completely sequenced
duplication (as applied to a gene or portion of chromosome)	Presence of an additional copy of part of a chromosome or of a gene
dysmorphology	The study of malformation syndromes
empiric risks	Risk estimates based on those actually observed, rather than on general principles
eugenics	The use of genetic measures to attempt to alter and improve the genetic nature of a whole population
exon	The segments of a gene whose sequence is expressed by formation of messenger RNA and (usually) protein
FISH	Fluorescence in-situ hybridization of DNA, allowing microscopic detection of abnormalities
gamete	Egg or sperm
gene	The unit of inheritance, consisting of a DNA sequence coding for a specific protein or component of a protein, arranged in a linear manner on chromosomes
genotype	The genetic constitution of an individual (either overall or referring to a specific gene locus)
germ line	The cell lineage resulting in eggs or sperm
gonadal (germ line) mosaicism	The occurrence of more than one genetic constitution in the precursor cells of eggs or sperm
haplotype	A series of alleles found at linked loci on a single chromosome
hemizygous	The presence of a gene in only a single copy, e.g. X-linked genes in males, but also autosomal genes where one copy is deleted
heritability	The proportion of variance of a characteristic due to genetic rather than environmental factors
heterogeneity (genetic)	The occurrence of a single phenotype due to mutation of more than one gene (usually implies more than one genetic locus)
heterozygote	An individual with two different alleles at a particular locus

HLA system	The major histocompatibility region, determined by a complex of genetic loci on chromosome 6
homozygote	An individual with identical alleles at a particular locus
imprinting (genomic/genetic)	The differential expression of a genetic characteristic or disease depending on parent of origin, often related to differences in methylation
in-situ hybridization	The technique of applying molecular probes to a chromosome spread or section
interphase	The stage of the nucleus between cell division
intron	The DNA sequences in a gene that are not converted into messenger RNA, and which separate the coding regions (exons)
inversion	The turning round of a chromosomal segment with consequent alteration of its fine structure and sometimes its function
isochromosome	An abnormal chromosome composed of two identical arms
karyotype	The chromosome constitution as displayed by a microscopic preparation of dividing chromosomes
linkage, genetic	The occurrence of two genetic loci close enough on the same chromosome to interfere with independent assortment at cell division
locus	The specific site of a gene on a chromosome
Lyon hypothesis	The principle of inactivation of one of the two X chromosomes in normal female cells (first proposed by Dr Mary Lyon)
lysosome	An intracellular body containing important enzymes involved in the breakdown of cell components
meiosis	The process of cell division leading to formation of eggs and sperm, with halving of the chromosome number
mendelian	Following the patterns of inheritance proposed originally by Gregor Mendel
microdeletion	A small or invisible loss of genetic material on a chromosome; often detectable by FISH techniques
mitochondrial inheritance	Exclusively maternal inheritance determined by DNA in the mitochondria, cytoplasmic bodies that also contain key enzymes
mitosis	The process of cell division of somatic cells, in which the daughter cells are normally genetically identical to the parent
monosomy	The occurrence of only a single member of a chromosome pair
monozygotic twins	Twins derived from a single fertilized egg
mosaicism	The occurrence in an individual of more than one genetic constitution, arising after fertilization (cf. chimaera)
mutation/mutant	The change from the normal to an altered form of a particular gene/the individual who has undergone such a change
non-disjunction	Failure of the normal separation of chromosomes at cell division, giving an unbalanced chromosome number (as in trisomy 21)
oncogene	A gene involved in cell proliferation whose abnormal activation or over-expansion is important in a normal cell into a tumorous cell

p	The short arm of a chromosome
penetrance	The proportion of individuals with a particular genetic constitution who show its effect
pericentric inversion	An inversion of genetic material around the centromere of a chromosome
phenotype	The visible expression of the action of a particular gene; the clinical picture resulting from a genetic disorder
polygenic/multifactorial	Determined by multiple genes and usually also by non-genetic factors
polymerase chain reaction (PCR)	The amplification of DNA using a specific technique, which allows analysis of minute original amounts of DNA
polymorphism	Frequent hereditary variations at a genetic locus
pre-mutation	A clinically insignificant change in a gene that predisposes to a subsequent full mutation
proband	The affected individual through whom a family with a genetic disorder is ascertained (also called propositus)
probe	A labelled DNA sequence that can be used to identify a corresponding sequence by hybridization
propositus, proposita	Proband (see above)
q	The long arm of a chromosome
recessive	A characteristic or disorder only expressed when both alleles at a genetic locus are altered
recombination	The separation of alleles that are close together on the same chromosome by crossing over of homologous chromosomes at meiosis
restriction enzyme	A group of bacterial enzymes that cleaves the DNA chain at sequence specific sites
RFLP	Restriction fragment length polymorphism: inherited variation in DNA detected by the cutting of DNA at different points by a restriction enzyme
ring chromosome	A chromosome in which breakage close to the ends has been followed by rejoining to form a ring
RNA	Ribonucleic acid: the nucleic acid for which DNA forms a template before protein is produced
Robertsonian translocation	The formation of a single abnormal chromosome by the joining of two chromosomes by their short arms
somatic	Involving the body cells rather than the germ line
Southern blotting	Transfer of DNA fragments from a electrophoretic gel to a membrane prior to DNA hybridization
syndrome	A combination of clinical features forming a recognizable entity
telomere	The terminal region of the chromosome arms
teratogen	An agent that can damage the developing embryo
translocation	Transfer and exchange of genetic material between different chromosomes, not members of the same pair
trinucleotide repeat	A repeated sequence of three bases (e.g. CAG) expanded and unstable in a group of genetic disorders

trisomy	The presence of three copies of a specific chromosome
X inactivation	Inactivation of one of the two X chromosomes in a normal female cell (see Lyon hypothesis)
Y chromosome	The small chromosome possessed by males only, whose principal function is involvement in sex determination
zygote	The fertilized egg

family tree (pedigree) 5–8, 146–7
  consanguinity and 132, 133
  constructing/recording 5–8, 146
  mendelian disorders 21, 22, 23
    autosomal dominant 22, 24, 25
    autosomal recessive 31
    mitochondrial DNA 47, 48
    X-linked *see* X-linked disorders
  symbols used 4–5
Fanconi pancytopenia 216
fatty acid metabolic defects 319
febrile convulsions 184
females (women and girls)
  mitochondrial disorders 48
  non-mendelian disorders, risk 56
  phenotypic
    infertility in, causes 308
    non-correspondence with
      chromosomal sex 307
  X-linked disorders 39
fertility problems *see* infertility
fetus
  diagnostic tests *see* prenatal diagnosis
    and specific tests
  hydrops 324
  sexing *see* sex determination
FGFR3 and achondroplasia 210
fibrillin 218
fibroblast growth factor receptor-3 and
    achondroplasia 210
fibroelastosis, endocardial 270
fibromatosis
  congenital 246
  gingival 232
fibrosis, congenital hepatic 289
first cousin marriages 133, 135, 137, 137–8
5p- syndrome 74
foot deformities 223–4
4p- syndrome 74
fragile chromosome sites 76
  X chromosome *see* X chromosome
François dyscephalic syndrome 234
Frax sites 201
Freeman–Sheldon syndrome 225
Friedreich's ataxia 180
frontonasal dysplasia 235
frontotemporal dementia 194, 195

galactosaemia 316
gallstones 285
Galton, Francis 4
gamete donation 152
  in Huntington's disease 177
  in infertility 309
Gardner's syndrome 334
gastric cancer 284
gastritis, atrophic 284
gastrointestinal tract 281–90
  polyposis 334–5
gastroschisis 283
gender *see* sex
gene(s)
  in development, dysfunction 92–3
  expression with autosomal dominant
    disorders, variable 26
  extensive trans-species homology 79
  see also mutations
gene therapy 157–8
generalized epilepsy, primary idiopathic
    184–5
Genetic Alliance 378
genetic counselling
  aims and outcome measures 372–3
  back-up to 151–4
  confidentiality *see* confidentiality
  definition 3–4
  development *see* historical
    perspectives
  increasing load of deleterious genes 361
  population aspects *see* population
  regional centres 377
genetic heterogeneity *see* heterogeneity
Genetic Interest Group 378
genetic registers 154–6
genetic relationships *see* relationships
genetic risk *see* risk
genetics and society *see* social issues
genetics nurse specialist 148–9
genomic imprinting 26–7, 75
germinal mosaicism 29
Gerstmann–Straussler syndrome 196
Gilbert's syndrome 288
gingival fibromatosis 232
girls *see* females
glaucoma 254–5